Mechanisms of Tumor Promotion

Volume I

Tumor Promotion in Internal Organs

Editor

Thomas J. Slaga, Ph.D.

Director
Science Park Research Division
UT System Cancer Center
Smithville, Texas

CRC Press, Inc.
Boca Raton, Florida

Library of Congress Cataloging in Publication Data
Main entry under title:

Tumor promotion in internal organs.

(Mechanisms of tumor promotion ; v. 1)
Includes bibliographical references and index.
Contents: Multistage hepatocarcinogenesis /
Carl Peraino, William L. Richards, and Fred J. Stevens —
Promotion of hepatic neoplasia by gonadal steroids /
James D. Yager, Jr. — Enhancement of tumor formation
in mouse lung / H. P. Witschi — [etc.]
1. Cocarcinogenesis. 2. Viscera—Cancer. I. Slaga,
Thomas J. II. Series.
RC268.52.M43 1983 vol. 1 616.99'4071s 83-6366
ISBN Q-8493-6521-X [616.99'4071]

Direct all inquiries to CRC Press, Inc., 2000 Corporate Blvd., N.W., Boca Raton, Florida, 33431.

International Standard Book Number 0-8493-6521-X

Library of Congress Card Number 83-6366
Printed in the United States

PREFACE

There has been increased interest in recent years in scientific investigations pertaining to the mechanisms of tumor promotion, and the resulting accumulation of new scientific data is receiving much attention. The promotion phase of carcinogenesis is widely investigated in a variety of systems and a presentation of these studies by the finest scientific minds is especially relevant.

With the increased attention being given to the daily exposure of man to low-level amounts of an assortment of cancer-causing chemicals, their scientific investigation is likewise increasing. Few of these agents are carcinogenic at very low levels; however, subthreshold amounts may become carcinogenic through an additive effect, cocarcinogenesis or by expression through both endogenous and/or natural tumor promoters. The role of these environmental chemicals, as well as diet, radiation, and viruses as possible modifying factors contributing to the increase of human cancers is of added importance. High caloric and high fat diets, cigarette smoking, asbestos, and alcohol are among the suggested promoting factors that may also play a significant part.

An in-depth examination of the phenomena of tumor promotion in various systems will help provide the scientific understanding of the cellular and biochemical mechanisms involved in these processes. As a more thorough comprehension of these mechanisms is developed, procedures can hopefully be devised to intervene in their course of events thereby inhibiting carcinogenesis. Better testing procedures may, in addition, be forthcoming that will be increasingly proficient in assessing the potential of various agents to act as modifiers of the process of carcinogenesis.

These four volumes will attempt to present the more recent accomplishments in the role of tumor promotion in internal organs (Volume I), investigations in the area of tumor promotion and skin carcinogenesis (Volume II), tumor promotion and cocarcinogenesis in vitro (Volumes III and IV). It will be the general aim of Volume I to carefully examine tumor promotion in various internal organs such as the liver, the lung, and the respiratory system, and in addition, studies on the colon, bladder, pancreas, and breast will be presented. The attainment of a better understanding of the two-stage system of carcinogenesis in these organs will be emphasized.

It is indeed hoped that these volumes will encourage further scientific investigations and therefore a better understanding of the multistage nature of tumor promotion, its role in the induction of cancer, and finally, the ultimate goal, its prevention. It should be of interest to all scientists as well as laymen interested in the pursuance of these goals.

THE EDITOR

Thomas J. Slaga, Ph.D., is the Director of The University of Texas System Cancer Center, Science Park — Research division in Smithville, Texas, an associate institute of the M. D. Anderson Hospital and Tumor Institute in Houston, Texas. In addition to his administrative duties at the Science Park-Research Division, Dr. Slaga continues to direct an extensive and highly productive research program on the mechanisms of chemical carcinogenesis both in vivo and in vitro.

Dr. Slaga received his Ph.D. in physiology/biophysics from the University of Arkansas Medical Center, Little Rock, Arkansas, in 1969. He then spent 3 years as a postdoctoral fellow in the laboratory of Dr. R. K. Boutwell at the McArdle Laboratory for Cancer Research, the University of Wisconsin, Madison, Wisconsin. This was indeed a significant period in his early career since it was under Dr. Boutwell's guidance that Dr. Slaga began his investigations of the carcinogenic effects of tumor promoters. In less than 10 years, he has assumed a position of leadership in this important area of investigative research, an area of study that may someday unravel the cancer puzzle.

CONTRIBUTORS

Samuel M. Cohen, M.D., Ph.D.
Professor and Vice Chairman
Department of Pathology and Laboratory Medicine
University of Nebraska Medical Center
Omaha, Nebraska

Leon B. Ellwein, Ph.D.
Senior Scientist Applied Research
Science Applications, Inc.
La Jolla, California

Robert E. Greenfield, M.D.,
Deputy Director
National Bladder Cancer Project
St. Vincent Hospital
Worcester, Massachusetts

Daniel S. Longnecker, M.D.
Professor of Pathology
Department of Pathology
Dartmouth Medical School
Hanover, New Hampshire

Gen'i Murasaki, M.D.
Research Associate
Department of Pathology and Laboratory Medicine
University of Nebraska Medical Center
Omaha, Nebraska

Paul Nettesheim, M.D.
Chief, Laboratory of Pulmonary Function and Toxicology
National Institute of Environmental Health Sciences
Research Triangle Park, North Carolina

Carl Peraino, Ph.D.
Senior Biochemist
Division of Biological and Medical Research
Argonne National Laboratory
Argonne, Illinois

Bandaru S. Reddy, D.V.M., Ph.D.
Member and Associate Chief
Division of Nutrition
American Health Foundation
Naylor Dana Institute for Disease Prevention
Valhalla, New York

William L. Richards
Research Associate
McArdle Laboratory
University of Wisconsin
Madison, Wisconsin

B. D. Roebuck
Assistant Professor of Toxicology
Department of Pharmacology and Toxicology
Dartmouth Medical School
Hanover, New Hampshire

Vernon E. Steele, Ph.D.
Senior Project Scientist
Genetic Toxicology Division
Northrop Services, Inc.
Research Triangle Park, North Carolina

Fred J. Stevens, Ph.D.
Postdoctoral Appointee
Division of Biological and Medical Research
Argonne National Laboratory
Argonne, Illinois

H. P. Witschi, M.D.
Senior Research Staff Member
Biology Division
Oak Ridge National Laboratory
Oak Ridge, Tennessee

James D. Yager, Jr., Ph.D.
Department of Anatomy
Dartmouth Medical School
Hanover, New Hampshire

Mechanisms of Tumor Promotion

Thomas J. Slaga

Volume I: Tumor Promotion in Internal Organs

Multistage Hepatocarcinogenesis
Promotion of Hepatic Neoplasia by Gonadal Steroids
Enhancement of Tumor Formation in Mouse Lung
Tumor Promotion in Respiratory Tract Carcinogenesis
Tumor Promotion in Colon Carcinogenesis
Tumor Promotion in Bladder Carcinogenesis
Initiation and Promotion in Pancreatic Carcinogenesis

Volume II: Tumor Promotion and Skin Carcinogenesis

Mechanisms Involved in Two-Stage Carcinogenesis in Mouse
Cancer Progression in Mouse Skin
Morphological Evaluation of Tumor Promoter Effects on Mammalian Skin
Ultraviolet Radiation Carcinogenesis
Phorbol Ester Tumor Promoter Receptors and their Down Modulation
The Role of Prostaglandins in Tumor Production
The Role of Polyamines in Tumor Promotion
Protein Phosphorylation and Tumor Promotion
Critical Protein Modifications During Skin Tumor Promotion in Mice
Multistage Skin Tumor Promotion and Specificity of Inhibition

Volume III: Tumor Promotion and Carcinogenesis In Vitro

Tumor Promotion in Epidermal Cells in Culture
Promotion and Other Interactions Between Agents in the Induction of Transformation In Vitro in Fibroblast-Like Cell Culture
Enhancement of Viral Transformation and Expression of the Transformed Phenotype by Tumor Promotors
Effects of Phorbol Ester Tumor Promoters on the Binding, Processing, and Biological Activity of Epidermal Growth Factor
Specific Receptors for Phorbol Ester Tumor Promoters and their Involvement in Biological Responses

Volume IV: Cellular Responses to Tumor Promoters

Modulation of Cell Differentiation by Tumor Promoters
Interaction of Phorbol Diesters and Other Tumor-Promoting Agents with Immunofunctional Cells In Vitro
The Relationship of Alterations in Phospholipid Metabolism to the Mechanism of Action of Phorbol Ester Tumor Promoters
Role of Intercellular Communication in Tumor Promotion

TABLE OF CONTENTS

Volume I

Chapter 1

MULTISTAGE HEPATOCARCINOGENESIS*

Carl Peraino, William L. Richards, and Fred J. Stevens

TABLE OF CONTENTS

* Submitted in August, 1981.

I. INTRODUCTION

As discussed in detail in Volume II, the concept of tumorigenesis as a multistage process originated from studies of the characteristics of skin tumor formation.[1-5] The multistage concept was first formalized by Rous,[4] who coined the now classic terms "initiation" and "promotion" to denote, respectively, (1) the production of potentially tumorigenic cells by limited exposure to carcinogen and (2) the completion of the neoplastic transformation as the result of subsequent treatment with appropriate agents that are not intrinsically carcinogenic.

Despite the definitiveness of the evidence for multistage skin tumorigenesis, the relevance of this mechanism to tumorigenesis in general did not have clear empirical support until the last decade, during which the additional initiation-promotion systems described in this volume have been developed. In this article we shall trace the evolution of the multistage carcinogenesis concept in liver, which is the first nonepidermal system in which this phenomenon was demonstrated unequivocally, and shall also provide an overview of the present state of the liver initiation-promotion system, including descriptions and evaluations of the various experimental models and methods that have been developed for the detection of preneoplastic changes. As part of this discussion, we shall identify what we consider to be conceptual ambiguities regarding the mechanistic boundaries between initiation and promotion that in our judgment are a product of experiments utilizing excessively severe tumorigenic protocols. Finally, we shall briefly discuss some of the possible insights into mechanisms of multistage hepatocarcinogenesis that can be gained from the examination of an important issue that has arisen with the newly acquired ability to detect preneoplastic hepatocyte foci, namely the fact that the numbers of such foci far exceed the numbers of hepatic tumors that ultimately appear.

II. HISTORICAL PERSPECTIVE

A. Indirect Evidence for Multistage Hepatocarcinogenesis

Since the first demonstration of chemically induced hepatocarcinogenesis in 1935,[6] the liver has become the focus of investigation by many experimental oncologists engaged in the analysis of tumorigenesis mechanisms. Indirect evidence that liver tumorigenesis occurs in stages was obtained several years ago in a number of these studies. Cole and Nowell[7] observed that administration of the hepatotoxin carbon tetrachloride (CCl_4) to previously X-irradiated mice substantially increased tumor incidence. Examination by Farber and coworkers[8,9] of various types of nodular hepatic lesions occurring during prolonged carcinogen treatment led to the suggestion that malignant liver tumors evolve from cells contained in certain of the characteristic lesions, termed "hyperplastic nodules," that precede tumor formation under these conditions. Circumstantial evidence for the role of hyperplastic nodules as tumor precursors was obtained by Teebor and Becker[10] who observed that the feeding of 0.06% dietary 2-acetylaminofluorene (AAF) to rats for three separate 3-week intervals, alternating with 1-week intervals on the basal diet, produced a high yield of hyperplastic nodules that regressed, with a low subsequent incidence of hepatic tumors. An additional 3-week interval of AAF treatment, however, yielded both nodules that persisted after carcinogen withdrawal and a high incidence of hepatic tumors. A later variant of this approach involved the administration of a single dose of dimethylnitrosamine (DMN) following the three AAF feeding intervals. This combined treatment produced a high tumor yield, though no tumors were generated by either treatment alone.[11] More recently, studies by Farber and associates have shown that the expression of the tumorigenic potential of hepatocytes exposed to diethylnitrosamine (DEN) is enhanced by subsequent administration of AAF as a cytotoxin, coupled with proliferative stimulation induced by partial hepatectomy or CCl_4 administration.[12-14]

The studies cited above indicated that limited carcinogen treatment produces preneoplastic hepatocytes that require subsequent additional stimuli in order to complete the transformation into frank tumor cells. However, these investigations suffered from a common methodological deficiency, namely the use of substances with carcinogenic and/or mutagenic activity as the additional stimuli. Under such conditions, it is not possible to determine whether progressive stages of tumorigenesis are qualitatively similar (involving, for example, the progressive accumulation of mutations) or dissimilar, as had been demonstrated for skin tumorigenesis. Moreover, the value of the earlier attempts (reviewed by Farber[8]) to identify stages of hepatic preneoplasia was vitiated by the severity of the carcinogenic treatments used in virtually all of the studies. Such procedures made it difficult to distinguish between hepatic responses causally related to neoplasia and those representing the response of the liver to the toxic effects of the prolonged exposure to high levels of carcinogen. This uncertainty was especially burdensome in attempts to evaluate the role of hyperplastic nodule development in the etiology of hepatic neoplasia.[8,15] Despite the exhaustive characterization of the cytological and biochemical properties of these lesions,[8] their identity as obligatory tumor precursors, as opposed to ancillary manifestations of regeneration from carcinogen-induced cytotoxicity, could not be established unequivocally. In view of these ambiguities, the types of protocols leading to the generation of hyperplastic nodules and the investigation of the characteristics of these lesions no longer appear to represent useful experimental approaches to the analysis of tumorigenesis mechanisms.

B. Direct Demonstration of Initiation-Promotion Phenomenon in Liver

The first definitive evidence that the onset of liver neoplasia proceeds in qualitatively distinct sequential stages emerged from an investigation of the effect of phenobarbital on AAF-induced hepatocarcinogenesis.[16] This study compared the effects of two different types of AAF-phenobarbital exposure modalities on tumor incidence. In the first instance, AAF (0.02%) and phenobarbital (0.05%) were present in the diet concurrently (simultaneous treatment protocol). Under these conditions, hepatic tumor incidence was substantially less than that produced by feeding AAF alone. A protective effect of phenobarbital also occurred when it was administered simultaneously with the hepatocarcinogens, 4-dimethylaminoazobenzene[17] and DEN.[18] Since phenobarbital is a potent inducer of enzymes that actively metabolize these carcinogens,[19] it may be concluded that the anticarcinogenic action of phenobarbital in these instances stems from a phenobarbital-mediated shift in the balance of carcinogen metabolism toward detoxification and degradation.

The second type of exposure involved the prolonged feeding of 0.05% dietary phenobarbital after the termination of a brief (2 to 3 week) interval of feeding 0.02% dietary AAF (sequential treatment protocol). This regimen produced a markedly greater tumor incidence than that observed in rats receiving only the brief AAF treatment.[16] Subsequent studies have verified and extended this observation.[20-23]

From a consideration of the contrasting effects of the simultaneous and sequential treatment protocols on tumorigenesis, it is evident that the enhancing effect of phenobarbital cannot be a consequence of increased metabolic activation of the carcinogen. The hypothesis most consistent with the data is that phenobarbital given according to the sequential treatment protocol facilitates the ultimate expression of tumorigenic changes initiated by prior exposure to the carcinogen. This interpretation implies the existence of at least two elements of the tumorigenic process that differ in mechanism as well as in temporal occurrence, and it comprises the basis for the argument that the initiation-promotion concept of tumorigensis applies to liver as well as to skin.

Because the overall carcinogen exposure in the AAF-phenobarbital studies[16,20-23] was greatly reduced in comparison with that in most of the earlier studies,[8,10,11] the AAF-phenobarbital treated livers exhibited none of the injury-related nodular hyperplasia that previously had been a common feature of carcinogen-treated liver.[8] As illustrated most clearly in a recent study of liver tumor promotion,[23] livers remained free of any nodular growth for approximately 4 months following cessation of carcinogen treatment, after which continually growing, nonregressing hepatic tumors began to appear.

Figure 1 shows a typical liver from a rat fed 0.02% dietary AAF during the first 18 days after weaning followed by the feeding of 0.05% dietary phenobarbital for 250 days. Note that the surface of the liver is smooth except for the occurrence of a large tumor in the left lobe. This appearance contrasts sharply with the grossly nodular surface seen prior to the appearance of tumors in rats on more severe carcinogen regimens,[8] and demonstrates clearly, in agreement with the conjecture of Foulds,[15] that hyperplastic nodules are not obligatory precursors of hepatic neoplasia.

III. METHODS FOR ANALYZING MULTISTAGE HEPATOCARCINOGENESIS

A. Treatment Protocols

1. Sequential Feeding of Carcinogen and Promoter

As indicated above, this approach has adapted the treatment strategies used for many years in studies of multistage skin tumorigenesis.[1-5] The main contribution of this procedure is the clarity with which it has revealed the existence of distinct stages of hepatic tumorigenesis and permitted the examination of several characteristics of the promotion stage,[16,20-23] as will be discussed in a subsequent section. Disadvantages of this system include (1) the retention of a significant interval of carcinogen treatment, thereby reducing the ability to detect and resolve the earliest stages of initiation, as well as blurring the distinction between the initiating and promoting action of the carcinogen, and (2) the slowness of the response, requiring a prolonged experimental duration in order to obtain useful information. Thus, whereas the sequential AAF-phenobarbital protocol has been useful as a means of examining the phenomenology of multistage hepatocarcinogenesis, the foregoing deficiencies severely limit its usefulness for more sophisticated mechanistic analyses of liver tumor initiation and promotion.

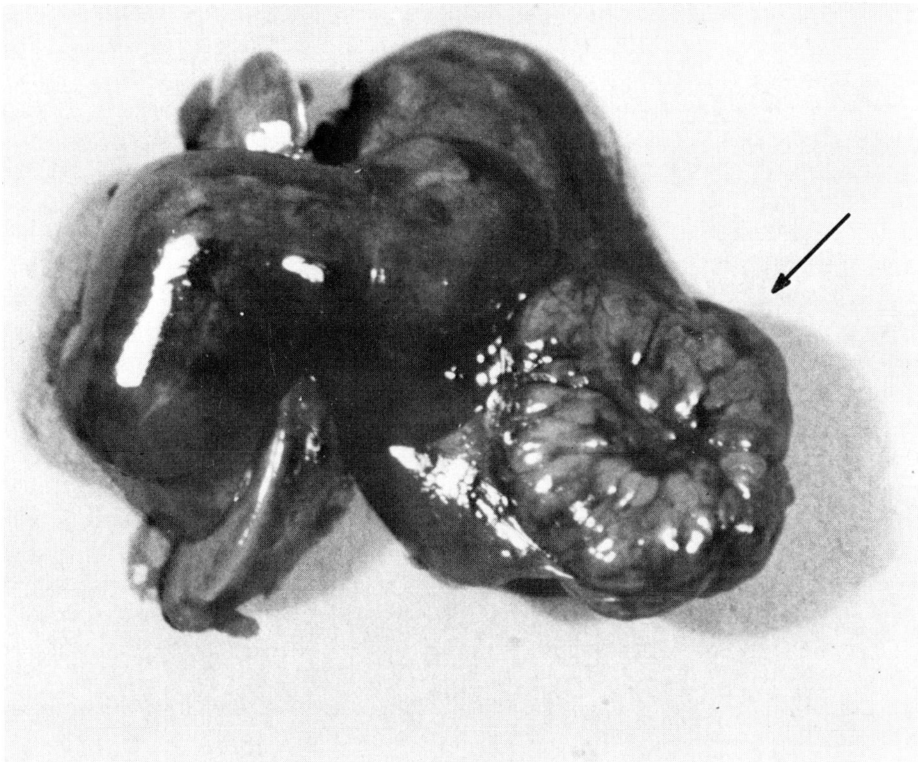

FIGURE 1. Tumor (arrow) in the left lobe of the liver from a rat fed a 0.02% AAF diet for 18 days followed by a 0.05% phenobarbital diet for 250 days. The largest diameter of the tumor is 2.5 cm. The remainder of the liver is free of nodular hyperplasia.

2. Single Treatment with Carcinogen Followed by Proliferative Stimulation in the Presence of a Growth Suppressant (Selection Model)

This procedure and the rationale on which it is based were discussed at length in a recent review by Farber.[14] Briefly, it was postulated that the neoplastic process involves, in part, the acquisition by preneoplastic cells of resistance to the cytotoxic and hence ''mitoinhibitory'' effects of the carcinogenic stimulus. The strategy for the early detection of such cells in experimental hepatocarcinogensis involves the creation of conditions fostering the selective growth of the putative preneoplastic hepatocytes. These hepatocytes are produced by prior treatment with a necrogenic dose of carcinogen such as DEN. The ''selection'' environment is produced by the generation of an intense proliferative stimulus, as a result of partial hepatectomy or CCl_4 administration,[24] in the midst of treatment with an agent, AAF, that inhibits the proliferation of normal hepatocytes. While the regeneration of the bulk of the liver is blocked, the hepatocytes rendered resistant by the prior DEN treatment proliferate rapidly and produce visible nodules within 1 week; tumors appear within 8 months. These responses are not observed in the absence of the initiating stimulus in adult rats, and the cells capable of responding to the ''selection'' procedure persist for at least 9 months.[24]

The major advantage of this procedure is the rapidity and intensity with which the initial response is produced (i.e., the appearance of histochemically altered foci and discrete nodules). This characteristic renders the procedure potentially useful as a rapid method for screening environmental contaminants for tumor initiating activity, as demonstrated in a recent study wherein 21 carcinogens, including polycyclic aromatic hydrocarbons, gave clear-cut positive responses.[25]

The procedure appears less satisfactory, however, as a means of analyzing mechanisms of multistage hepatocarcinogenesis. The basis for this reservation is the severity of both the initiation and "selection" steps, and the use of AAF as the selecting agent. Thus the administration of a necrogenic dose of initiating agent (DEN), justified on the basis of the need to juxtapose the production of regenerative hyperplasia with the creation of the initial tumorigenic lesion,[26-28] undoubtedly increases the number of tumorigenic molecular lesions borne by the initiated cells, thereby reducing the proportion of those initiated cells bearing the minimum number of changes essential for the acquisition of tumorigenic potential. Moreover, since the probability that the promoting action of an initiator will be expressed increases with increasing initiator dosage,[16] the high DEN level used in the selection procedure raises the possibility, as acknowledged by Solt et al.,[24] that a significant proportion of the response to this treatment is the result of the coincidental interplay of initiation and promotion mechanisms.

The use of AAF in conjunction with partial hepatectomy or CCl_4 administration as the selection procedure also compromises attempts at mechanistic interpretation, since one is inescapably faced with the possibility that the 2-week AAF treatment introduces additional molecular changes into the DEN-initiated cells (in essence exerting additional initiating effects), thereby influencing their growth rates, phenotypic characteristics, and tumorigenic potential. Fully cognizant of this problem, Tsuda et al.[25] have presented evidence that the AAF-CCl_4 treatment does not produce presumptive preneoplastic foci in the absence of the prior initiation treatment unless the AAF feeding interval is extended for 4 weeks or longer.[25] The significance of this observation is undermined, however, by the fact that the livers were examined 1 week after the cessation of AAF feeding, thereby eliminating the possibility of detecting later-emerging lesions. In any case, the occurrence of numerous altered foci per square centimeter of liver after 6 weeks of AAF treatment alone in these rats,[25] strengthens the possibility that the 2-week AAF exposure may subtly influence the character of the previously initiated cells.

Evidence that the AAF selection treatment might exert extraneous initiating effects also derives from studies in which this AAF treatment served as a potent initiator of tumorigenesis when fed to weanling rats,[23] or of altered hepatocyte foci when fed to older animals.[29] Moreover, it has clearly been demonstrated that hepatocytes, altered by prior carcinogen treatment, are subject to further tumorigenic modification by subsequent exposure to the same or different carcinogens.[10,11,30]

Finally, concern must be raised about the interchangeable use of CCl_4 and partial hepatectomy as methods for stimulating hepatocyte proliferation during AAF administration in the selection procedure.[14,24,25] The hepatotoxic effects of CCl_4 undoubtedly generate complex biochemical changes that interact in as yet unknown ways with those produced by hepatocarcinogens; in any case, the spectrum of interactions could very likely be considerably different from that engendered by combining carcinogen treatment with partial hepatectomy. Evidence for the complexity of CCl_4-hepatocarcinogen interactions is provided by several studies in which variable enhancing effects of CCl_4 on tumorigenesis were produced, depending on the nature of the hepatocarcinogen used and the temporal relationships of the carcinogen-CCl_4 treatments.[31-33]

Overall, therefore, the selection procedure appears to represent a valuable method for the rapid production of carcinogen-altered hepatocytes that can then be subjected to further study.[34] However, the multiplicity of complex overlapping effects generated by the various elements of this protocol reduces its value for distinguishing the characteristics of the sequential stages of hepatocarcinogenesis.

3. Single Treatment with Carcinogen During Liver Regeneration, Followed by Phenobarbital Feeding

This highly useful protocol[35-37] was synthesized from elements of a variety of published procedures and has significantly advanced our capacity to examine the stages of hepatic neoplasia. Basically, the protocol involves first, the gastric intubation of a nonnecrogenic dose of DEN (approximately 10 mg/kg body weight) 24 hr after partial hepatectomy; this aspect of the protocol derives from prior observations that such treatment produces foci of presumptive preneoplastic hepatocytes[30,38-40] and liver tumors if the DEN dosage is sufficiently high.[41] The second element of the protocol utilizes prolonged exposures to dietary phenobarbital[20-23] following the DEN intubation to enhance the production of foci and tumors. Finally, the development of altered hepatocyte foci is monitored by the application of histochemical tests to detect the absence of glucose-6-phosphatase[42-44] and canalicular ATPase,[30,38-40] and the presence of γ-glutamyltranspeptidase[44] in foci contained in adjacent frozen liver sections. By superimposing the images of these sections, foci with one to three of the foregoing marker changes are scored,[44] permitting the assessment of the occurrence of seven different focus phenotypes.[36,44]

The advantages of this procedure are (1) the use of a single carcinogen treatment at a relatively low dosage level minimizes uncertainties regarding the possible overlapping of initiating and promoting actions of the carcinogen that may occur with higher dosages or more prolonged administration of carcinogen; (2) the carcinogen treatment regimen allows precise control of carcinogen intake, an important consideration in carcinogen dose-response studies; and (3) the use of histochemical techniques permits the monitoring of relatively early hepatic changes during the onset of neoplasia. However, the protocol suffers from the requirement that carcinogen treatment be preceded by partial hepatectomy, a relatively impractical procedure for large-scale studies. In addition, the experimental duration required for the attainment of a definitive end point, namely the appearance of tumors,[36] is as long as those in other protocols.[16,20-23,45]

4. Production of Lipotrope Deficiency Prior to or Following Exposure to Carcinogen

As reviewed by Rogers and Newberne,[46] a number of studies have shown that the hepatocarcinogenicity of several agents, including aflatoxin, DEN, dibutylnitrosamine, and AAF, is increased in rats previously fed a diet marginally deficient in the lipotropes, choline, methionine, and folic acid. Despite substantial differences between the control and deficient diets with respect to protein composition, fat composition and content, and carbohydrate composition and content, the increase in liver tumorigenesis is largely reversed by lipotrope supplementation of the deficient diet,[46] supporting the role of lipotrope deficiency in tumorigenic enhancement. Thus, far, attempts to determine whether the lipotrope deficient diet alters carcinogen metabolism in a manner consistent with the diet's tumorigenic enhancing effect, have yielded inconclusive results (e.g., aflatoxin activation was not increased in livers of lipotrope deficient rats although urinary excretion of mutagenic aflatoxin metabolites was higher in these animals), raising the possibility that other factors such as diet-induced changes in host susceptibility (e.g., increased proliferation of target cells) may play a role in the enhancement process.[46]

Enhancement of hepatocarcinogenesis was also observed in rats fed a choline-devoid diet during[47-49] or after[50,51] exposure to the carcinogenic stimulus. In the latter instance, the addition of phenobarbital to the choline-devoid diet at a concentration of 0.06% produced a significantly greater enhancement than the sum of the responses to the choline-devoid and phenobarbital diets given individually, indicating a synergistic interaction of the two promoting stimuli.[51] In an investigation of the basis of this synergism, Abanobi et al.[52] reported that the feeding of a choline-devoid diet stimulated liver DNA synthesis and hepatocyte mitosis (as had been reported previously in the case of lipotrope deficiency[53]), whereas dietary phenobarbital suppressed both end points by 50% in control and choline-deficient rats. On the basis of these opposing effects of the two treatments in rats not treated with carcinogen, it is postulated that the promoting action of the choline-devoid diet involves proliferative stimulation of both initiated and noninitiated hepatocytes, whereas phenobarbital feeding primarily suppresses the proliferation of noninitiated cells.[52] This speculation follows the logic of the selection model outlined earlier (Section III.A.2) and places the choline-devoid diet in the role of proliferative stimulus, currently occupied in the model by partial hepatectomy or CCl_4 treatment,[12-14] with phenobarbital serving as the "selecting" agent instead of AAF. However, Farber and colleagues have, on the basis of preliminary data, suggested that the choline-devoid diet might substitute for AAF as the "selecting" agent in their model.[25] Should this substitution prove feasible, the rationale for the selection protocol would be compromised if the current interpretation[52] of the effect of the choline-devoid diet is correct, since the necessity for the selective "mitoinhibition" of noninitiated cells would be eliminated. The absence of such a requirement would in turn undermine the argument that the promoting action of phenobarbital stems from its selective proliferative suppression of noninitiated cells.[52]

It must be noted that the experimental end point reported in the studies of the promoting effect of choline deficiency, and its interaction with phenobarbital, was restricted to the occurrence of hepatic foci positive for γ-glutamyltranspeptidase with the assumption that this end point represents a valid early indication of the subsequent carcinogenic response.[51] The tentative nature of this assumption should be kept in mind, however, in view of the paucity of information on the constancy of the relationship between focus frequency and tumor frequency under various experimental conditions, especially in view of the fact that focus frequency exceeds tumor frequency by more than three orders of magnitude.[36]

With regard to its utility as a means of investigating multistage hepatocarcinogenesis, the induction of lipotrope deficiency would appear to suffer from the same limitation that characterized most of the early prior experimental hepatocarcinogenesis systems, namely the severity of the treatment, which in this case produces profound disruptions in lipoprotein metabolism, accompanied by fatty infiltration of the liver, leading to hepatic cirrhosis.[54-57] Under such circumstances, the observed hyperplasia[52,53] would be expected as part of the well-known compensatory regeneration that characterizes the response of the liver to chemically or physically induced injury. Thus, in terms of its enhancement of hepatocarcinogenesis, the induction of lipotrope deficiency may act in part as a means of stimulating hepatocyte proliferation, which may in turn play a role in tumorigenic enhancement both during and after carcinogen treatment (see below). In any case, in view of the complex biochemical manifestations of hepatic damage induced by lipotrope deficiency, it is difficult to see how events causally related to tumorigenic enhancement can be distinguished from extraneous injury-related responses; consequently, the value of this approach for mechanistic studies would appear to be limited.

5. *Tumorigenic Enhancement by Proliferative Stimulation*

a. Proliferative Stimulation Concurrent with Initiation

In this section we shall be concerned only with artificially induced hepatocyte proliferative stimulation at the time of initiation. Initiation of inherently rapidly proliferating hepatocytes in newborn animals will be discussed later (Section III.A.8).

Several studies have shown that the hepatocarcinogenic potential of various agents is greatly enhanced if the agents are administered to animals undergoing liver regeneration as a result of partial hepatectomy.[40,41,58-64] Such enhancement could stem from an increase in the vulnerability of replicating DNA to alteration by carcinogen,[63] and subsequently to fixation of the carcinogen-induced DNA lesions by replication of the modified DNA prior to repair.[65] In any case, preinitiation partial hepatectomy has become an important part of recent experimental protocols aimed at analyzing mechanisms of multistage hepatocarcinogenesis,[36,40] since, by improving the sensitivity of the carcinogenic response, this procedure has permitted the use of subtoxic initiating dosages of carcinogen. Moreover, this increase in sensitivity has also made possible the detection of hepatocarcinogenic activity in agents such as urethan and 7,12-dimethylbenz[a]anthracene that are virtually ineffective in quiescent hepatic tissues.[58-63]

Replacement of the preinitiation partial hepatectomy by a single necrogenic CCl_4 treatment also enhances subsequent hepatic tumor incidence,[66-68] and the mechanism of this enhancement is presumed to be strictly analogous to that underlying the enhancing effect of partial hepatectomy, namely the stimulation of regenerative hyperplasia.[67] However, as pointed out earlier, there exists the inescapable possibility that the complex biochemical changes accompanying CCl_4-induced hepatotoxicity also influence the response to the carcinogen. The virtual impossibility of assessing the magnitude of this influence vitiates the usefulness of CCl_4 treatment as a substitute for partial hepatectomy in such studies.

b. Proliferative Stimulation Following Initiation

Repeated partial hepatectomies have been performed following carcinogen treatment in an effort to determine whether the repeated proliferative stimulation of hepatocytes exerts a promoting effect on hepatocarcinogenesis.[64] Marginal enhancement of tumorigenesis by this procedure suggests, but does not demonstrate convincingly, that regenerative hyperplasia promotes hepatic tumorigenesis. The equivocal results suggest either that proliferative stimulation does not constitute a potent promoting stimulus, or that surgical removal of clones of dividing initiated cells masks what might be in fact a strong response.

An alternative approach, involving repeated postinitiation treatments with CCl_4 in place of multiple partial hepatectomy, has produced a substantially larger increase in tumor yield.[32,68] It is argued that the greater promoting effectiveness of the CCl_4 treatment stems from a higher proliferative response to this treatment than to partial hepatectomy.[68] However, it is equally likely that other biochemical effects unrelated to proliferative stimulation are predominantly responsible for the promoting activity of CCl_4. This possibility is supported by evidence that phenobarbital, a potent promoter of hepatocarcinogenesis,[16,20-23] produces only a single early transient increase in hepatocyte proliferation,[16,21,69,70] despite prolonged administration, although many other phenobarbital-mediated hepatic changes are sustained as long as this treatment continues.[19] Since extended exposure to phenobarbital, far beyond that required for manifestation of its limited proliferative effect, is required for expression of phenobarbital's promoting activity,[20,22] it is probable that factors other than proliferative stimulation are primary contributors to the mechanism of liver tumor promotion.

6. Hybrid Treatment Protocols

In efforts to develop rapid bioassays for tumor initiators and promoters using liver as the test system, various treatment protocols have been assembled from elements of the procedures described above. Ito and colleagues[71,72] describe a system (based on the selection system discussed in Section III.A.2) in which rats are given a necrogenic dose of DEN (200 mg/kg) by i.p. injection, followed after 2 weeks by administration of the test agent for 2 weeks, with partial hepatectomy performed midway through the latter treatment. Rats killed at the end of the latter 2-week interval are examined histochemically and histologically for the presence of "hyperlastic nodules". In a later variant of this procedure,[29] rats are fed AAF for 2 weeks, followed by an 8-week feeding of the test chemical, the rats being subjected to partial hepatectomy after 1 week of the latter treatment. At the end of the 10-week experiment, livers are examined histologically for hyperplastic nodule formation. Most recently, these workers have reverted to their DEN-initiation protocol in comparing its efficacy with that of the AAF-initiation protocol[73] and in examining the issue of hyperplastic nodule reversibility.[74]

The foregoing studies of Ito and colleagues have not convincingly demonstrated the utility of their treatment protocol, either as the basis for a rapid screening procedure for carcinogens and tumor promoters or as a means of examining hepatocarcinogenesis mechanisms. With respect to the development of a screening procedure, their protocol, which requires the performance of partial hepatectomies, is no less troublesome to implement than those described by several other investigators. Moreover, the test end points, namely hyperplastic nodule formation and subsequent liver tumor incidence,[74] are not attained more rapidly than with the other protocols. Finally, the protocol tests only the ability of an agent to produce an effect in animals with previously altered hepatocytes, thereby virtually eliminating the possibility of discriminating between initiators and promoters.

The inadequacy of the protocols of Ito and co-workers for mechanistic studies, in common with several of the protocols discussed above, stems primarily from the severity of the treatments used. Thus, the monitoring of the emergence and turnover characteristics of hyperplastic nodules produced under such conditions[74] appears fruitless in view of the undecipherable contributions of hepatotoxicity and regenerative hyperplasia to the occurrence and behavior of these lesions.

Recently, Ford and Pereira[75] described a treatment protocol developed as the basis for a short-term bioassay for liver tumor initiators and promoters. The protocol is basically similar in design to that developed by Solt and Farber[12] with the substitution of phenobarbital for AAF in the "selection" phase of the treatment, a modification also introduced by Ito and colleagues in some of their procedures.[29,73] This substitution eliminates the problems of interpretation associated with the use of AAF as the selecting agent, as discussed earlier, and provides a valid initiation-promotion system, resembling that described earlier by Pitot and colleagues,[35-37] with the exception that the partial hepatectomy is shifted from the initiation phase to the promotion phase of the protocol. Ford and Pereira argue[75] that this shift increases the utility of the system for initiator dose response studies and simplifies the analysis of the mechanism of initiation. However, it is also apparent that this temporal relocation of the partial hepatectomy step correspondingly reduces the utility of the system for measuring promoter dose effects and complicates the analysis of promotion mechanisms.

A possible solution to the problem of locating the partial hepatectomy step appropriately would be to perform the operation during the promotion phase when the initiation phase is under investigation and during the initiation phase when promotion is being studied. The enhancing effects of partial hepatectomy on the whole system could thereby be exploited while retaining the capacity to examine each phase of the initiation-promotion process without the disrupting influence of this surgical procedure.

7. Carcinogen In Vivo, Promoter In Vitro

In an important study, Kitagawa et al.[76] recently demonstrated that phenobarbital enhances the production in vitro of malignantly transformed colonies in epithelial cell cultures from the livers of rats fed AAF. Cells obtained from these livers after collagenase treatment were cultured in the presence or absence of phenobarbital, and the numbers and sizes of transformed foci were scored at the end of 12 weeks. The malignancy of these foci was verified by their ability to grow in softer agar and by the appearance of tumors after inoculation of these cells into syngeneic newborn rats.

Under these conditions, phenobarbital induced a sevenfold increase in the total number of foci per culture dish and also caused a marked shift in the size distribution of foci toward those with the smallest diameters. It is clear, therefore, that phenobarbital increased the occurrence of foci exhibiting the transformed phenotype without increasing their growth rates. These data are in agreement with in vivo studies showing that phenobarbital increases the numbers but not the growth rates of hepatic tumors in rats previously fed AAF[23] and represent a valuable contribution to our understanding of tumor promotion mechanisms, as will be discussed in a later section. Moreover, the procedure may well serve as the basis for the development of a useful in vitro assay for tumor promoters, although at present the long total experimental duration (at least 24 weeks) does not endow this system with any temporal advantage over in vivo procedures currently in use.

8. Initiation at Birth, Promotion after Weaning

Several studies have shown that newborn mice and rats are more susceptible than older animals to chemically induced hepatocarcinogenesis.[77-88] Since a major component of the mechanism for this increased sensitivity in newborns is apparently the same as that in partially hepatectomized rats, and involves enhanced hepatocyte proliferative activity,[61] it would appear that the use of newborn animals might substitute for partial hepatectomy at the time of initiation, thereby eliminating a cumbersome experimental manipulation. The feasibility of this approach for the study of liver tumor initiation and promotion was demonstrated by Uchida and Hirono[89] who administered a single i.p. injection of dimethylnitrosamine to newborn mice (approximate dose, 30 mg/kg) and fed phenobarbital in the drinking water (concentration, 0.05%) to a proportion of the carcinogen-treated animals, beginning at the time of weaning. At the end of 16 weeks the mice receiving both the dimethylnitrosamine and phenobarbital had a significantly higher incidence of liver tumors than those given only the carcinogen, indicating that the experimental conditions used constituted a valid initiation-promotion system.

In a recent study from our laboratory,[90] the foregoing procedure was adapted to rats as part of an effort to develop a rapid and reliable method of assessing environment contaminants for tumorigenic potential. The shift to rats was prompted by our preliminary data suggesting that rats are considerably more susceptible than mice to chemically induced hepatic tumorigenesis under these experimental conditions. This indication of differential sensitivity is corroborated by our observation of more rapid liver tumor formation at lower carcinogen dosage in rats[90] as opposed to mice.[89] The reported data indicate incidences of γ-glutamyltranspeptidase-positive hepatocyte foci and liver tumors in rats given a single i.p. injection of DEN, benzo(a)pyrene (BaP) or benzo(e)pyrene (BeP) 1 day after birth; all rats received etary phenobarbital (0.05%) after weaning to maximize the tumorigenic response. Results from the first 16 weeks of this study, which is still in progress, permit the following conclusions:

1. The protocol used renders the liver highly responsive to carcinogenic polycyclic aromatic hydrocarbons, as well as known hepatocarcinogens.
2. Putative preneoplastic changes, represented by the appearance of γ-glutamyltranspeptidase-positive hepatocyte foci, can be detected within 1 week after weaning[391] and appear to be reasonably accurate indicators of subsequent tumorigenesis, as suggested by the positive correlations between foci incidence and tumor formation in the various treatment groups.
3. The protocol used produces tumors earlier than any other known procedure and is sufficiently sensitive that subhepatotoxic doses of the test agent can be administered.
4. Newborn female rats are far more sensitive than newborn males to tumor initiators. These results differ from those in an earlier study, which did not indicate a sex

difference in tumor incidence in rats treated with urethan at birth.[80] In addition, newborn male mice were found to be more susceptible than females to chemically induced hepatocarcinogenesis in some experiments,[84-86,91] whereas others showed no sex difference.[89] Clearly, the nature of the sex effect and the reason for its inconsistency require further investigation.

B. Analyses for the Presence of Neoplastic and/or Preneoplastic Hepatocytes

1. Detection In Vivo

a. Areas of Atypia in Histologic Sections

During hepatocarcinogenesis in rats, mice, and other experimental animals, histologic studies on liver sections stained with hematoxylin and eosin, toluidine blue, or other routine histologic stains reveal progressive microscopic alterations that precede or accompany the development of liver neoplasms. Such alterations are often manifested as foci of altered hepatocytes of at least four types: (1) clear cell; (2) acidophilic, eosinophilic, or ground glass cell; (3) vacuolated cell; (4) basophilic cell. It has been recommended that groups of these altered cells be termed "foci or areas of cellular alteration" when less than one liver lobule in size and "neoplastic nodules" (rather than "hyperplastic nodules") when occupying an area equivalent in size to that of several liver lobules.[92] Most studies in experimental hepatocarcinogenesis have utilized either rats or mice. The morphology of preneoplastic and neoplastic liver lesions has been detailed for rats,[92-96] mice,[97-99] and other animal species.[100] Using routine histologic sections as research tools, investigators have described the progressive changes in parenchymal tissue that culminate in the development of liver neoplasms.[6,8-11,14,94,96,101-118] Farber and Cameron[113] have provided a list of hepatocarcinogenesis ". . . studies designed to clarify the sequence of changes possibly important in cancer development . . . performed as a function of time after beginning a carcinogenic regimen." Hunt and Laishes[118] have provided a table listing carcinogens for which early focal hyperplasia has been observed. Evaluation of histologic liver sections continues to be the principal method for pathologic diagnosis. Studies of hepatocarcinogenesis in which routine histologic sections serve as the primary objects of study are evident today,[12,73,119,120] but are encountered less and less frequently. Instead, most recent investigations on multistage hepatocarcinogenesis have used a combination of histologic and histochemical techniques, the former to provide detailed information on morphologic changes and the latter to provide data on the association of enzymatic and other biochemical changes with specific types of lesions or cells. Histochemical changes in specific lesions or cells can also be related to the deviations from normalcy discovered through biochemical studies on preneoplastic and neoplastic livers and minimal deviation hepatomas.[121-124]

b. Markers of Altered Hepatocyte Foci

In 1948, Mellors and Sugiura[125] applied a histochemical technique to the study of alkaline phosphatase activity in the livers of rats that had been administered the carcinogen butter yellow. Using serial liver sections, they demonstrated uniformly low alkaline phosphatase activity in normal rat liver cells, but increased alkaline phosphatase activity in foci of basophilic hyperplastic and proliferating hepatocytes of carcinogen-treated rats.

Table 1 lists many of the subsequently identified histochemical markers that aid in the detection of neoplastic and/or preneoplastic hepatocytes. Emphasis has been placed on marker studies because of their actual or potential usefulness in all other types of analyses for the presence of neoplastic and/or preneoplastic hepatocytes. References included in the table were discovered through computer searches of indexed literature and through examining the literature cited by recent reviews on enzyme-altered liver foci[14,37,40,102,118,126,127] and by primary research papers on this subject. We apologize if any important references were inadvertently omitted. The literature searches extended through May 1981. Table 1 provides

Table 1
HISTOCHEMICAL DEMONSTRATIONS OF NEOPLASTIC AND/OR PUTATIVE PRENEOPLASTIC HEPATOCYTE FOCI

Animals	Administered substance(s)[a] or procedure(s)	Marker changes[b]	Ref.
Male Wistar rats	DAB	RNase (−)	128
BDI and BDII rats	NNM	Glycogen (+), (−)	96
Rats	NNM	Glycogen (+), (−)	103
Rats	NNM	Glycogen (+)	111
Monkeys	DEN	Glycogen (+)	
Rats	NNM	Glycogen (+) G6Pase (+), (−)	129
Male Sprague-Dawley rats	NNM	Glycogen (+), (−) G6Pase (−)	130
Rats	NNM	Glycogen (+), (−) G6Pase (−)	102
Mice	ENU	Glycogen (+)	
Male Wistar rats	DMN + P.H.	Glycogen (+) M.I.	131
Male Wistar rats	DEN + P.H.	Glycogen (+) M.I.	132
Male Wistar rats	DEN	Glycogen (+)	133
Male Wistar rats	DEN	Glycogen (+) M.I.	134
Male Wistar rats	DEN + P.H.	Glycogen (+) M.I.	135
Female Sprague-Dawley rats	P.H. + DEN	ATPase (−) Ferritin (+)	136
Sprague-Dawley rats	DEN	Succinic dehydrogenase (−) Alkaline phosphatase (+) Glycogen (+) Acid phosphatase (−) G6Pase (−) ATPase (−)	137
Weanling C3H mice	PB	Glycogen (+) G6Pase (−) Succinic dehydrogenase (−) Aniline hydroxylase (−) ATPase (−), (+) Alkaline phosphatase (−), (+)	138
Male Fischer 344 rats	2-AAF, DEN	GGT (+)	139
Male Wistar rats	3′-Me-DAB	α-Fetoprotein (+) Fetal liver antigen (+)	140
Male Fischer 344 rats	MNU + P.H. + (CCl_4 or αHCH)	GGT (+)	26
Male Fischer 344 rats	1,2-DMH + P.H. + choline-deficient diet	GGT (+)	141
Male Wistar rats	DAB, 3′-Me-DAB	RNase (−)	142
Male Wistar rats	DAB	RNase (−) ATPase (−)	143
Female Sprague-Dawley (Neuherberg) rats	DEN + PCB mixture, NNM, DEN	Glutathione (+) GGT (+) ATPase (−)	144
Female Sprague-Dawley rats	DEN + P.H.	ATPase (−)	40
Male Wistar rats	Ethionine, 2-AAF	Glycogen (+) G6Pase (−)	145
Male Sprague-Dawley rats	DEN	RNase (−)	146
Male Sprague-Dawley rats	DEN + PB + P.H.	GGT (+)	75

Table 1 (continued)
HISTOCHEMICAL DEMONSTRATIONS OF NEOPLASTIC AND/OR PUTATIVE PRENEOPLASTIC HEPATOCYTE FOCI

Animals	Administered substance(s)[a] or procedure(s)	Marker changes[b]	Ref.
Male Wistar rats	DAB	Glycogen (+), (−)	147
Female Sprague-Dawley rats	DEN	Glycogen (+) G6Pase (−)	42
Female Sprague-Dawley rats	DEN, TAA	G6Pase (−). Several other markers were studied in hepatocellular carcinomas.	148
Male Sprague-Dawley rats	3′-Me-DAB	G6Pase (−) Glycogen (−) Butyrocholinesterase (−) Nonspecific esterase (+) ATPase (−)	149
Male Sprague-Dawley rats	DAB, 2-AAF + PB	GGT (+) ATPase (−) G6Pase (−) L.I.	126
Male Sprague-Dawley rats	2-AAF + PB	GGT (+) ATPase (−) G6Pase (−) L.I. Enzyme histochemical phenotypes of hepatocellular carcinomas, reported here, can be compared to phenotype distributions in altered foci (Pugh and Goldfarb[44])	150
Female Swiss Webster mice	Griseofulvin	Alkaline phosphatase (+) GGT (+) in some cell clusters L.I.	151
Infant male C57BLx C3H F1 mice	DEN	G6Pase (−) L.I. Serial section reconstruction of foci	152
Male Sprague-Dawley rats	3′-Me-DAB	Glycogen (+)	153
Rats	P.H. + DEN + PB	GGT (+) ATPase (−) G6Pase (−)	154
Female Sprague-Dawley rats	DEN, NNM	G6Pase (−)	155
Male Sprague-Dawley rats	N-OH-AAF + aflatoxin B_1	GGT (+)	156
Male Wistar rats	DAB	Intercellular cations L.I.	157
Male Fischer rats	2-AAF	GGT (+) Iron accumulation (−) ATPase (−) G6Pase (−)	158
Male F344 rats	2-AAF	GGT (+) Iron accumulation (−)	159

Table 1 (continued)
HISTOCHEMICAL DEMONSTRATIONS OF NEOPLASTIC AND/OR PUTATIVE PRENEOPLASTIC HEPATOCYTE FOCI

Animals	Administered substance(s)[a] or procedure(s)	Marker changes[b]	Ref.
Fischer F344 rats were treated with a carcinogenic regimen (donor rats); liver cell suspensions, obtained by collagenase perfusion of donor rat livers, were injected into the mesenteric vein of WF × F344 F_1 hybrid host rats administered a two thirds hepatectomy during short-term 2-AAF feeding		Histochemistry of presumptive donor foci as compared to host parenchymal cells: GGT (+), fluorescence of alloantisera specific for the WF haplotype (−)	160
Male Sprague-Dawley rats	DEN + P.H. + PB	ATPase (−)	65
Male Wistar rats	3′-Me-DAB	Catalase (−)	161
Male Fischer 344 rats	2-AAF, DEN, and many others	GGT (+)	73
Female C3H/A/BOM mice	*o*-AT	α-Fetoprotein (+) GGT (+)	162
Male Wistar R rats	Aflatoxin B_1	Glycogen (+), (−) Alkaline phosphatase (+), (−) ATPase (−) G6Pase (−) DNase (−) RNase (−) Acid phosphatase (−) 5′-Nucleotidase (−) G6PDH (+), (−) Succinic dehydrogenase (−)	163,164
Rats	Aflatoxin B_1	G6Pase (−) GGT (+) α-fetoprotein (+)	165
Rats	Aflatoxin B_1	GGT (+)	166
Male Wistar R rats	Aflatoxin B_1	GGT (+)	167
Male Wistar rats	DAB	ATPase (−)	168
Male Wistar rats	DAB	Alkaline phosphatase (+), (−)	169
Male Donryu rats	2-AAF	β-Glucuronidase (−) Acid phosphatase (−) ATPase (−) Alkaline phosphatase (−), (+) G6Pase (−) Phosphorylase (−), (+) Glycogen (−), (+) Succinic dehydrogenase (−) Lactic dehydrogenase (−)	170
Male Donryu and Sprague-Dawley rats	2-AAF	β-Glucuronidase (−), (+) G6Pase (−) Serine dehydratase (−), (+) L.I.	171
Male Sprague-Dawley rats	2-AAF, DEN	G6Pase (−), (+) Serine dehydratase (−), (+) β-Glucuronidase (−)	172
Weanling male Donryu rats	2-Me-DAB + PB	ATPase (−)	173
Male Donryu rats	2-AAF + P.H.	β-glucuronidase (−) ^{3}H-TdR labeling	174
Male Donryu rats	2-AAF + P.H.	β-Glucuronidase (−) G6Pase (−) ATPase (−) ^{3}H-TdR labeling	175

Table 1 (continued)
HISTOCHEMICAL DEMONSTRATIONS OF NEOPLASTIC AND/OR PUTATIVE PRENEOPLASTIC HEPATOCYTE FOCI

Animals	Administered substance(s)[a] or procedure(s)	Marker changes[b]	Ref.
Weanling male Donryu rats	3′-Me-DAB + PB	ATPase (−)	176
Weanling male Donryu rats	3′-Me-DAB + PB	ATPase (−)	177
Male C3H/HeMs NRS mice	DEN, PB	G6Pase (−), (+) ATPase (−), (+) Glycogen (+) GGT (+)	178
Male Donryu rats	2-AAF in vivo, PB in vitro, s.c. injection of cells into syngeneic newborns	GGT (+)	76
Female Lewis rats	NNM	ATPase (−) Epoxide hydrolase (+) GGT (+)	179
Female Wistar rats	DEN + PB	ATPase (−)	180
Newborn Wistar rats	Vinyl chloride Trichloroethylene	ATPase (−) No foci detected	181
Male F344 rats	Carcinogen-altered hepatocytes from donor rats were transferred by i.v. injection to the livers of suitably-treated syngeneic hosts	GGT (+)	182
Male rats	As above	GGT (+) L.I.	183
Male F344 rats	Hepatocytes from carcinogen-treated rats were examined in vivo and in vitro	GGT (+)	184
Male F344 rats	See Laishes and Farber[182]	GGT (+) L.I.	34
Male F344 rats	2-AAF + P.H.	GGT (+)	185
BD II rats	Methyl-allyl-nitrosamine	Glycogen (+), (−)	186
Male BALB/c mice	Safrole	Iron accumulation (−)	187
Male BALB/c mice	Safrole	GGT (+)	188
Female Fischer 344 rats	DEN + 2-AAF + P.H.	Chorionic gonadotropin (+)	189
Male Sprague-Dawley rats	2-AAF	Iron accumulation (−) G6Pase (−) Glycogen (+) M.I.	190
Sherman rats	DAB	Alkaline phosphatase (+)	125
Newborn male and female CD-1 and B6C3F$_1$ mice	DEN	G6Pase (−)	91
Weanling male Donryu rats	3′-Me-DAB + PB	ATPase (−)	191
Male Sprague-Dawley rats	2-AAF	Epoxide hydrase (+)	192
Male Wistar rats	3′-Me-DAB	ATPase (−) G6Pase (−) Glycogen (+)	193
Male Fischer F344 rats	DEN + 2-AAF + P.H.	GGT (+) D-T diaphorase (+) G6Pase (−) ATPase (−)	194
Female Wistar rats	DEN + (α-HCH or CPA)	GGT (+) L.I.	195
Male Charles River CDF rats	2-AAF then transplantation of neoplastic module fragments	Iron accumulation (−)	196
Male Wistar rats	2-AAF	α-Fetoprotein (+)	197

Table 1 (continued)
HISTOCHEMICAL DEMONSTRATIONS OF NEOPLASTIC AND/OR PUTATIVE PRENEOPLASTIC HEPATOCYTE FOCI

Animals	Administered substance(s)[a] or procedure(s)	Marker changes[b]	Ref.
CFN, F344, and BUF rats	2-AAF, ethionine, 3′-Me-DAB, DMN, DEN	PN antigen (+)	198
Rats	DAB	Succinic dehydrogenase (−)	199
Newborn female Sprague-Dawley rats	(DEN, BAP, or BEP) + PB	GGT (+)	90
Rats	P.H. + DEN + PB	GGT (+) ATPase (−) G6Pase (−)	35,200, 201
Rats	P.H. + DEN + (PB, TCDD, or BHA)	GGT (+) ATPase (−) G6Pase (−) Iron accumulation (−)	202
Female Sprague-Dawley rats	P.H. + DEN + PB	GGT (+) ATPase (−) G6Pase (−)	36
Rats	P.H. + DEN + PB	GGT (+) ATPase (−) G6Pase (−)	203
Female Charles River rats	P.H. + DEN + (TCDD or PB)	GGT (+) ATPase (−) G6Pase (−)	204
Male Buffalo rats	2-AAF + PB	GGT (+) ATPase (−) G6Pase (−) L.I.	44
Rats	DEN + P.H.	ATPase (−) G6Pase (−) L.I.	205
Male Wistar AF/Han rats	DEN	ATPase (−) G6Pase (−) L.I. (in vivo and in vitro)	43
Male Wistar AF/Han rats	DEN	ATPase (−) G6Pase (−) L.I. Cell kinetic parameters	206
Male Fischer rats	Lipotrope-deficient diet + aflatoxin B_1	G6Pase (−)	53
Male rhesus monkeys	DEN	Glycogen (+) G6Pase (−) Succinic dehydrogenase (−) ATPase (entire cell surface)	207
Chickens	Choline-deficient diet	Iron accumulation (−)	208
Female Sprague-Dawley rats	DEN	ATPase (−) G6Pase (−) Glycogen (+), (−) L.I.	209
Female Sprague-Dawley rats	P.H. + DEN	ATPase (−)	30
Female Sprague-Dawley rats	P.H. + DEN	ATPase (−) G6Pase (−) Glycogen (+)	210
Female Sprague-Dawley rats	P.H. + DEN	ATPase (−) G6Pase (−) Glycogen (+) Glycogen phosphorylase (−) Arylesterase (+)	39

Table 1 (continued)
HISTOCHEMICAL DEMONSTRATIONS OF NEOPLASTIC AND/OR PUTATIVE PRENEOPLASTIC HEPATOCYTE FOCI

Animals	Administered substance(s)[a] or procedure(s)	Marker changes[b]	Ref.
Female Sprague-Dawley rats	P.H. + DEN	ATPase (−) L.I.	211
Female Sprague-Dawley rats	P.H. + DEN	ATPase (−) G6Pase (−) Glycogen (+)	38
Male & female Sprague-Dawley & BDIX rats	DEN, P.H. + DEN	G6Pase (−) ATPase (−)	212
Male & female Wistar rats	DEN	Acid phosphatase (−) Nonspecific esterase (−) β-Glucuronidase (−) G6PDH (−) Isocitric dehydrogenase (−) Succinic dehydrogenase (−) Glycerophosphate dehydrogenase (−) Lactic dehydrogenase (−) Monoamine oxidase (−) DPN diaphorase (−) TPN diaphorase (+) G6Pase (−)	213
Rats	DEN + 2-AAF + P.H.	D-T diaphorase (+)	214
Male Fischer rats	2-AAF	α-Fetoprotein (+)	215
Male Sprague-Dawley rats	(P.H. + DEN + choline-devoid diet) or (DEN + choline-devoid diet + P.H.)	GGT (+)	50
Male Sprague-Dawley rats	P.H. + DEN + choline-devoid diet + PB	GGT (+)	51
Female Sprague-Dawley rats	P.H. + DEN + PB	GGT (+) ATPase (−) G6Pase (−)	216
Male F-344 rats	(DEN + 2-AAF + P.H.) or (P.H. + MNU + 2-AAF + CCl_4)	GGT (+)	24
Male Fischer 344 rats	DEN + 2-AAF + P.H.	GGT (+) L.I.	13
Female Wistar rats	3′-Me-DAB	α-Fetoprotein (+)	217
Male Wistar rats	(P.H. + azaserine + choline-devoid diet) or (azaserine + 2-AAF + choline-devoid diet)	GGT (+)	218
Male Sprague-Dawley rats	NNM	Glycogen (+) DNase (−) RNase (−)	219
Male Wistar R rats	NNM	DNase (−) RNase (−)	220
Male Sprague-Dawley rats	Many	GGT (+) Acid phosphatase (−) G6Pase (−) ATPase (−)	71
Male Fischer rats	DEN + (2-AAF or −HCH) + P.H.	GGT (+) ATPase (−)	74
Fischer 344 rats	Carcinogen (many tested) + 2-AAF + proliferative stimulus	GGT (+)	25
Male Riv:Tox [M] rats	DEN + 2-AAF + P.H.	Glycogen (+)	119

Table 1 (continued)
HISTOCHEMICAL DEMONSTRATIONS OF NEOPLASTIC AND/OR PUTATIVE PRENEOPLASTIC HEPATOCYTE FOCI

Animals	Administered substance(s)[a] or procedure(s)	Marker changes[b]	Ref.
Male Wistar/RIV rats	DEN + 2-AAF + P.H.	Glycogen (+) GGT (+) ATPase (−) G6Pase (−)	120
Male Wistar rats	Ethionine	ATPase (−) Alkaline phosphate (−) (+)	221
F344 rats	2-AAF + PB	Iron accumulation (−)	222
Male Wistar rats	3′-Me-DAB	Aldolases A and C (+) in oval cells	223
BDI rats	DAB	Liver-specific antigen (−)	224
Male Wistar rats	2-AAF	Iron accumulation (−) Glycogen (+) M.I.	225
Male Fischer 344 rats	2-AAF	Iron accumulation (−)	226
Male Fischer 344 rats	2-AAF	Iron accumulation (−) GGT (+)	127
Male C3H/HeN and (C57BL/6 × C3Hf)F_1 hybrid mice	Spontaneous nodule formation	Iron accumulation (−)	229
Male Wistar rats	2-AAF	Iron accumulation (−) Glycogen (+) M.I.	228
Male & female C3HfB/HeN mice	PB	GGT (+) G6Pase (−) ATPase (−) Iron accumulation (−)	229
Male Charles River F344 CDF rats	2-AAF + nodule fragment transplantation	Iron accumulation (−)	230
F344 rats	2-AAF	Iron accumulation (−) Glycogen (+)	231
Male Fischer F344 rats	DEN, 2-AAF	Iron accumulation (−)	232
Female Sprague-Dawley rats	DEN, + PB or contraceptive steroids	GGT (+)	233
Male Fischer F344 rats	2-AAF	Iron accumulation (−)	234

[a] 2-AAF, 2 acetylaminofluorene; *o*-AT, *o*-aminoaxotoluene; BAP, benzo[a]pyrene; BEP, benzo[e]pyrene; BHA, butylated hydroxyanisole; CPA, cyproterone acetate; DAB, dimethylaminoazobenzene; DEN, diethylnitrosamine; 1,2-DMH, 1,2-dimethylhydrazine; DMN, dimethylnitrosamine; ENU, ethylnitrosourea; α-HCH, α-hexachlorocyclohexane; 2-Me-DAB, 2-methyl-*N,N*-dimethyl-4-aminoazobenzene; 3′-Me-DAB, 3′-methyl-4-dimethylaminoazobenzene; MNU, *N*-methyl-*N*-nitrosourea; NNM, *N*-nitrosomopholine; *N*-OH-AAF, *N*-hydroxy-acetylaminofluorene; PB, phenobarbital; PCB, polychlorinated biphenyls; P.H., partial hepatectomy; TAA, thioacetamide; and TCDD, 2,3,7,8-tetrachloro-dibenzo-*p*-dioxin.

[b] (+), increased and (−), decreased in neoplastic and/or putative preneoplastic hepatocyte foci; ATPase, adenosine triphosphatase; DNase, deoxyribonuclease; GGT, γ-glutamyltranspeptidase; G6Pase, glucose 6-phosphatase; G6PDH, glucose 6-phosphate dehydrogenase; L.I., labeling index (% of hepatocyte nuclei labeled by ^{3}H-thymidine); M.I., mitotic index; PN antigen, preneoplastic antigen; and RNase, ribonuclease.

information on markers that were studied simultaneously in individual investigations. Other recent reviews have presented tables of marker information in different organizational styles.[14,37,118]

The following section summarizes information on the histochemical and biochemical properties of the markers shown in Table 1. There are four valuable general references on histochemical methods.[235-238]

1. Acid Phosphatase

Detection — Histochemical method of Gomori[239] or of Barka and Anderson.[240] Thompson[238] has listed specific precautions to take when applying these methods. In normal rat liver, strong acid phosphatase activity was present in hepatocytes and weak activity was observed in Kupffer cells.[241] Hepatocyte acid phosphatase granules were typically found in a pericanalicular arrangement,[242,243] with a slightly stronger reaction in periportal cells.[242] Rodent liver acid phosphatase was primarily associated with lysosomes and to a lesser extent with the endoplasmic reticulum.[123,244]

Biochemistry — An orthophosphoric monoester + H_2O = an alcohol + H_3PO_4.[244] Acid phosphatase liberates phosphate from many alcoholic or phenolic phosphomonoesters. The activities of the multiple forms of acid phosphatase in hepatocytes tend to increase during aging.[245]

Significance in hepatic neoplasia — Acid phosphatase was an equivocal marker during hepatocarcinogenesis in rats. In one study,[71] the acid phosphatase activity of the neoplastic nodules produced by a variety of carcinogenic regimens was consistently reduced compared to that of the normal rat liver parenchymal cells. Others reported reduced or unchanged activity of this enzyme in many preneoplastic altered foci or neoplastic nodules,[137,164,170,213] and Kitagawa found increased acid phosphatase activity in 14% of the neoplastic nodules examined.[170] In rat hepatocellular carcinomas, the acid phosphatase activities were decreased or absent,[123,148,164,170,213] unchanged,[123,148,170,213] or increased.[148,170,213] compared with activity in host liver.

2. Adenosine Triphosphatase (ATPase)

Detection — Histochemical method of Wachstein and Meisel.[238,246] This method detects Mg^{2+}-Ca^{2+}-dependent ATPase activity expressed as an intense staining of hepatocyte bile cancaliculi and a weaker staining of nuclei and microsomes.[247] Activity is also seen in the lining of blood vessels and bile ducts.[238] The usual formol-calcium fixative inhibits mitochondrial ATPase.[247] Calcium ions can replace magnesium ions in this procedure[246] without diminution of staining intensities in the plasma membrane/bile canaliculi.[247]

Biochemistry — ATP + H_2O = ADP + orthophosphate.[244] Regulation of liver-calcium-ion concentration by calcitonin and other hormones may be mediated by Ca^{2+}-ATPase.[248] Peterson et al. concluded that rat liver surface membrane Mg^{2+}-ATPase was not involved in hepatic uptake or biliary excretion of ouabain.[249] Membrane-bound Mg^{2+}-Ca^{2+}-ATPase may also function in pinocytosis, exocytosis, membrane fusion, or microvilli formation.[169,250]

Significance in hepatic neoplasia — Canalicular ATPase activity was reduced in most human,[251] mouse,[178,229] and rat[148,150,164] hepatomas in comparison with surrounding liver parenchymal tissue. Occasionally, however, ATPase activity was increased in hepatomas of the mouse[138,178] and rat.[148] Consistent with the results in hepatomas, canalicular ATPase activity was also reduced in most preneoplastic enzyme-altered liver cell foci.[44,126,202] Primarily using data on ATPase-negative altered foci, Emmelot and Scherer[40] have provided an elegant review on the kinetics of induction and growth of foci and on the precursor-product relationships between altered foci and malignant liver tumors.

3. Aldolases

Detection — Immunoperoxidase and immunofluorescence techniques.[223]

Biochemistry — A ketose 1-phosphate = dihydroxyacetone phosphate + an aldehyde[244] (or) fructose 1,6-diphosphate = dihydroxyacetone phosphate + D-glyceraldehyde 3-phosphate.[244]

Significance in hepatic neoplasia — During hepatocarcinogenesis induced in rats by 3′-methyl-4-(dimethylamino)azobenzene, the aldolase enzymes did not serve to delineate the boundaries of preneoplastic enzyme-altered foci.[224] In normal liver, aldolase B was present in parenchymal cells, aldolase A was in sinusoidal cells, and aldolase C was not detected. During neoplasia, aldolase B was observed in normal and megalocytic hepatocytes, while aldolases A and C were found in small oval and transient cells.[223]

4. Alkaline Phosphatase (AP)

Detection — Histochemical methods of Gomori,[252] Burstone,[253,254] and Mayahara et al.[255] The latter method has been modified by Karasaki[169] for simultaneous demonstration of alkaline phosphate localization and ^{3}H-thymidine-labeled nuclei distribution. In adult liver parenchymal cells, AP activity in the bile canaliculi was low in rats[148,163,242] and negligible in mice.[151] AP activity was also detected in occasional capillaries and in connective tissue surrounding the bile ducts. In rat hepatocytes, some cytoplasmic and nucleolar staining was evident.[169] High bile canalicular AP activity occurred in the livers of fetal and neonatal mice.[151]

Biochemistry — An orthophosphoric monoester + H_2O = an alcohol + H_3PO_4.[244] Fishman[256] has reviewed the biochemical and physical properties of AP and the relation of this enzyme to tissue development and neoplasia. The physiological functions of AP are not known,[256] but several proposed functions have been discussed by Fishman[256] and Karasaki.[169]

Significance in hepatic neoplasia — During hepatocarcinogenesis in rats, increased alkaline phosphatase activity in bile canaliculi and over the entire cell surface was often a feature of advanced lesions[125,137,148,164,169,170,221] (hyperbasophilic hepatocytes, neoplastic nodules, hepatocellular carcinomas), but was infrequently cited as a feature of preneoplastic altered foci.[170] Altered foci can exhibit decreased AP activity relative to surrounding parenchyma.[170] In a study of hepatic neoplasia induced by any of several carcinogenic regimens, the AP activity of neoplastic nodules was unchanged compared to the activity of nonhyperplastic areas.[71] In biochemical assays, the AP activities of transplantable hepatomas were increased, unchanged, or decreased compared with host livers.[123]

During griseofulvin-induced mouse hepatocarcinogenesis, hepatocytes in all types of foci and nodules showed increased amounts of plasma membrane AP activity.[151] AP activity was also increased in the liver nodules of C3H mice treated with phenobarbital but the AP activity of the spontaneous nodules in untreated C3H mice was less than that of the surrounding liver.[138]

5. Aniline Hydroxylase (AH)

Detection — Histochemical method of Gangolli and Wright.[257] AH activity was present in all parenchymal cells of the adult rat[257] and mouse[138] liver, but some lobular heterogeneity of enzyme intensity was evident. In adult rat livers, no reaction was observed in the bile ducts, endothelial cells, or connective tissue.[257] In newborn rats, AH activity was similarly distributed but considerably weaker.[257] Histochemically, AH was confined to the cytoplasm of hepatocytes,[138,257] and upon subcellular fractionation AH activity was detected predominantly in the microsomal fraction/endoplasmic reticulum.

Reaction — Aniline is converted to *p*-aminophenol by a mixed function oxidase reaction.[257] The detailed molecular mechanism of this reaction is under investigation.[258]

Significance in hepatic neoplasia — In a study of mouse hepatocarcinogenesis, reduction of AH activity relative to liver parenchyma activity served as a marker only of advanced lesions or neoplasms.[138] In studies of several Morris hepatomas, AH activity was reduced to 50% of normal liver activity or less in all but one tumor.[121]

6. Antigens [PN (Epoxide Hydrase), Fetal Liver, Liver Specific, Neo-]

Detection — Immunohistochemical methods.[259]

Biochemistry — A biochemical function has not been discovered for most of these antigens. One exception, PN antigen,[192,198,260] has been identified as epoxide hydrase.[261]

Significance in hepatic neoplasia — Antigens that have been studied as markers of altered foci in preneoplastic livers include (1) antigens that, compared to a normal adult, were reduced in foci (liver-specific antigen[224] and antigen studied by Hunt et al.[160] in the colony forming unit assay); or (2) antigens that were increased in foci (fetal liver antigen[140] and PN antigen[179,192,198]). PN antigen (or epoxide hydrolase) was found in every rat neoplastic nodule and hepatoma examined in one study,[198] but was absent from the rat hepatocellular carcinomas examined by other investigators.[179] Baldwin has reviewed the types of neoantigens expressed during rat hepatic neoplasia and in hepatic tumors.[262]

7. Catalase

Detection — Histochemical method of Novikoff and Goldfischer.[161,263] Reaction-positive granules, representing peroxisomes, were observed in normal hepatocytes.[161]

Biochemistry — $H_2O_2 + H_2O_2 = O_2 + 2H_2O$.[244]

Significance in hepatic neoplasia — In the single reference on catalase in Table 1, most of the altered foci and some of the neoplastic nodules of rats showed quite reduced catalase activity compared with the activity in surrounding parenchymal cells.[161] Most hepatic tumors in rats also had reduced catalase activity.[264]

8. Chorionic Gonadotropin (CG)

Detection — Immunoperoxidase method of Malkin et al.[189] CG was absent from fetal, regenerating, and adult rat liver.

Biochemistry — CG, a glycopeptide hormone, is a normal product of the syncitiotrophoblast.[189]

Significance in hepatic neoplasia — CG or an antigenically related substance was absent from normal rat liver but was present in preneoplastic altered foci and in hepatomas.[189]

9. Dehydrogenases — Glycerophosphate (GDH), Isocitric (IDH), Lactic (LDH), and Succinic (SDH)

Detection — See discussion by Thompson[238] on the histochemical demonstration of dehydrogenases.

Biochemistry — Substrate + acceptor = oxidized substrate + reduced acceptor.[238]

Significance in hepatic neoplasia — These four dehydrogenases are grouped because of their uniformity of change during early hepatic neoplasia. Thus, in comparison to activity in normal liver parenchymal cells, the activity of GDH,[213] IDH,[213] and LDH[170,213] was reduced in most rat liver preneoplastic foci, and the activity of SDH was reduced in most liver preneoplastic foci of rats[137,164,170,199,213] and monkeys[207] and in most nodular lesions of neoplastic mouse livers.[138] In neoplastic nodules and hepatocellular carcinomas, the activities of the dehydrogenases were often reduced with respect to those of normal liver, but many cases of increased activity were also reported.[170,213]

10. DPN-TPN Diaphorase or D-T Diaphorase (DTD)

Detection — Histochemical method of Schor.[214] The methodology is discussed in detail by Thompson.[238] DPN diaphorase activity was found in all rat liver parenchymal cells, with stronger staining in centrilobular areas. Activity was primarily in mitochondria, but there was also diffuse cytoplasmic staining. The Kupffer cells, vessel walls, cytoplasm of bile ducts, and stroma of periportal fields also exhibited activity.[242] TPN diaphorase activity was marked in hepatocytes surrounding periportal fields and slight in bile ducts.[242]

Biochemistry — The reduced coenzymes DPNH and TPNH are oxidized to DPN and TPN, by their respective diaphorases (DPN-diaphorase and TPN-diaphorase), which are flavoproteins.[238]

Significance in hepatic neoplasia — DTD activity was increased in preneoplastic foci and hyperplastic nodules of rat liver in one study.[214] In another report in which the DPN-diaphorase and TPN-diaphorase activities of preneoplastic liver foci were studied separately, the former enzyme was reduced and the latter enzyme was reduced, normal, or increased in activity compared to normal parenchymal cell activity.[213] In rat hepatocellular carcinomas, DPN-diaphorase activity was normal or reduced,[213] TPN-diaphorase activity was reduced,[213] and D-T diaphorase activity was increased[214] with respect to normal liver. Apparently, the methodology used for demonstration of DTD activity can significantly affect results (see discussion by Schor[214]).

11. Esterases (Arylesterase, Butyrocholinesterase, Nonspecific Esterase)

Detection — Thompson[238] thoroughly discusses methods for the histochemical detection of esterase activity and methods for distinguishing among the various esterases by means of inhibitors. Several esterases are involved in hydrolysis of the substrates that demonstrate nonspecific esterases. In a summary of studies on adult rat and mouse liver, Thompson[238] reported that nonspecific esterase activity was present in the hepatocytes, Kupffer cells, and biliary epithelium, but was absent from the portal vessels and connective tissue.

Biochemistry — Ester + water = acid + alcohol. The true esterases hydrolyze simple esters of monohydric alcohols; the cholinesterases hydrolyze esters of choline.[238]

Significance in hepatic neoplasia — In the only cited study of arylesterase (Table 1), the activity of this enzyme was elevated in a preneoplastic altered focus of rat liver.[39] In one case, nonspecific esterase activity was elevated in neoplastic nodules but markedly deficient in hepatocellular carcinomas,[149] while in another case, this enzymatic activity was reduced in neoplastic nodules but unchanged or reduced in hepatocellular carcinomas.[213] Butyrocholinesterase activity was decreased both in neoplastic nodules and hepatocellular carcinomas.[149]

12. Ferritin

Detection — Immunoperoxidase method of Beaumont et al.[136] In adult rat liver, ferritin was found throughout the cytoplasm of the parenchymal cells.[136]

Biochemistry — Each molecule of ferritin, the major cellular iron storage protein, can associate with up to 5000 atoms of iron.[265] Frieden[266] recently reviewed the relationship between iron transport and iron storage.

Significance in hepatic neoplasia — In a study of hepatocarcinogenesis induced by diethylnitrosamine, all ATPase-deficient liver cell foci and neoplastic nodules displayed a strong staining for ferritin imposed upon a background of moderate staining for ferritin in surrounding parenchymal cells.[136] This increased ferritin in the early lesions contrasts with the reduced levels observed in six transplantable rat hepatomas.[265,267] However, the study on foci was performed with an antibody that did not distinguish between ferritin and its subunits,[136] while the study on hepatomas used specific ferritin antiserum.[267]

13. α-Fetoprotein (AFP)

Detection — Fluorescence immunohistochemistry.[268] AFP was absent from the livers of adult rats and mice, but was present in nearly all the hepatocytes of newborns.[269,270]

Significance in hepatic neoplasia — During rodent hepatocarcinogenesis, serum AFP concentrations increased as a function of the duration of carcinogen treatment.[162,215] In the transplantable Morris hepatoma series, slowly-growing well-differentiated hepatomas generally did not produce elevated serum AFP concentrations, but poorly differentiated fast-growing tumors produced high serum AFP concentrations.[271] The reports in Table 1 regarding AFP seem to indicate that AFP may be a marker of advanced lesions (neoplastic nodules), but only under certain conditions. Thus, with intermittent feeding of 2-acetylaminofluorene, Okita et al. found that virtually all the hepatocytes of a given neoplastic nodule were either quite uniformly stained, or unstained, in male Wistar rats,[197] while Sell showed that none of the 1078 neoplastic nodules examined in male Fischer rats had any AFP-containing cells.[215] In other reports, AFP was present only in isolated cells or small patches of cells within larger lesions that had been delineated by other markers.[162,165] Thus, in most cases, AFP did not clearly delimit the boundaries of preneoplastic enzyme-altered liver foci.

14. Glucose 6-Phosphatase (G6Pase)

Detection — Histochemical method of Wachstein and Meisel.[246,272] In adult rat and mouse liver, G6Pase activity was found only in parenchymal cells, with more intense activity in periportal areas.[246] In subcellular distribution studies, G6Pase was located mainly in the microsomal fraction.[244]

Biochemistry — Glucose 6-phosphate + H_2O = glucose + Pi. Cleavage of glucose 6-phosphate by G6Pase is a vital step in the conversion of liver glycogen to blood glucose.[273]

Significance in hepatic neoplasia — In 1955, Weber and Cantero showed that the G6Pase activity of rat liver decreased progressively during carcinogenesis produced by 4-dimethylaminoazobenzene.[274] This biochemical study set the stage for the discovery, in 1961, that nodules of G6Pase-deficient hydropic cells appeared and persisted in rat liver after discontinuation of methyl butter yellow feeding, but prior to tumor induction.[153] The authors[153] concluded that there ". . . may be an association between these nodules and induced hepatocellular carcinomas." This conclusion is strengthened by the findings that G6Pase activity was significantly reduced in most or all hepatocellular carcinomas of the rat,[121,148,150,164,170,274] human,[251] and mouse,[138,229] and in a significant proportion of the preneoplastic enzyme-altered liver foci of rats[44,126,154,158,170,202] and mice.[91,152] In a report by Pugh and Goldfarb,[44] loss of G6Pase from preneoplastic liver foci served as the best marker for foci with the highest labeling indexes after ^{3}H-thymidine injection.

15. Glucose 6-Phosphate Dehydrogenase (G6PDH)

Detection — Histochemical methods of Hess et al.[275] and Karnovsky and Himmelhoch[276] as modified by Kalengayi and Desmet.[163] In adult rat liver, G6PDH activity was exclusively in the cytoplasm of hepatocytes that were more intensely stained in the periportal region of the liver lobule.[163]

Biochemistry — Glucose 6-phosphate + NADP = 6-phosphoglucono-δ-lactone + NADPH + + H^+.[277] G6PDH is the first enzyme of the pentose phosphate pathway.[277]

Significance in hepatic neoplasia — G6PDH was normally increased in primary hepatomas and experimental hepatocellular carcinomas compared to levels in normal or host liver,[121,164] but exceptions were found.[121,123,164,213] In preneoplastic enzyme-altered foci, G6PDH was unchanged,[164,213] increased,[102,164] or decreased.[213] In the Morris hepatomas, G6PDH exhibited abnormal responses to environmental stimuli.[278]

16. β-Glucuronidase (βG)

Detection — Histochemical method of Hayashi et al.[279] Autoradiography can be used in combination with this method.[175] In adult rat liver, βG activity was detected as small positive granules in the pericanalicular cytoplasm of hepatocytes in the periportal zone of the lobule. Diffuse cytoplasmic staining was also noted.[279] This enzyme was primarily localized in lysosomes.[123,243]

Biochemistry — This enzyme hydrolyzes and synthesizes glucuronic acid conjugates and is specific for the β-glycoside linkage of a number of glucuronides.[238] A β-D-glucuronide + H_2O = an alcohol + D-glucuronic acid.[244]

Significance in hepatic neoplasia — Compared to the activity of βG in the parenchyma of normal rat liver, the activity of this enzyme was generally reduced in preneoplastic altered foci of in neoplastic nodules,[170-172,174,175,213] but cases of unchanged[170,213] or increased[170] activity were occasionally noted. βG activity was also reduced in most rat hepatocellular carcinomas.[170,213]

17. γ-Glutamyltranspeptidase (GGT)

Detection — Histochemical method of Rutenberg et al.[280] using the modification of Ogawa et al.[194] or, typically, of Kalengayi et al.[167] Vanderlaan et al.[281] have described a histochemical method suitable for fluorometric detection of cells having GGT activity. In adult rat[167,280] and mouse[178,229] liver, GGT activity was essentially absent from parenchymal cells (with one exception[282]), but present in bile ductular cells. Bile ducts are readily identified by their shape and proximity to the portal vein and hepatic artery. In developing liver, GGT activity was present at high levels until 3 to 10 days post partum[139,283-285] in parenchymal cell plasma membranes and bile canaliculi.[139,167]

Biochemistry — γ-Glutamyl-cysteinyl-glycine + amino acid, peptide, or H_2O = cysteinyl-glycine + γ-glutamyl-amino acid, γ-glutamyl-peptide, or glutamic acid.[285] GGT may be involved in amino acid transport as part of a 6-enzyme γ-glutamyl cycle,[285] in peptide transport,[285,286] in regulation of glutathione levels,[287] or in acid-base balance by acting as a glutaminase during metabolic acidosis.[288]

Significance in hepatic neoplasia — GGT is one of the most important and widely studied markers of preneoplastic enzyme-altered liver foci (Table 1). Elevated GGT activity was found in most hepatocellular carcinomas of the rat[150,289,290] and human.[251] In the mouse, most neoplastic lesions had GGT activities close to that of normal liver.[151,289] If mice were treated with phenobarbital, however, the GGT activity of the neoplastic lesions was considerably greater than that of the surrounding parenchyma.[178,229] Elevated GGT activity was also found in enzyme-altered mouse liver foci during safrole-induced hepatocarcinogenesis.[188] The biochemical activity of GGT in rat liver increased as a function of duration of carcinogen administration,[209,291] but part of this increase may be due to a disproportionate increase in the number of GGT-positive bile duct cells.[292] When serial sections from preneoplastic rat livers were treated with different histochemical stains and superimposed in order to assign a histochemical phenotype to each altered cell focus, increased GGT activity served to mark a greater proportion of foci than other markers examined.[44,126,202]

Following two thirds hepatectomy, the total GGT activity of rat liver remained at a normal level, but reciprocal changes occurred in enzymatic forms differing in sialic acid content.[293] This indicates that GGT elevation is not obligatorily linked to hepatocyte proliferation.

GGT activity varied cyclically in the mouse hair follicle, increasing markedly in each successive growth/maturation stage of the hair growth cycle.[294] GGT activity increased markedly in rat hepatocytes cultured on collagen gels[295] or in endothelial cells co-cultured with glial cells.[296] These considerations open the possibility that the increased activity of GGT in enzyme-altered liver foci and liver neoplasms can be influenced by cell-cell or cell-extracellular matrix interactions.

Elevated GGT activity was also associated with neoplasia of the colon,[297] breast,[298] lung,[299] skin,[294] and lymphoid cells.[300]

18. Glutathione, Reduced (GSH)

Detection — Histochemical method of Asghar et al.[301] as modified by Deml and Oesterle.[144]

Biochemistry — GSH participates in a multitude of biochemical reactions in liver and other tissues[302-304] serving to detoxify xenobiotics, protect -SH groups of essential proteins and other molecules, inactivate free radicals, and support amino acid and peptide transport.

Significance in hepatic neoplasia — The significance of GSH as a marker of preneoplastic enzyme-altered liver foci is unclear. Continual administration of any of several hepatocarcinogens to rats led to an early increase in total liver GSH followed by a return to normal or subnormal levels at the time of appearance of neoplastic nodules. The subsequently appearing hepatic neoplasms also had normal GSH levels (in well-differentiated, slowly-growing hepatomas) or subnormal GSH levels (in nondifferentiated, slowly-growing hepatomas) or subnormal GSH levels (in nondifferentiated, rapidly-growing hepatomas).[290] Other investigators[287] found that fetal liver and the Novikoff hepatoma contained similar GSH levels, and that these levels were significantly lower than that of adult liver. The activities of enzymes involved in GSH metabolism have been studied in liver as a function of the duration of the hepatocarcinogenesis regimen.[291] Though unexpected from the results reported above, Deml and Oesterle[144] reported that histochemically detected GSH was markedly elevated in enzyme-altered liver foci of rats treated with either of the two different carcinogens. GSH, administered by gavage to rats bearing aflatoxin β_1-induced liver tumors, caused regression of tumor growth and increased animal survival.[305] In this study, however, it was not clear whether GSH or the products of its cleavage by digestive enzymes served as the active agent(s).

19. Glycogen

Detection — Histochemical method of McManus.[306] The choice of fixative and fixation method are critical to the retention of tissue glycogen.[307,308] The lobular distribution of liver glycogen is subject to marked diurnal variation.[308]

Biochemistry — Liver glycogen functions as a carbohydrate reserve that stabilizes the blood glucose level in the interval between meals.[273] Rhythmic changes in liver glycogen are associated with diurnal variations of glycogen synthetase, which catalyzes the rate-limiting step in glycogen synthesis, and of glycogen phosphorylase, which initiates the breakdown of glycogen.[309]

Significance in hepatic neoplasia — In a major review, Bannasch et al.[102] described two stages of liver carcinogenesis that could be distinguished by the histochemical demonstration of glycogen. The first stage was characterized by excessive storage of glycogen in foci of preneoplastic hepatocytes. Such changes were reported for the preneoplastic livers of rats, mice, pigs, *Mastomys,* and monkeys.[102] This excessive focal storage of glycogen was especially apparent when the surrounding parenchyma was depleted of glycogen during a period of fasting.[38,145] Biochemical and histochemical studies on some enzymes related to carbohydrate metabolism have not revealed clear-cut enzymatic changes that might account for excessive glycogen storage in preneoplastic liver foci.[102] The second stage was marked by a gradual reduction of the glycogen initially stored in excess; this reduction was accompanied by morphologic cellular changes characteristic of progression toward hepatocellular carcinoma.[102]

20. Glycogen Phosphorylase

Detection — Histochemical method of Takeuchi as modified by Korsgaard and Wulff.[235,310]

Biochemistry — Glycogen phosphorylase initiates the breakdown of glycogen.[309] (α-1,4-glucosyl)$_n$ + orthophosphate = (α-1,4-glucosyl)$_{n-1}$ + D-glucose 1-phosphate.[244]

Significance in hepatic neoplasia — Compared to the activity in normal liver parenchyma, phosphorylase activity was reduced in most preneoplastic altered foci,[39,102,170] neoplastic nodules,[145,170] and hepatomas[170] of the rat. However, examples of unchanged or increased phosphorylase activity were also reported.[102,107] Farber[8] has suggested that the altered phosphorylase activity might account, in part, for altered glycogen metabolism during hepatocarcinogenesis. This possibility has been further discussed by Bannasch et al.[102]

21. Iron, Resistance to Accumulation

Detection — After induction of hepatic siderosis by dietary iron loading with hydroxyquinoline and ferrous gluconate[232] or by rapid iron loading produced by multiple subcutaneous injections of iron dextran,[227] iron is detected in liver sections by the Prussian blue method.[311]

Significance in hepatic neoplasia — Williams[127] has reviewed the advantages of iron-resistance as a marker for altered liver foci. Color photographs of such foci have been published.[228] Although some studies have found that iron resistance characterizes all hepatocellular lesions at all stages of development in both rats and mice,[127,227] another study showed that iron resistance was a property of only 28% of all the foci that could be detected by all combinations of four markers.[202] Since iron overload may result in delayed growth and morphologic abnormalities of liver mitochondria,[312] hepatocarcinogenesis studies that employ iron loading as a technique for detecting iron-resistant lesions may require additional controls to determine whether iron loading itself has an effect on tumor progression. The mechanism of the resistance of preneoplastic and neoplastic liver lesions to iron accumulation is unknown.[227] In normal liver about 60% of the nonheme iron present is found in the form of ferritin.[265] In comparison with the ferritin content of normal adult rat liver, the ferritin protein content of six transplantable rat hepatomas was reduced by more than 50%.[267] In the same study, the ferritin iron content of the hepatomas decreased with increasing growth rate. In contrast to the finding of decreased ferritin in hepatomas, ferritin protein was increased in enzyme-altered rat liver foci.[136] In the latter study, the antibody used did not distinguish between ferritin or its subunits.

22. Monoamine Oxidase (MAO)

Detection — Histochemical method of Glenner et al.[238] In adult rat liver, activity was seen in parenchymal cells without much difference between periportal and central areas of the lobule.[242]

Biochemistry — MAO oxidatively deaminates primary aliphatic amines to aldehydes.[238] $RCH_2NH_2 + O_2 + H_2O = RCHO + NH_3 + H_2O_2$.[238,244]

Significance in hepatic neoplasia — The MAO activity of preneoplastic altered foci and hepatocellular carcinomas of the rat was considerably reduced compared to the activity in normal liver parenchymal cells.[213]

23. Nucleases

Detection — RNase activity by the substrate-film method of Daoust.[313] Acid nucleases by the method of Aronson et al. as modified by Vorbrodt.[314] Alkaline nucleases, method of Taper.[315] Thompson[238] has discussed these methods. Activity of the acid nucleases was intense in hepatocyte nuclei and weak in peribiliary granules (lysosomes). Compared with the acid nucleases, activity of the alkaline nucleases was less intense in hepatocyte nuclei and more intense in canaliculi (and sinusoids for the RNase). Alkaline RNase activity was more intense in centrilobular canaliculi but the activity of the other nucleases was evenly distributed throughout the liver lobule.[163]

Biochemistry — DNase and RNase catalyze the depolymerization of DNA and RNA, respectively.[238]

Significance in hepatic neoplasia — In every histochemical study of acid or alkaline nuclease activity changes during rat hepatocarcinogenesis, the activity of these enzymes was considerably reduced or absent in altered foci, neoplastic nodules, and malignant hepatocellular tumors.[128,142,143,146,164,219,220] Altered foci, hyperbasophilic foci, and hepatocellular carcinomas were simultaneously deficient in both RNase and canalicular ATPase activities.[143] Foci having reduced nuclease activity developed later than foci of excessive glycogen storage.[219]

24. 5'-Nucleotidase

Detection — Histochemical method of Wachstein and Meisel.[246] In normal liver of adult rats, bile canaliculi and sinusoids of the centrilobular area showed a more marked activity than those of the periportal zone.[163,242,246] In the portal tract the blood vessel walls, basal membrane of bile ductular cells, and the fibrous stroma also showed activity.[163]

Biochemistry — This enzyme hydrolyzes nucleotides containing phosphate esterified at carbon five or ribose.[242] 5'-ribonucleotide + H_2O = ribonucleoside + H_3PO_4.[244]

Significance in hepatic neoplasia — In the rat the altered foci, hyperplastic nodules and liver cell carcinomas showed a loss or variable decrease of 5'-nucleotidase activity as compared with the activity of normal parenchyma.[164]

25. Serine Dehydratase (SerDH)

Detection — Immunohistochemical method of Kitagawa and Pitot.[316] In normal adult rat liver, SerDH was demonstrated diffusely in the cytoplasm of hepatocytes in the periportal zone.[172,316] Activity was not demonstrated in nonparenchymal cells.[316]

Biochemistry — L-serine + H_2O = pyruvate + NH_3 + H_2O.[244]

Significance in hepatic neoplasia — Compared with normal rat liver SerDH levels, the enzyme was deficient and not inducible in neoplastic nodules during their developing phase. Later, however, there was an elevation of SerDH and its inducibility in the majority of nodules.[171,172] Extensive variability of SerDH activity was demonstrated in a number of transplantable rat hepatocellular carcinomas.[121]

c. Biochemical Studies

Biochemical investigations on the "minimal deviation" hepatomas, other transplantable hepatomas, and primary hepatocellular carcinomas,[121-124,278,317,318] in conjunction with studies on adult, regenerating, developing, and preneoplastic liver[274,319,320] have shown that numerous changes in the complement, activity, or concentration of liver enzymes, proteins, and other cellular components can be specifically associated with hepatic neoplasia. A few of the biochemically identified hepatocarcinogenesis-associated changes have been studied by histochemical or immunohistochemical techniques (Table 1), but the majority serve as a reservoir of potential markers of preneoplastic and neoplastic hepatocytes.

d. Transplantation

Liebelt and Liebelt[321] have discussed in general terms the applicability of tissue transplantation techniques to the identification of stages of tumor progression. Hepatocellular carcinomas of the rat[114,322,323] or mouse[324] will grow upon transplantation to the liver or various other sites in syngeneic hosts. In contrast, neoplastic nodule and normal liver transplants persist but will not grow.[114,196,230,324,325] Thus, after donor rats have been exposed to hepatocarcinogenesis regimens, the transplantation of liver fragments to syngeneic hosts will reveal neoplastic cells by their growth at the transplantation site, but will not distinguish between normal hepatocytes and preneoplastic hepatocytes because neither displays progressive growth. Normal transplantation procedures can be employed to analyze for the presence of neoplastic cells in hepatocyte cultures that have been treated in vitro by hepatocarcinogens.[326,327] The tumorigenicity of liver epithelial-like cell line transplants in newborn rats[328,329] or in nude mice[330] was a criterion of malignant transformation that correlated with cytochemical activity of γ-glutamyltranspeptidase,[328,329] growth in soft agar,[329,330] and growth in low calcium medium.[329] Jirtle et al.[331] are investigating the transplantation of rat hepatocyte suspensions into the dorsal fascia of syngeneic hosts as a potential tool in the study of survival and neoplastic transformation of hepatocytes as a result of exposure to X-radiation and chemical carcinogens.

Recently, Laishes et al. developed a novel transplantation system that can be termed the liver colony-forming unit assay.[34,160,182,183,185] The three elements of this assay are (1) induction of presumptive preneoplastic lesions in donor rats by hepatocarcinogenic regimen; (2) dissociation of the donor rat liver into component cells by collagenase perfusion; and (3) transfer of viable putative premalignant donor hepatocytes, via mesenteric vein injection, to the livers of host rats given a two thirds hepatectomy during short-term feeding of 2-acetylaminofluorene.

2. Detection In Vitro

a. Characterization of Surgically Excised Preneoplastic and/or Neoplastic Lesions

After gross separation, neoplastic nodules have been subjected to direct biochemical analysis[145] or have been cultured in vitro and then subjected to biochemical and other analyses.[43,332-334]

b. Selective Survival and/or Growth

Morphologic transformation — In long-term cell cultures derived from primary liver cell cultures, carcinogen treatment resulted in morphologic transformation accompanied by increased growth in soft agar and an increased frequency of 8-azaguanine-resistant mutants.[335] In contrast, malignant transformation occurred in aflatoxin B_1-treated rat hepatocyte cell (RL-PR-C) cultures, as demonstrated by carcinoma formation upon back injection of the treated cells into isogenic animals, without evidence of in vitro cytopathological morphology.[326] These authors[326] concluded that ". . . parameters commonly used to monitor fibroblast cultures for transformation in vitro were not applicable for assessing the tumorigenic potential of these epithelial cells."

Growth in soft agar — San et al., in an extensive survey of adult rat liver epithelial-like cell lines, found that the combined assessment of growth in soft agar, cytochemical assay of γ-glutamyltranspeptidase, and growth in low-calcium medium provided a reliable means of identifying transformation in an epithelial cell system.[329,330] Increased growth in soft agar can be accompanied by morphologic transformation and an increased frequency of 8-azaguanine-resistant mutants.[335] In epithelial cell cultures established from normal rat liver, only the tumorigenic cells grow in soft agar,[336] but tumorigenicity can develop independently of the ability to grow in soft agar.[326,327]

Growth on living cell layers — In a comparison of normal and transformed rat liver epithelial cells in vitro, the control cells grew on tissue culture plates, but not on a base layer of living parent cells, while transformed cells formed distinct colonies under either condition. Colony formation over a base layer of living parent cells thus identified transformed cells.[337]

Resistance to toxic chemicals — Compared to cultures of hepatocytes from normal rat livers, cultures of cells from rat liver neoplastic nodules or cells from the livers of rats fed 0.02% 2 AAF for 8 to 12 weeks are relatively resistant to the toxic effects of carcinogens and of some nonhepatocarcinogenic drugs.[183,334,338]

Promoter in vitro — In Section III.A.7 we discussed the study of Kitagawa et al. in which phenobarbital enhanced the production, in vitro, of malignantly transformed colonies in epithelial cell cultures from the livers of rats fed AAF.[76] Phenobarbital also has biological effects that mimic the transformation of adult rat liver epithelial cells in culture.[339] The tumor promoters phenobarbital, saccharin, and 12-*O*-tetradecanoylphorbol-13-acetate can stimulate DNA synthesis in calcium-deprived T51B liver cells.[340]

Selective media — Growth of rat liver epithelial-like cell lines in low-calcium medium correlated with tumorigenicity in nude mice or newborn rats and with growth in soft agar and cytochemical assay of γ-glutamyltranspeptidase activity.[329] Swierenga et al. have shown that calcium and cyclic AMP control the proliferation of nontumorigenic liver cells, but that calcium has little or no effect on the proliferation of tumorigenic cells in vitro.[341]

c. Isolation, Enrichment, or Detection, by Physical or Biochemical Techniques

Affinity reagents — Iype and Pontzer found that increased attachment of Con A:agarose to cell colonies was a characteristic of transformed or malignant rat liver cells. They have utilized this property for quantitating transformed colonies in a mixed population of transformed and untransformed cells.[342]

Differential sedimentation — Wanson et al. isolated hepatocytes from control and carcinogen-treated rats by collagenase perfusion. Five distinct hepatic subpopulations were separated by elutriation or counterflow centrifugation. In liver cell populations from the carcinogen-treated rats, hypertrophic parenchymal cells with a high degree of ploidy were concentrated in two elutriated fractions and ". . . constitute interesting material for further studies on biochemical changes of hepatocytes treated with carcinogens."[343]

Cell sorting/cytophotometry — Vanderlaan et al.[281] have used flow microfluorometry to identify liver cells with elevated GGT activity after exposure to a hepatocarcinogen. Five weeks after carcinogen injection, the number of GGT (+) cells from the carcinogen-treated rats was more than 20 times that from the control rats. Cytochemical stains for alkaline phosphatase and acid arylamidase, suitable for flow microfluorometry, have also been developed.[344]

Perfusion technique — DeGerlache et al.[345] treated rats with a hepatocarcinogen until liver neoplastic nodules appeared. They then subjected the livers to collagenase perfusion. The neoplastic nodules remained essentially nondissociated and could be separated by filtration from the well-dissociated cells of the surrounding parenchyma.

d. Other In Vitro Detection Methods

Iype et al.[346] and Montesano et al.[347] have reviewed markers for transformation in rat liver epithelial cells in culture.

IV. CHARACTERISTICS OF MULTISTAGE HEPATOCARCINOGENESIS

A. Known Initiators and Promoters of Liver Tumorigenesis

Following the initial observation of the promotion of AAF hepatocarcinogenesis by phenobarbital,[16] several reports have demonstrated that initiation and promotion in liver can each be produced by a wide variety of agents (Table 2) administered according to the sequential treatment protocol. It is noteworthy that the use of a promoting stimulus has increased the sensitivity of the liver system to the extent that agents heretofore considered to have virtually no hepatocarcinogenic activity (benzo[a]pyrene, 7,12-dimethylbenz[a]anthracene, and 2-methyl-*n*,*n*-dimethyl-4-aminobenzene) were unequivocally identified as initiators.

It is clear that phenobarbital is not an initiator of hepatocarcinogenesis in mice[18] or rats,[23] and in fact barbiturates can exert a protective effect against hepatic tumorigenesis when administered simultaneously with a known carcinogen,[16,17] as indicated above (Section II.B). Therefore, the observation that phenobarbital increased the incidence of liver tumors in mice subject to a "spontaneous" incidence of such tumors[360-363] suggests that phenobarbital was promoting the phenotypic expression of tumorigenic lesions induced by an as yet unknown initiator. This explanation presumably also applies to a similar observation made recently in rats.[364] In view of this type of tumorigenic effect by the clear-cut promoter, phenobarbital, it appears reasonable to question the validity of the practice of classifying agents such as DDT as carcinogens simply on the basis of their ability to increase liver tumor incidence,

Table 2
INITIATION-PROMOTION EXPERIMENTS IN LIVER

Initiator	Promoter	Ref.
2-Acetylaminofluorene	Phenobarbital	16,20—23,29, 44,73,348
Diethylnitrosamine	Phenobarbital	35,51,177,233, 349—351
Dimethylnitrosamine	Phenobarbital	352
N-Butyl-*N*(4-hydroxybutyl)-nitrosamine	Phenobarbital	353
Benzo[a]pyrene	Phenobarbital	354
7,12-Dimethylbenz[a]anthracene	Phenobarbital	355
N,*N*-dimethyl-4-aminoazobenzene	Phenobarbital	356
3-Methyl-*N*,*N*-dimethyl-4-aminoazobenzene	Phenobarbital	177
2-Methyl-*N*,*N*-dimethyl-4-aminoazobenzene	Phenobarbital	173
2-Acetylaminofluorene	Dichlorodiphenyltrichloroethane	21
Diethylnitrosamine	Dichlorodiphenyltrichloroethane	351
Diethylnitrosamine	Polychlorinated biphenyls	350,351
2-Acetylaminofluorene	Butylated hydroxytoluene	357
Diethylnitrosamine	2,3,7,8-Tetrachlorodibenzo-*p*-dioxin	204
Diethylnitrosamine	Contraceptive steroids	233
Diethylnitrosamine	Choline deficiency	51
Diethylnitrosamine	α-Hexachlorocyclohexane	359
Diethylnitrosamine	Hepatic peroxisome proliferators	358

when fed at high dietary concentrations for long intervals to mice[365-369] or rats[370,371] susceptible to such tumors. Tumor promoting activity might also be assigned to certain plant resins, since prolonged exposure to such substances in softwood bedding has increased hepatic tumor incidence in susceptible mice.[372]

B. Characteristics of Liver Tumor Promotion by Phenobarbital

In analyzing the characteristics of liver tumor promotion using the sequential AAF-phenobarbital treatment protocol we have examined the effects on tumorigenesis of: (1) separating the carcinogen and phenobarbital treatments by various intervals, (2) varying the duration of exposure to phenobarbital, and (3) varying the dietary concentration of phenobarbital. We have observed that the promoting effect of phenobarbital occurs despite the interposition of a 120-day interval between the termination of the carcinogen treatment and the onset of exposure to phenobarbital.[22] These findings indicate that carcinogen-modified hepatocytes with tumorigenic potential (i.e., "initiated" hepatocytes) persist long after the initiating event. Such persistence is in accord with skin tumorigenesis studies suggesting that the initiation stage of tumorigenesis is irreversible.[5,373] In addition, an increase in the duration of the phenobarbital treatment interval following AAF exposure was accompanied by parallel increases in tumor yield;[20,22] prolonged exposure to phenobarbital was required for maximal promoting effectiveness.[20,22]

Our most recent investigations[23] compared the promoting effects of different dietary levels of phenobarbital. When fed at dietary concentrations that did not affect body weight gain, phenobarbital elicited dose-dependent increases in the final incidence (plateau level) of hepatic tumors in rats previously fed AAF. However, these phenobarbital treatments did not affect the time to onset or to cessation (attainment of the plateau phase) of tumorigenesis. The highest dietary concentration of phenobarbital retarded tumor promotion initially, but ultimately had the strongest promoting effect; rats on this regimen also showed a reduction in growth rate. None of the dietary levels of phenobarbital affected the growth rates or the morphological characteristics (degree of differentiation) of the tumors that were produced. The foregoing observations suggest that (1) phenobarbital has no initiating activity and (2) tumor promotion by phenobarbital involves primarily an increase in the probability that initiated hepatocytes will express the neoplastic phenotype and does not influence the character of this phenotype or the kinetics of its expression.

The current experimental evidence suggests that the tumor promoting effect of phenobarbital is specific for the liver. In CF1 mice, phenobarbital feeding increased the spontaneous incidence of hepatic tumors, but had no effect on the spontaneous incidence of other tumors such as lymphomas, lung adenomas, and osteomas.[362] Likewise, phenobarbital increased the subsequent incidence of liver tumors in mice treated with DEN at birth, but had no effect on DEN-induced lung tumors in these animals.[352] Phenobarbital feeding also failed to enhance skin tumorigenesis in mice subjected to prior skin painting with 7,12-dimethylbenz[a]anthracene.[374] Other barbiturate derivatives may exhibit broader organ specificities, however, as indicated by the observation that chronic sodium barbiturate administration promoted intestinal tumorigenesis in rats previously exposed to dimethylhydrazine.[375]

With respect to the consequence of human exposure to phenobarbital, the evidence concerning the effects of barbiturates on tumorigenesis in liver or other tissue is ambiguous. In a study of patients receiving long-term treatment with phenobarbital, a slightly greater than expected incidence of liver tumors was observed[376] (the significance of which has been debated[377,378]), but no increase occurred in other types of tumors.[376] Additional epidemiological studies suggest that chronic barbiturate treatment may increase the risk of brain tumorigenesis in children,[380] although this conclusion is also disputed.[380,381]

V. CRITIQUE OF CURRENT SPECULATIONS ON MECHANISMS OF MULTISTAGE HEPATOCARCINOGENESIS

In view of the recent publication of reviews covering a spectrum of viewpoints on mechanisms of liver tumor initiation and promotion,[14,35,38,382] we shall restrict our remarks on mechanisms to what we perceive as a conceptual problem common to most current discussions of multistage hepatocarcinogenesis, namely the ambiguity associated with the identification of the mechanistic boundaries between initiation and promotion. The following discussion compares the two alternative initiation-promotion models that we presently visualize as defining this issue.

A. Model I — Initiation produces phenotypically altered cells that acquire a selective growth advantage through promoter action.

The underlying premise in this case is that the process of initiation encompasses events related both to the creation of the primary tumorigenic molecular lesion and to aspects of its expression. Thus, histochemically detectable foci of phenotypically and behaviorally altered hepatocytes are categorized as clones of initiated cells.[14,35,38,382] In this context promoters presumably confer a selective growth advantage on such cells, encouraging their accumulation to a critical mass that is then intrinsically resistant to host-imposed growth constraints. Postulated mechanisms for such promoter action include: (1) the direct and selective proliferative stimulation of the cells within these foci,[14,195,383] (2) interference with the flow of growth regulatory information by disruption of intercellular communication,[382,384] and (3) the creation of conditions in which generalized proliferative stimulation is signaled in a mitoinhibitory environment to which initiated cells are relatively resistant, thereby favoring the differential proliferation of the initiated cells.[14,50]

The two central predictions emerging from the foregoing arguments are (1) initiated cells should embody detectable phenotypic alterations that render them uniquely responsive to direct or indirect promoter action, and (2) the chief manifestation of promoter action should be an acceleration of tumorigenesis (rather than a *de novo* increase in tumor incidence) as exemplified by increases in the growth rates of preneoplastic hepatocyte foci, with consequent reductions in tumor latency and possible increases in tumor growth rates.

B. Model II — Initiation is restricted to the creation of a tumorigenic molecular lesion; initiated cells are phenotypically normal until stimulated to express their altered phenotypes and neoplastic potential through promoter action.

In this model the sequence of events involved in the acquisition of neoplastic potential (initiation) is mechanistically completely distinct and isolatable from the processes involved in the phenotypic expression of this potential (promotion). Following such expression, promotion per se has ended, and subsequent events involve progression of the neoplastic cells and/or the dynamics of their interaction with the host. Predictions generated by this model include: (1) an initiated cell would be directly detectable only through the identification of the tumorigenic molecular lesion that it carries (e.g., site-specific carcinogen binding and/or DNA modification) and not by any criteria based on phenotypic change; indirect identification would be possible on the basis of promotion-mediated expression of the transformed phenotype; and (2) promotion would be manifested only as an increase in the incidence rates for tumors and preneoplastic hepatocytes and would not involve an acceleration of the growth rates of these entities.

C. Evaluation of Models I and II

Although Model I currently dominates considerations of hepatic tumorigenesis mechanisms,[14,38,50,204,382,383] we believe that the weight of evidence accumulating from recent in vivo studies of skin and liver tumorigenesis, and from in vitro initiation-promotion experiments, would appear to necessitate a reevaluation of this position. The basis for this viewpoint derives from an evaluation of the degree to which the foregoing predictions generated by each of the models coincides with existing experimental evidence.

A systematic assessment of the validity of the first prediction for each model has not yet been undertaken in the liver system, possibly in part as a result of the prevailing presupposition that initiated hepatocytes are phenotypically altered, and also because detection of phenotypically unaltered initiated hepatocytes might be prohibitively difficult. At present, therefore, the most feasible approach would appear to be an indirect evolutionary one involving the development and application of increasingly sensitive tests for phenotypic change in concert with the use of progressively milder initiating stimuli (to approach as closely as possible ''pure'' initiating conditions) and an optimum promoting regimen that maximizes the expression of the tumorigenic lesions without introducing such extraneous effects as cytotoxicity or additional initiating activity. Under such sensitive conditions, the first prediction of Model I would require that the incidence of the minimal detectable phenotypic change associated with the expression of neoplasia be dependent only on initiator dosage, and should be unaffected by promoter treatment. On the other hand, the first prediction under Model II suggests that the inclusion of promoter treatment would significantly lower the initiatior dose required for the production of the first detectable phenotypic changes associated with neoplasia.

Although experiments of this nature remain to be conducted in liver, evidence accumulating from skin tumorigenesis studies indicates that initiator dosages can be reduced to the extent that no phenotypic changes are detected in initiated skin; the presence of initiated cells under such conditions can be revealed only following the application of promoter with the consequent emergence of phenotypic changes characteristic of neoplasia.[385] These observations are in accord with the first prediction generated by Model II.

In contrast to the experimental difficulties associated with the first prediction, the second prediction generated by each of the models has been relatively accessible to investigation, and consequently a somewhat more definitive evaluation of the alternative viewpoints is possible. Recent liver tumorigenesis studies have shown, as indicated earlier (Section IV.B), that tumor promotion by phenobarbital involves an increased incidence of tumors without an increase in growth rate or a decrease in latency. This indication that tumor promotion does not involve an acceleration of neoplasia, but only an increase in the probability of its expression, is in accord with the second prediction from Model II. Additional support for this position comes from a study cited earlier (Section III.A.7) that showed that phenobarbital added in vitro, to cultured hepatocytes from in vivo AAF-initiated livers, increased the incidence but not the growth rates of the malignantly transformed hepatocyte foci appearing in the cultures.[76]

Data in apparent disagreement with the foregoing observations, and in apparent agreement with the second prediction from Model I, include indications that phenobarbital and other liver tumor promoters directly stimulate proliferative activity in histochemically altered (GGT-positive) hepatocyte foci in rats treated previously with DEN.[195,383] However, the treatment protocols used in these studies involved single[383] or widely spaced (3 weeks) multiple[195] injections of the test agents, as opposed to continuous administration. Prior experience has shown that a prolonged and continuous exposure to phenobarbital, such as that used in the tumor promotion studies, is accompanied by a transient episode of hepatocyte proliferation that occurs only during the first 3 days of the phenobarbital treatment;[16,21] subsequent proliferative activity is at or below normal levels.[16,21,50] Feeding phenobarbital only long enough for this proliferative effect to be exerted (5 days) does not promote liver tumorigenesis;[20,22] the duration of exposure for promotion must be extended far beyond the interval during which phenobarbital is mitogenic for normal hepatocytes.[22] In fact, repeated phenobarbital treatments, sufficiently widely spaced (2 weeks) so that each treatment would be expected to induce proliferative stimulation (on the basis of the rapid reversion of the liver to its normal state between treatments[19]), are much less effective in tumor promotion than the nonmitogenic continuous treatment with an equivalent total phenobarbital dosage.[154] Thus, the experiments examining the mitogenic effects of liver tumor promoters on putative preneoplastic hepatocyte foci[195,383] were inappropriately designed for assessing the degree of causality in the relationship between the mitogenicity of these promoters and their capacity to enhance hepatic tumorigenesis. A more relevant study would measure proliferative activity in the preneoplastic foci during continuous promoter administration, at a time long after the mitogenic effect of the agent on normal hepatocytes had ended.

An alternative method for assessing promoter effects on the incidence and growth of putative preneoplastic hepatocyte foci involves the use of mathematical techniques for measuring the numbers and volumes of those foci per unit volume of liver; application of these techniques provided apparent evidence that tumor promoters, such as phenobarbital and 2,3,7,8-tetrachlorodibenzo-*p*-dioxin (TCDD) increase both the numbers and volumes of GGT-positive foci.[154,204] Such results would raise the possibility that tumor promotion encompasses mechanisms proposed in Models I and II, as described above, involving both an increase in the expression of the transformed phenotype and a subsequent stimulation of growth of the transformed cells. Ambiguities in the data from these studies suggest, however, that the relationship between the behavior of GGT-positive hepatocyte foci and hepatocarcinogenesis may not yet be sufficiently clear to permit this level of mechanistic interpretation. Thus, comparisons of phenobarbital and TCDD effects on the generation of altered foci and hepatocellular carcinomas in DEN-initiated rats show an apparent lack of correlation between foci and tumor formation.[204] Specifically, a regimen of TCDD sufficient to cause a 13-fold increase in the percentage of liver volume occupied by foci did not promote the appearance of hepatocellular carcinomas in any of the treated animals, whereas phenobarbital treatment promoted such tumors in 80% of the animals, although it caused only a 9-fold increase in the percentage focal volume. A dosage of TCDD sufficient to promote tumors in 70% of the rats produced a 61-fold increase in percentage focal volume, a 7-fold greater increase than that produced by the phenobarbital treatment that was equivalently effective in promoting tumorigenesis. On balance, therefore, the studies of promoter effects on the growth of GGT-positive hepatocyte foci do not provide convincing support for the argument that the mechanism of tumor promotion involves the proliferative stimulation of initiated hepatocytes.

A number of in vitro initiation-promotion studies also bear on the relationship between proliferative stimulation and the promotion of transformation. In experiments establishing the initiation-promotion phenomenon in cultured C3H/10T1/2 mouse embryo cells, it was determined that the promotiong effect of TPA on cells initiated by prior exposure to polycyclic aromatic hydrocarbons could not be explained in terms of TPA's mitogenic activity.[386,387] Additional studies with these cells, utilizing X-radiation as the initiating stimulus, have shown that the promotion of transformation by TPA involves the enhancement of expression of the transformed phenotype in a given initiated cell rather than the creation of a selective growth advantage for the progenitors of transformed clones.[388] Evidence that TPA induces the expression of the tumor cell phenotype (manifested as the acquisition of anchorage independence), as opposed to providing a selective growth stimulation for preexisting transformants, was also obtained with JB6 mouse epidermal cell cultures.[389]

On the basis of the foregoing collective evidence from liver, skin, and cell culture studies, we suggest that the initiation-promotion Model II described above is superior to Model I as a working hypothesis defining the mechanistic limits of initiation and promotion and is as applicable to liver carcinogenesis as to skin carcinogenesis and in vitro transformation. Moreover, we are convinced that much of the current ambiguity regarding the demarcation of these processes in liver carcinogenesis has arisen from the retention, by investigators in this area, of treatment protocols (long outmoded in studies of skin tumorigenesis) involving excessive exposure to carcinogens, thereby truncating the tumorigenic process to the degree that the resolution of successive intermediate stages is virtually precluded. The use of additional heroic procedures such as CCl_4 administration, the production of choline deficiency, and the postinitiation administration of AAF, produce myriad hepatic changes, most of which are probably unrelated to whatever effects these agents have on the tumorigenic process. Such approaches have probably retarded the identification of those processes that are causally related to neoplasia by obscuring them within a melange of extraneous hepatic responses, and have also engendered the inappropriate classification of the stages of liver tumorigenesis by including promotional events within the initiation category and by mislabeling as promotion later events concerned with the interaction of the transformed cell with the host.

VI. APPROACHES TO THE FURTHER CHARACTERIZATION OF MULTISTAGE HEPATOCARCINOGENESIS

Of the several systems in which evidence for initiation and promotion has been obtained, the liver offers a unique combination of advantages for mechanistic studies. These advantages include: (1) the responsiveness of the liver to a broader spectrum of initiators and promoters than any other single tissue (Table 2); (2) the abundance, relative homogeneity, and ready accessibility of hepatic tissue; (3) the already vast accumulation of information on hepatic parenchymal cell biochemistry and the relative ease with which biochemical studies can be conducted in liver; (4) the high probability that the aforementioned biochemical information can have mechanistic relevance to tumorigenesis, on the basis of the evidence that hepatic parenchymal cells are the progenitors of hepatocellular carcinomas; (5) the retention of the cells representing the various stages of tumorigenesis at their sites of origin in contrast to epithelial systems in which altered cells are lost by sloughing; and (6) the availability of histochemical techniques for identifying putative clones of early preneoplastic hepatocytes (Section III.B, Table 1).

The liver, therefore, constitutes one of the best available systems in which to characterize the sequence of events involved in the expression of the neoplastic phenotype. It is becoming increasingly apparent that such an analysis requires the examination of relationships between tumor incidence kinetics and phenotypes, on the one hand, and the numbers, incidence kinetics, sizes, and histochemical phenotypes of putative preneoplastic hepatocyte foci on the other. Approaches to the coherent organization and evaluation of data from such studies include the development of models of liver tumor initiation and promotion that serve as the basis for computer simulations of relationships against which the empirical data can be compared. Continuing iterative comparisons of the simulated and experimental data permit the progressive refinement of the mechanistic assumptions upon which the tumorigenesis models are based and also reveal new questions that can be addressed by appropriate experiments.

An example of an important issue that can be examined by this type of approach is the marked discrepancy between the numbers of histochemically altered foci and tumors that appear in the livers of animals undergoing hepatocarcinogenesis (foci exceed tumors by several orders of magnitude).[36] This high ratio of foci to tumors raises the following alternative possibilities that are amenable to testing:

1. Most of the foci represent early stages in tumorigenesis, but have not yet undergone the full complement of changes necessary for expression of the tumor phenotype.
2. Most of the foci were initially tumor progenitors, but have subsequently undergone changes that preclude their further development into tumors.

Alternative 1 may be described in a model formulation as the accumulation of appropriate events, perhaps at one or more regulatory loci, resulting in a focus, followed by specific subsequent transitions (stages) which may or may not depend upon additional mutations. If the subsequent transitions require mutations, these mutations are either not dependent upon the presence of the carcinogen, and occur spontaneously during clonal proliferation, or are accumulated during prior exposure to the initiator.

Alternative 2 addresses the issue of the possible existence of nontumorigenic foci, as well as the origins of foci with diverse histochemical phenotypes. If initiation results from a genetic lesion at a specific regulatory locus, then the observation of heterogeneity in focus phenotypes implies that the phenotypes are dependent upon additional mutations that may be positive, negative, or neutral with respect to tumorigenesis, since no single histochemical alteration appears in every focus. On the other hand, if the production of a focus is itself only dependent upon the genetic lesion that gives rise to the distinctive phenotypic marker, then no separate initiation event need be postulated for focus formation, and initation in the sense of tumor formation may simply reflect the accumulation of the appropriate essential lesions during exposure to the carcinogen.

To formulate a model of initiation and promotion, it is therefore necessary to consider the role of multiple mutations, whether resulting directly from the action of the carcinogen or occurring spontaneously during focus development. The generally accepted working hypothesis, as embodied in Alternative 1 above, is that a tumor results from the accumulation of many mutations, affecting loci specifically involved in the transformation process. According to this scheme, the majority of foci, which do not develop into tumors, represent cells that did not acquire sufficient lesions to complete the transformation process. However, assuming mutation to be a random process and assuming that the loci essential to the transformation process comprise a small fraction of the total genome, it would be expected that many mutations would not contribute to transformation but could, in fact, block the process. Therefore, in developing the hypothetical framework of initiation and promotion in a manner suitable for computer simulation, it is necessary to consider the possibility that some foci that do not develop into tumors may have sustained an excess rather than an insufficiency of mutations, and consequently may no longer have tumorigenic potential (Alternative 2).

Alternatives 1 and 2 may be distinguished by the predictions that they generate, as follows. Alternative 1 predicts monotonic, though not necessarily linear, responses to increased carcinogen dose. These responses include increased frequency of foci, increased proportion of foci with multiple phenotypic changes, increased tumor frequency, and an increased ratio of tumors to foci. The process predicted by Alternative 2 is biphasic; at low* carcinogen dose ranges, increased tumor and focus frequency would be expected with increasing carcinogen levels. At high* carcinogen dose ranges a decreased proportion of foci with multiple phenotypic changes, a decreased ratio of tumors to foci, and a decreased tumor frequency would be expected with increasing carcinogen levels. The decline in tumor frequency at high carcinogen dose observed by Scherer and Emmelot[390] and attributed to toxicity is also consistent with the predictions generated by Alternative 2. Testing the validity of these inferred predictions clearly requires a mathematical formulation supported by computer simulation, in conjunction with the acquisition of experimental data.

VII. SUMMARY AND CONCLUSIONS

Although early studies of hepatocarcinogenesis justifiably used high carcinogen dosage levels as a means of maximizing the tumorigenic response, the continued application of this basic experimental approach by many investigators in recent years has retarded progress toward an understanding of hepatocarcinogenesis mechanisms. Exposure of the test animals to excessive dosages of carcinogens compresses the successive stages of hepatic neoplasia to a degree that virtually precludes their resolution, and also obscures essential tumorigenic events within a host of extraneous changes accompanying the production of hepatotoxicity and regenerative hyperplasia. Departures from such an approach in favor of the milder treatment procedures long since adopted by investigators of skin tumorigenesis have led to the observation that hepatocarcinogenesis proceeds via a multistage process analogous to that occurring in skin tumor formation.

Use of the liver system for the further characterization of the stages of tumorigenesis appears especially promising in view of the burgeoning development of sensitive techniques for the detection of putative preneoplastic hepatocytes. Realization of this potential requires that the evolution in the sensitivity of these detection methods be coupled with the progressive refinement (reduction in severity) of tumorigenic treatment protocols, the ultimate objective being the identification of the minimal sequence of changes essential for the neoplastic transformation. However, the continued use of inappropriately severe tumorigenic protocols in conjunction with the more sensitive indicators of putative preneoplasia is perpetuating, and possibly magnifying, the problems of interpretation associated with earlier studies. The importance of this issue is illustrated by the current uncertainty regarding the mechanistic boundaries between the initiation and promotion stages of liver tumorigenesis, two major alternative viewpoints being (1) initiation encompasses events related both to the creation of the primary tumorigenic molecular lesion and to aspects of its expression, thereby leading to the production of phenotypically and behaviorally altered hepatocytes that acquire a selective growth advantage through promoter action, and (2) initiation involves only the creation of the primary tumorigenic molecular lesion; initiated cells are phenotypically normal until stimulated to express their altered phenotypes through promoter action.

We suggest that the first alternative arose as the result of experiments utilizing excessive

* The functional criteria for "low" or "high" dose are undefined. Dosages commonly used experimentally may already approach high levels in the sense used here.

carcinogen dosage and represents the inappropriate inclusion of promotional events within the initiation category as well as the mislabeling, as promotion, of later events concerned with the progression of transformed cells and their interaction with the host. The second alternative, on the other hand, is increasingly favored by evidence accumulating from appropriately designed tumorigenesis experiments in liver and skin as well as from in vitro transformation studies.

In exploiting the tests for putative preneoplastic hepatocytes as an approach to the further characterization of multistage hepatocarcinogenesis, it is important to understand the basis for the much greater incidence of altered hepatocyte foci in comparison with the yield of liver tumors. The examination of this issue, as well as the assessment of the developmental kinetics of the various focus phenotypes, should permit the characterization of the sequential phenotypic changes occurring in hepatocytes during the early stages of neoplasia and should also provide useful information on the involvement of multiple mutations in tumorigenesis.

The establishment of initiation-promotion systems in a variety of tissues not only supports the general applicability of the multistage concept of tumorigenesis, but also suggests an approach to the development of a more systematic analysis of possible tumorigenesis mechanisms than has been possible thus far. The approach envisioned would involve comparisons among different systems in which tumor production or cell transformation has been optimized through the use of the most effective system-specific agents, administered according to the most appropriate protocols. When each tumor system was operating optimally, intersystem comparisons could then be undertaken with respect to carefully selected biochemical parameters (e.g., ornithine decarboxylase induction). Such comparisons would permit the identification of those responses that are common to the various systems and hence potentially relevant to the tumorigenic process; responses that are system-specific could be eliminated from further consideration in this context. Since, as a rule, each of the tumorigenesis systems is under study in a different laboratory, cross-comparisons among different systems would require cooperative interactions among several research groups.

ACKNOWLEDGMENT

This work was supported by the U.S. Department of Energy under Contract No. W-31-109-ENG-38. We are indebted to Ms. N. Dast for her assistance in proofreading references.

REFERENCES

1. **Deelman, H. T.,** The part played by injury and repair in the development of cancer; with remarks on the growth of experimental cancers, *Br. Med. J.*, 1, 872, 1927.
2. **Rous, P. and Kidd, J. G.,** Conditional neoplasms and subthreshold neoplastic states. A study of the tar tumors of rabbits, *J. Exp. Med.*, 73, 356, 1941.
3. **Berenblum, I.,** The cocarcinogenic action of croton resin, *Cancer Res.*, 1, 44, 1941.
4. **Friedewald, W. F. and Rous, P.,** The initiating and promoting elements in tumor production. An analysis of the effects of tar, benzpyrene, and methylcholanthrene on rabbit skin, *J. Exp. Med.*, 80, 101, 1944.
5. **Berenblum, I. and Shubik, P.,** The persistence of latent tumour cells induced in the mouse's skin by a single application of 9,10-dimethyl-1,2-benzanthracene, *Br. J. Cancer*, 3, 384, 1949.
6. **Sasaki, T. and Yoshida, T.,** Experimentelle Erzeugung des Lebercarcinoma durch Futterung mit o-Amidoazotoluol, *Virchow Arch. Pathol. Anat. Physiol.*, 295, 175, 1935.
7. **Cole, L. J. and Nowell, P. C.,** Radiation carcinogenesis: the sequence of events, *Science*, 150, 1782, 1965.
8. **Farber, E.,** Hyperplastic liver nodules, in *Methods in Cancer Research*, Vol. 7, Busch, H., Ed., Academic Press, New York 1973, chap. 8.

9. **Farber, E.,** Carcinogenesis — cellular evolution as a unifying thread: presidential address, *Cancer Res.*, 33, 2537, 1973.
10. **Teebor, G. W. and Becker, F. F.,** Regression and persistence of hyperplastic nodules induced by N-2-fluorenylacetamide and their relationship to hepatocarcinogenesis, *Cancer Res.*, 31, 1, 1971.
11. **Becker, F. F.,** Alteration of hepatocytes by subcarcinogenic exposure to N-2-fluorenylacetamide, *Cancer Res.*, 35, 1734, 1975.
12. **Solt, D. and Farber, E.,** New principle for the analysis of chemical carcinogenesis, *Nature (London)*, 263, 701, 1976.
13. **Solt, D. B., Medline, A., and Farber, E.,** Rapid emergence of carcinogen-induced hyperplastic lesions in a new model for the sequential analysis of liver carcinogenesis, *Am. J. Pathol.*, 88, 595, 1977.
14. **Farber, E.,** The sequential analysis of liver cancer induction, *Biochim. Biophys. Acta*, 605, 149, 1980.
15. **Foulds, L.,** *Neoplastic Development*, Vol. 2, Academic Press, New York, 1975, chap. 5.
16. **Peraino, C., Fry, R. J. M., and Staffeldt, E.,** Reduction and enhancement by phenobarbital of hepatocarcinogenesis induced in the rat by 2-acetylaminofluorene, *Cancer Res.*, 31, 1506, 1971.
17. **Ishidate, M., Watanabe, M., and Odashima, S.,** Effect of barbital on carcinogenic action and metabolism of 4-dimethylaminoazobenzene, *Gann.* 58, 267, 1967.
18. **Kunz, W., Schaude, G., and Thomas, C.,** The effect of phenobarbital and halogenated hydrocarbons on nitrosamine carcinogenesis, *Z. Krebsforsch.*, 72, 291, 1969.
19. **Schulte-Hermann, R.,** Induction of liver growth by xenobiotic compounds and other stimuli, *Crit. Rev. Toxicol.*, 3, 97, 1974.
20. **Peraino, C., Fry, R. J. M., Staffeldt, E., and Kisieleski, W. E.,** Effects of varying the exposure to phenobarbital on its enhancement of 2-acetyl-aminofluorene-induced hepatic tumorigenesis in the rat, *Cancer Res.*, 33, 2701, 1973.
21. **Peraino, C., Fry, R. J. M., Staffeldt, E., and Christopher, J. P.,** Comparative enhancing effects of phenobarbital, amobarbital, diphenylnydantoin, and dichlorodiphenyltrichloroethane on 2-acetylaminofluorene-induced hepatic tumorigenesis in the rat, *Cancer Res.*, 35, 2884, 1975.
22. **Peraino, C., Fry, R. J. M., and Staffeldt, E.,** Effects of varying the onset and duration of exposure to phenobarbital on its enhancement of 2-acetylaminofluorene-induced hepatic tumorigenesis, *Cancer Res.*, 37, 3623, 1977.
23. **Peraino, C., Staffeldt, E. F., Haugen, D. A., Lombard, L. S., Stevens, F. J., and Fry, R. J. M.,** Effects of varying the dietary concentration of phenobarbital on its enhancement of 2-acetylaminofluorene-induced hepatic tumorigenesis, *Cancer Res.*, 40, 3268, 1980.
24. **Solt, D. B., Cayama, E., Sarma, D. S. R., and Farber, E.,** Persistence of resistant putative preneoplastic hepatocytes induced by N-nitrosodiethylamine or N-methyl-N-nitrosourea, *Cancer Res.*, 40, 1112, 1980.
25. **Tsuda, H., Lee, G., and Farber, E.,** Induction of resistant hepatocytes as a new principle for a possible short-term in vivo test for carcinogens, *Cancer Res.*, 40, 1157, 1980.
26. **Cayama, E., Tsuda, H., Sarma, D. S. R., and Farber, E.,** Initiation of chemical carcinogenesis requires cell proliferation, *Nature (London)*, 275, 60, 1978.
27. **Columbano, A., Rajalakshmi, S., and Sarma, D. S. R.,** Requirement of cell proliferation for the initiation of liver carcinogenesis as assayed by three different procedures, *Cancer Res.*, 41, 2079, 1981.
28. **Ying, T. S., Sarma, D. S. R., and Farber, E.,** Role of acute hepatic necrosis in the induction of early steps in liver carcinogenesis by diethylnitrosamine, *Cancer Res.*, 41, 2096, 1981.
29. **Tatematsu, M., Nakanishi, K., Murasaki, G., Miyata, Y., Hirose, M., and Ito, N.,** Enhancing effect of inducers of liver microsomal enzymes on induction of hyperplastic liver nodules by N 2-fluorenylacetamide in rats, *J. Natl. Cancer Inst.*, 63, 1411, 1979.
30. **Scherer, E. and Emmelot, P.,** Foci of altered liver cells induced by a single dose of diethylnitrosamine and partial hepatectomy: their contribution to hepatocarcinogenesis in the rat, *Eur. J. Cancer*, 11, 145, 1975.
31. **Ueda, Y.** The relation between experimental liver carcinoma and liver cirrhosis induced by simultaneous administration of p-dimethylaminoazobenzene and carbon tetrachloride, *Tohoku J. Exp. Med.*, 92, 83, 1967.
32. **Ueda, Y.,** The relation between experimental liver carcinoma and liver cirrhosis induced by successive administration of p-dimethylaminoazobenzene and carbon tetrachloride, *Tohoku J. Exp. Med.*, 92, 109, 1967.
33. **Kozuka, S. and Sassa, R.,** Acceleration of hepatocarcinogenesis of 2,7-bis(acetamido)fluorene by carbon tetrachloride and time relation of treatment, *Gann*, 67, 141, 1976.
34. **Laishes, B. A. and Rolfe, P. B.,** Quantitative assessment of liver colony formation and hepatocellular carcinoma incidence in rats receiving intravenous injections of isogeneic liver cells isolated during hepatocarcinogenesis, *Cancer Res.*, 40, 4133, 1980.
35. **Pitot, H. C.,** The natural history of neoplasia. Newer insights into an old problem, *Am. J. Pathol.*, 89, 402, 1977.

36. **Pitot, H., Barsness, L., Goldsworthy, T., and Kitagawa, T,.** Biochemical characterisation of stages of hepatocarcinogenesis after a single dose of diethylnitrosamine, *Nature (London)*, 271, 456, 1978.
37. **Pitot, H. C. and Sirica, A. E.,** The stages of initiation and promotion in hepatocarcinogenesis, *Biochim. Biophys. Acta*, 605, 191, 1980.
38. **Scherer, E., Hoffmann, M., Emmelot, P., and Friedrich-Freksa, M.,** Quantitative study on foci of altered liver cells induced in the rat by a single dose of diethylnitrosamine and partial hepatectomy, *J. Natl. Cancer Inst.*, 49, 93, 1972.
39. **Scherer, E. and Emmelot, P.,** Kinetics of induction and growth of enzyme-deficient islands involved in hepatocarcinogenesis, *Cancer Res.*, 36, 2544, 1976.
40. **Emmelot, P. and Scherer, E.,** The first relevant cell stage in rat liver carcinogenesis. A quantitative approach, *Biochem. Biophys. Acta*, 605, 247, 1980.
41. **Craddock, V. M.,** Effect of a single treatment with the alkylating carcinogens dimethylnitrosamine, diethylnitrosamine, and methyl methanesulphonate on liver regenerating after partial hepatectomy, *Chem. Biol. Interactions*, 10, 313, 1975.
42. **Friedrich-Freksa, H., Gossner, W., and Borner, P.,** Histochemische Untersuchungen der Cancerogenese in der Rattenleber nach Dauergaben von Diathylnitrosamin, *Z. Krebsforsch.*, 72, 226, 1969.
43. **Rabes, H. M., Scholze, P., and Jantsch, B.,** Growth kinetics of diethylnitrosamine-induced, enzyme-deficient "preneoplastic" liver cell populations in vivo and in vitro, *Cancer Res.*, 32, 2577, 1972.
44. **Pugh, T. D. and Goldfarb, S.,** Quantitative histochemical and autoradiographic studies of hepatocarcinogenesis in rats fed 2-acetylaminofluorene followed by phenobarbital, *Cancer Res.*, 38, 4450, 1978.
45. **Farber, E.,** Response of liver to carcinogens: a new analytical approach, in *Toxic Liver Injury*, Farber, E. and Fisher, M. M., Eds., Marcel Dekker, New York, 1979, 445.
46. **Rogers, A. E. and Newberne, P. M.,** Lipotrope deficiency in experimental carcinogenesis, *Nutr. Cancer*, 2, 104, 1980.
47. **Shinozuka, H., Lombardi, B., Sell, S., and Iammarino, R. M.,** Early histological and functional alterations of ethionine liver carcinogenesis in rats fed a choline deficient diet, *Cancer Res.*, 38, 1092, 1978.
48. **Shinozuka, H., Lombardi, B., Sell, S., and Iammarino, R. M.,** Enhancement of DL-ethionine-induced liver carcinogenesis in rats fed a choline-devoid diet, *J. Natl. Cancer Inst.*, 61, 813, 1978.
49. **Shinozuka, H., Katyal, S. L., and Lombardi, B.,** Azaserine carcinogenesis: organ susceptibility change in rats fed a diet devoid of choline, *Int. J. Cancer*, 22, 36, 1978.
50. **Sells, M. A., Katyal, S. L., Sell, S., Shinozuka, H., and Lombardi, B.,** Induction of foci of altered, γ-glutamyltranspeptidase-positive hepatocytes in carcinogen-treated rats fed a choline-deficient diet, *Br. J. Cancer*, 40, 274, 1979.
51. **Shinozuka, H. and Lombardi, B.,** Synergistic effect of a choline-devoid diet and phenobarbital in promoting the emergence of foci of γ-glutamyltranspeptidase-positive hepatocytes in the liver of carcinogen-treated rats, *Cancer Res.*, 40, 3846, 1980.
52. **Abanobi, S. E., Lombardi, B., and Shinozuka, H.,** Possible mechanism(s) of action of a choline-devoid diet and phenobarbital as promoters of hepatocarcinogenesis, *Proc. Am. Assoc. Cancer Res.*, 22, 130, 1981.
53. **Rogers, A. E. and Newberne, P. M.,** Aflatoxin B_1 carcinogenesis in lipotrope-deficient rats, *Cancer Res.*, 29, 1965, 1969.
54. **Best, C. H.,** Protection of liver and kidneys by dietary factors choline and its precursors as lipotropic agents, *Fed. Proc.*, 9, 506, 1950.
55. **Olson, R. E.,** Scientific contributions of Wendell H. Griffith to our understanding of the function of choline, *Fed. Proc.*, 30, 131, 1971.
56. **Lombardi, B.,** Effects of choline deficiency on rat hepatocytes, *Fed. Proc.*, 30, 139, 1971.
57. **Mookerjea, S.,** Action of choline in lipoprotein metabolism, *Fed. Proc.*, 30, 143, 1971.
58. **Chernozemski, I. N. and Warwick, G. P.,** Liver regeneration and induction of hepatomas in $B6AF_1$ mice by urethan, *Cancer Res.*, 30, 2685, 1970.
59. **Marquardt, H., Sternberg, S. S., and Philips, F. S.,** 7,12-Dimethylbenz(a)anthracene and hepatic neoplasia in regenerating rat liver, *Chem. Biol. Interactions*, 2, 401, 1970.
60. **Hollander, C. F. and Bentvelzen, P.,** Enhancement of urethan induction of hepatomas in mice by prior partial hepatectomy, *J. Natl. Cancer Inst.*, 41, 1303, 1968.
61. **Lane, M., Liebelt, A., Calvert, J., and Liebelt, R. A.,** Effect of partial hepatectomy on tumor incidence in BALB/c mice treated with urethan, *Cancer Res.*, 30, 1812, 1970.
62. **Warwick, G. P.,** Effect of the cell cycle on carcinogenesis, *Fed. Proc.*, 30, 1760, 1971.
63. **Pound, A. W. and Lawson, T. A.,** Effects of partial hepatectomy on carcinogenicity, metabolism, and binding to DNA of ethyl carbamate, *J. Natl. Cancer Inst.*, 53, 423, 1974.
64. **Pound, A. W. and McGuire, L. J.,** Repeated partial hepatectomy as a promoting stimulus for carcinogenic response of liver to nitrosamines in rats, *Br. J. Cancer*, 37, 585, 1978.

65. **Ishikawa, T., Takayama, S., and Kitagawa, T.,** Correlatin between time of partial hepatectomy after a single treatment with diethylnitrosamine and induction of adenosinetriphosphatase-deficient islands in rat liver, *Cancer Res.*, 40, 4261, 1980.
66. **Ueda, Y.,** Experimental liver carcinoma and liver cirrhosis induced by ρ-dimethylaminoazobenzene after preliminary carbon tetrachloride injections, *Tohoku J. Exp. Med.*, 92, 175, 1967.
67. **Pound, A. W., Lawson, T. A., and Horn, L.,** Increased carcinogenic action of dimethylnitrosamine after prior administration of carbon tetrachloride, *Br. J. Cancer*, 27, 451, 1973.
68. **Pound, A. W.,** Influence of carbon tetrachloride on induction of tumours of the liver and kidneys in mice by nitrosamines, *Br. J. Cancer*, 37, 67, 1968.
69. **Japundzic, M., Knezevic, B., Djordjevic-Camba, V., and Japundzic, I.,** The influence of phenobarbital-Na on the mitotic activity of parenchymal liver cells during rat liver regeneration, *Exp. Cell Res.*, 48, 163, 1967.
70. **Argyris, T. S. and Magnus, D. R.,** The stimulation of liver growth and demethylase activity following phenobarbital treatment, *Dev. Biol.*, 17, 187, 1968.
71. **Tatematsu, M., Shirai, T., Tsuda, H., Miyata, Y., Shinohara, Y., and Ito, N.,** Rapid production of hyperplastic liver nodules in rats treated with carcinogenic chemicals: a new approach for an in vivo short-term screening test for hepatocarcinogens, *Gann*, 68, 499, 1977.
72. **Tatematsu, M., Murasaki, G., Nakanishi, K., Miyata, Y., Shinohara, Y., and Ito, N.,** Sequential quantitative studies on hyperplastic nodules in the liver of rats treated with carcinogenic chemicals, *Gann*, 70, 125. 1979.
73. **Ito, N., Tatematsu, M., Nakanishi, K., Hasegawa, R., Takano, T., Imaida, K., and Ogiso, T.,** The effects of various chemicals on the development of hyperplastic liver nodules in hepatectomized rats treated with N-nitrosodiethylamine or N-2-fluorenylacetamide, *Gann*, 71, 832, 1980.
74. **Tatematsu, M., Takano, T., Hasegawa, R., Imaida, K., Nakanowatari, J., and Ito, N.,** A sequential quantitative study of the reversibility or irreversibility of liver hyperplastic nodules in rats exposed to hepatocarcinogens, *Gann*, 71, 843, 1980.
75. **Ford, J. O. and Pereira, M. A.,** Short-term in vivo initiation/promotion bioassay for hepatocarcinogens, *J. Environ. Pathol. Toxicol.*, 4, 39, 1980.
76. **Kitagawa, T., Watanabe, R., Kayano, T., and Sugano, H.,** in vitro carcinogenesis of hepatocytes obtained from acetylaminofluorene-treated rat liver and promotion of their growth by phenobarbital, *Gann*, 71, 747, 1980.
77. **Liebelt, R. A., Yoshida, R., and Gray, G. F.,** Enhancement of liver tumorigenesis in Zb mice injected with urethan at newborn age, *Proc. Am. Assoc. Cancer Res.*, 3, 245, 1961.
78. **Chieco-Bianchi, L., De Benedictis, G., Tridente, G., and Fiore-Donati, L.,** Influence of age on susceptibilty to liver carcinogenesis and skin initiating action by urethane in Swiss mice, *Br. J. Cancer*, 17, 672, 1963.
79. **Toth, B., Magee, P. N., and Shubik, P.,** Carcinogenesis study with dimethylnitrosamine administered orally to adult and subcutaneously to newborn BALB/c mice, *Cancer Res.*, 24, 1712, 1964.
80. **Vesselinovitch, S. D. and Mihailovich, N.,** The induction of benign and malignant liver tumors by urethan in newborn rats, *Cancer Res.*, 28, 881, 1968.
81. **Chernozemski, I. N. and Warwick, G. P.,** Production of hepatomas in suckling mice after single application of β-propiolactone, *J. Natl. Cancer Inst.*, 45, 709, 1970.
82. **Kommineni, V. R. C., Greenblatt, M., Vesselinovitch, S. D., and Mihailovich, N.,** Urethan carcinogenesis in rats, importance of age and dose, *J. Natl. Cancer Inst.*, 45, 687, 1970.
83. **Kommineni, V. R. C., Greenblatt, M., Mihailovich, N., and Vesselinovitch, S. D.,** The significance of perinatal age periods and the dose of urethan on the tumor profile in the MRC rat, *Cancer Res.*, 30, 2552, 1970.
84. **Vesselinovitch, S. D., Rao, K. V. N., Mihailovich, N., Rice, J. M., and Lombard, L. S.,** Development of broad spectrum of tumors by ethylnitrosourea in mice and the modifying role of age, sex, and strain, *Cancer Res.*, 34, 2530, 1974.
85. **Vesselinovitch, S. D., Kyriazis, A. P., Mihailovich, N., and Rao, K. V. N.,** Conditions modifying development of tumors in mice at various sites by benzo(a)pyrene, *Cancer Res.*, 35, 2948, 1975.
86. **Vesselinovitch, S. D., Rao, K. V. N., and Mihailovich, N.,** Neoplastic response of mouse tissues during perinatal age periods and its significance in chemical carcinogenesis, *Natl. Cancer Inst. Monogr.*, 51, 239, 1979.
87. **Vesselinovitch, S. D.,** Infant mouse as a sensitive bioassay system for carcinogenicity of N-nitroso compounds, in *N-Nitroso Compounds: Analysis, Formation and Occurrence*, IARC Sci. Publ. No. 31, Walker, E. A., Griciute, L., Castegnaro, M., and Borzonyi, M., Eds., International Agency for Research on Cancer, Lyon, 1980, 645.
88. **Vesselinovitch, S. D.,** Factors modulating response to carcinogenic mutagens, in *Progress in Environmental Mutagenesis*, Alacevic, M., Ed., Elsevier/North Holland Biomedical Press, Amsterdam, 1980, 281.

89. **Uchida, E. and Hirono, I.,** Effect of phenobarbital on induction of liver and lung tumors by dimethylnitrosamine in newborn mice, *Gann,* 70, 639, 1979.
90. **Peraino, C., Staffeldt, E. F., and Ludeman, V. A.,** Early appearance of histochemically altered hepatocyte foci and liver tumors in female rats treated with carcinogens one day after birth, *Carcinogenesis,* 2, 463, 1981.
91. **Moore, M. R., Drinkwater, N. R., Miller, E. C., Miller, J. A., and Pitot, H. C.,** Quantitative analysis of the time-dependent development of glucose-6-phosphate-deficient foci in the livers of mice treated neonatally with diethylnitrosamine, *Cancer Res.,* 41, 1585, 1981.
92. **Squire, R. A. and Levitt, M. H.,** Report of a workshop on classification of specific hepatocellular lesions in rats, *Cancer Res.,* 35, 3214, 1975.
93. **Stewart, H. L., Williams, G. M., Keysser, C. H., Lombard, L. S., Montali, R. J., Burek, J. D., Kimbrough, R. D., Murchison, T. E., Ruebner, B. H., and Strandberg, J. D.,** Histologic typing of liver tumors of the rat, *J. Natl. Cancer Inst.,* 64, 177, 1980.
94. **Stewart, H. L. and Snell, K. C.,** The histopathology of experimental tumors of the liver of the rat, in *The Physiopathology of Cancer,* 2nd ed., Homburger, F. and Fishman, W. H., Eds., Paul B. Hoeber, New York, 1959, 85.
95. **Schauer, A. and Kunze, E.,** Tumours of the liver, in *Pathology of Tumours in Laboratory Animals, Tumours of the Rat, Part 2,* Vol. 1, IARC Sci. Publ. No. 6, Turusov, V. S., Ed., International Agency for Cancer Research, Lyon, 1976, 41.
96. **Bannasch, P.,** *The Cytoplasm of Hepatocytes During Carcinogenesis, Recent Results in Cancer Research,* Springer-Verlag, New York, 1968, 19.
97. **Turusov, V. S. and Takayama, S.,** Tumours of the liver, in *Pathology of Tumours in Laboratory Animals, Tumours of the Mouse,* Vol. 2, IARC Sci. Publ. No. 23, Turusov, V. S., Ed., International Agency for Cancer Research, Lyon, 1979, 193.
98. **Frith, C. H. and Ward, J. M.,** A morphologic classification of proliferative and neoplastic hepatic lesions in mice, *J. Environ. Pathol. Toxicol.,* 3, 329, 1980.
99. **Jones, G. and Butler, W. H.,** Morphology of spontaneous and induced neoplasia, in *Mouse Hepatic Neoplasia,* Butler, W. H. and Newberne, P. M., Eds., Elsevier, Amsterdam, 1975, 21.
100. **Squire, R. A., Goodman, D. G., Valerio, M. G., Fredrickson, T. N., Strandberg, J. D., Levitt, M. H., Lingeman, C. H., Harshbarger, J. C., and Dawe, C. J.,** Tumors, in *Pathology of Laboratory Animals,* Vol. 2, Benirschke, K., Garner, F. M., and Jones, T. C., Eds., Springer-Verlag, New York, 1978, 1051.
101. **Bannasch, P.,** Cytology and cytogenesis of neoplastic (hyperplastic) hepatic nodules, *Cancer Res.,* 36, 2555, 1976.
102. **Bannasch, P., Mayer, D., and Hacker, H.-J.,** Hepatocellular glycogenesis and hepatocarcinogenesis, *Biochim. Biophys. Acta,* 605, 217, 1980.
103. **Daoust, R.,** Cellular populations and nucleic acid metabolism in rat liver parenchyma during azo dye carcinogenesis, *Can. Cancer Conf.,* 5, 225, 1963.
104. **Price, J. M., Harman, J. W., Miller, E. C., and Miller J. A.,** Porgressive microscopic alterations in the livers of rats fed the hepatic carcinogens 3′-methyl-4-dimethylaminoazobenzene and 4′-fluoro-4-dimethylaminoazobenzene, *Cancer Res.,* 12, 192, 1952.
105. **Bannasch, P., Hacker, H.-J., and Mayer, D.,** Early biological markers during liver carcinogenesis, *Arch. Toxicol.,* Suppl. 2, 145, 1979.
106. **Tomatis, L., Partensky, C., and Montesano, R.,** The predictive value of mouse liver tumour induction in carcinogenicity testing — a literature survey, *Int. J. Cancer,* 12, 1, 1973.
107. **Daoust, R. and Calamai, R.,** Hyperbasophilic foci as sites of neoplastic transformation in hepatic parenchyma, *Cancer Res.,* 31, 1290, 1971.
108. **Briere, N. and Daoust, R.,** Histochemical studies on rat liver proteins during 4-dimethylaminoazobenzene carcinogenesis, *Cancer Res.,* 30, 1370, 1970.
109. **Daoust, R. and Molnar, F.,** Cellular populations and mitotic activity in rat liver parenchyma during azo dye carcinogenesis, *Cancer Res.,* 24, 1898, 1964.
110. **Farber, E.,** The pathology of experimental liver cell cancer, in *Liver Cell Cancer,* Cameron, H. M., Linsell, D. A., and Warwick, G. P., Eds., Elsevier, Amsterdam, 1976, 243.
111. **Bannasch, P.,** Cellular and subcellular pathology of liver carcinogenesis, in *Primary Liver Tumors,* Remmer, H., Bolt, H. M., Bannasch, P., and Popper, H., Eds., University Park Press, Baltimore, 1978, 87.
112. **Farber, E. and Ichinose, H.,** On the origin of malignant cells in experimental liver cancer, *Acta Unio Int. Contra Cancrum,* 15, 152, 1959.
113. **Farber, E. and Cameron, R.,** The sequential analysis of cancer development, *Adv. Cancer Res.,* 31, 125, 1980.
114. **Reuber, M. D.,** Evolution of hyperplasia, hyperplastic nodules, and carcinomas of the liver induced in rats by N-2-fluorenyldiacetamide, *Gann Monogr.,* 17, 301, 1975.

115. **Farber, E.,** On the pathogenesis of experimental hepatocellular carcinoma, in *Hepatocellular Carcinoma*, Okuda, K. and Peters, R. L., Eds., John Wiley & Sons, New York 1976, 3.
116. **Firminger, H. I.,** Histopathology of carcinogenesis and tumors of the liver in rats, *J. Natl. Cancer Inst.*, 15, 1427, 1955.
117. **Gellatly, J. B. M.,** The natural history of hepatic parenchymal nodule formation in a colony of C57BL mice with reference to the effect of diet, in *Mouse Hepatic Neoplasia*, Butler, W. H. and Newberne, P. M., Eds., Elsevier, Amsterdam, 1975, 77.
118. **Hunt, J. M. and Laishes, B. A.,** New hepatocyte phenotypes as early indicators of carcinogenicity, in *Target Organ Toxicity: Liver*, Hewitt, W. R. and Plaa, G. L., Eds., Raven Press, New York, 1981.
119. **Van der Heijden, C. A. and Dormans, J. A. M. A.,** Short-term induction of neoplastic nodules in the rat liver. II. Study of their development and the effects of withdrawal of 2-acetylaminofluorene, *Carcinogenesis*, 2, 147, 1981.
120. **Van der Heijden, C. A., Dormans, J. A. M. A., and Van Nesselrooij, J. H. J.,** Short-term induction of preneoplastic nodules in the rat liver. I. The role of 2-AAF as selecting agent, *Eur. J. Cancer*, 16, 1389, 1980.
121. **Goldfarb, S. and Pitot, H. C.,** Enzymology of highly differentiated hepatocellular carcinomas, in *Frontiers of Gastrointestinal Research*, Vol. 2, Van der Reis, L., Eds., S. Karger, Basel, 1976, 194.
122. **Criss, W. E.,** A review of isozymes in cancer, *Cancer Res.*, 31, 1523, 1971.
123. **Shamberger, R. J., Hozumi, M., and Morris, H. P.,** Lysosomal and nonlysosomal enzyme activities of Morris hepatomas, *Cancer Res.*, 31, 1632, 1971.
124. **Morris, H. P. and Criss, W. E., Eds.,**, *Morris Hepatomas, Mechanisms of Regulation*, Plenum Press, New York, 1978.
125. **Mellors, R. C. and Sugiura, K.,** Alkaline phosphatase activity and basophilia in hepatic cells following administration of butter yellow to rats, *Proc. Soc. Exp. Biol. Med.*, 67, 242, 1948.
126. **Goldfarb, S. and Pugh, T. D.,** The origin and significance of hyperplastic hepatocellulr islands and nodules in hepatic carcinogenesis, *J. Am. Coll. Toxicol.*, 1, 119, 1982.
127. **Williams, G. M.,** The pathogenesis of rat liver cancer caused by chemical carcinogens, *Biochim. Biophys. Acta*, 605, 167, 1980.
128. **Amano, H. and Daoust, R.,** The distribution of ribonuclease activity in rat liver during azo-dye carcinogenesis, *J. Histochem. Cytochem.*, 9, 161, 1961.
129. **Bannasch, P.,** Dose-dependence of early cellular changes during liver carcinogenesis, *Arch. Toxicol.*, Suppl. 3, 111, 1980.
130. **Bannasch, P. and Angerer, H.,** Glycogen and glucose-6-phosphatase during cancerization of rat liver cells by N-nitrosomorpholine, *Arch. Geschwulstforsch.*, 43, 105, 1974.
131. **Barbason, H., Fridman-Manduzio, A., and Betz, E. H.,** Long term effects of a single dose of dimethylnitrosamine on the rat liver, *Z. Krebsforsch.*, 84, 135, 1975.
132. **Barbason, H., Fridman-Manduzio, A., Lelievre, P., and Betz, E. H.,** Variations of liver cell control during diethylnitrosamine carcinogenesis, *Eur. J. Cancer*, 13, 13, 1977.
133. **Barbason, H., Smoliar, V., Fridman-Manduzio, A., and Betz, E. H.,** Effects of discontinuation of chronic feeding of diethylnitrosamine on the development of hepatomas in adult rats, *Br. J. Cancer*, 40, 260, 1979.
134. **Barbason, H., Smoliar, V., and Van Cantfort, J.,** Correlation of liver growth and function during liver regeneration and hepatocarcinogenesis, *Arch. Toxicol.*, Suppl. 2, 157, 1979.
135. **Barbason, H. and Betz, E. H.,** Liver cell control after discontinuation of DENA feeding in hepatocarcinogenesis, *Eur. J. Cancer*, 17, 149, 1981.
136. **Beaumont, C., Le Rumeur, E., Guillouzo, C., Latinier, M.-F., Bourel, M., and Guillouzo, A.,** Ferritin is increased in diethylnitrosamine-altered rat hepatocytes, *Biochem. Biophys. Res. Commun.*, 99, 879, 1981.
137. **Borner, P. and Gossner, W.,** Enzymhistochemische Untersuchungen der Adenosin-Triphosphatase, der alkalischen und sauren Phosphatase sowie der Succinodehydrogenase im Leberparenchym der Ratte wahrend der Einwirkung des Cancerogens Diathylnitrosmin, *Z. Naturforsch.*, 23b, 1085, 1968.
138. **Butler, W. H. and Hempsall, V.,** Histochemical observations on nodules induced in the mouse liver by phenobarbitone, *J. Pathol.*, 125, 155, 1978.
139. **Cameron, R., Kellen, J., Kolin, A., Malkin, A., and Farber, E.,** γ-Glutamyltransferase in putative premalignant liver cell populations during hepatocarcinogenesis, *Cancer Res.*, 38, 823, 1978.
140. **Cauchi, M. N., Halley, J. B. W., Irving, M. G., and Williams, J. F.,** Hepatocellular localization of fetal antigens during induction of rat liver tumors by 3′-methyl-4-dimethylaminoazobenzene, *Cancer Res.*, 34, 1808, 1974.
141. **Columbano, A., Rajalakshmi, S., and Sarma, D. S. R.,** Requirement of cell proliferation for the induction of presumptive preneoplastic lesions in rat liver by a single dose of 1,2-dimethylhydrazine, *Chem. Biol. Interactions*, 32, 347, 1980.
142. **Daoust, R.,** Focal loss of ribonuclease activity in preneoplastic rat liver, *Cancer Res.*, 32, 2502, 1972.

143. **Daoust, R.,** Histochemical comparison of focal losses of RNase and ATPase activities in preneoplastic rat livers, *J. Histochem. Cytochem.*, 27, 653, 1979.
144. **Deml, E. and Oesterle, D.,** Histochemical demonstration of enhanced glutathione content in enzyme-altered islands induced by carcinogens in rat liver, *Cancer Res.*, 40, 490, 1980.
145. **Epstein, S., Ito, N., Merkow, L., and Farber, E.,** Cellular analysis of liver carcinogenesis: the induction of large hyperplastic nodules in the liver with 2-fluorenylacetamide or ethionine and some aspects of their morphology and glycogen metabolism, *Cancer Res.*, 27, 1702, 1967.
146. **Fontaniere, B. and Daoust, R.,** Histochemical studies on nuclease activity and neoplastic transformation in rat liver during diethylnitrosamine carcinogenesis, *Cancer Res.*, 33, 3108, 1973.
147. **Forget, A. and Daoust, R.,** Histochemical study on rat liver glycogen during DAB carcinogenesis, *Int. J. Cancer*, 5, 404, 1970.
148. **Friedrich-Freksa, H., Papadopulu, G., and Gossner, W.,** Histochemical investigations of carcinogenesis in rat liver after time-limited application of diethnitrosamine, *Z. Krebsforsch.*, 72, 240, 1969.
149. **Goldfarb, S.,** A morphological and histochemical study of carcinogenesis of the liver in rats fed 3′-methyl-4-dimethylaminoazobenzene, *Cancer Res.*, 33, 1119, 1973.
150. **Goldfarb, S. and Pugh, T. D.,** Enzyme histochemical phenotypes in primary hepatocellular carcinomas, *Cancer Res.*, 41, 2092, 1981.
151. **Goldfarb, S., Pugh, T. D., and Cripps, D. J.,** Increased alkaline phosphatase activity — a positive histochemical marker for griseofulvin-induced mouse hepatocellular nodules, *J. Natl. Cancer Inst.*, 64, 1427, 1980.
152. **Goldfarb, S., Vesselinovitch, S. D., Pugh, T. D., Mihailovich, N., Koen, H., and He, Y.,** Tumor progression during diethylnitrosamine (DEN) induced mouse hepatocarcinogensis, *Proc. Am. Assoc. Cancer Res.*, 22, 124, A491, 1981.
153. **Goldfarb, S. and Zak, F. G.,** Role of injury and hyperplasia in the induction of hepatocellular carcinoma, *JAMA*, 178, 729, 1961.
154. **Goldsworthy, T., Moran, S., Weeks, J., Campbell, H. A., and Pitot, H. C.,** The effect of dose and dosage regimen on phenobarbital (PB) promotion of hepatocarcinogenesis by diethylnitrosamine (DEN), *Proc. Am. Assoc. Cancer Res.*, 22, 130, A517, 1981.
155. **Gossner, W. and Friedrich-Freksa, H.,** Histochemische Untersuchungen uber die Glucose-6-Phosphatase in der Rattenleber wahrend der Kanzerisierung durch Nitrosamine, *Z. Naturforsch.*, 19b, 862, 1964.
156. **Harada, M., Okabe, K., Shibata, K., Masuda, H., Miyata, K., and Enomoto, M.,** Histochemical demonstration of increased activity of γ-glutamyltranspeptidase in rat liver during hepatocarcinogenesis, *Acta Histochem. Cytochem.*, 9, 168, 1976.
157. **Heidcamp, W. H. and Karasaki, S.,** Intracellular cations and basophilia in rat liver parenchyma during azo dye carcinogenesis, *Cancer Res.*, 36, 3086, 1976.
158. **Hirota, N. and Williams, G. M.,** The sensitivity and heterogeneity of histochemical markers for altered foci involved in liver carcinogenesis, *Am. J. Pathol.*, 95, 317, 1979.
159. **Hirota, N. and Williams, G. M.,** Persistence and growth of rat liver neoplastic nodules following cessation of carcinogen exposure, *J. Natl. Cancer Inst.*, 63, 1257, 1979.
160. **Hunt, J. M., Buckley, M. T., Onnink, P. A., Rolfe, P. B., and Laishes, B. A.,** Liver-cell membrane alloantigens as cellular markers in genotypic mosaic rat livers undergoing chemically induced hepatocarcinogenesis, *Cancer Res.*, 42, 227, 1982.
161. **Itabashi, M., Mochizuki, Y., and Tsukada, H.,** Changes in peroxisomes in preneoplastic liver of rats induced by 3′-methyl-4-dimethylaminoazobenzene, *Cancer Res.*, 37, 1035, 1977.
162. **Jalanko, H. and Ruoslahti, E.,** Differential expression of alpha-fetoprotein and gamma-glutamyltranspeptidase in chemical and spontaneous hepatocarcinogenesis, *Cancer Res.*, 39, 3495, 1979.
163. **Kalengayi, M. M. R. and Desmet, V. J.,** Sequential histological and histochemical study of the rat liver after single-dose aflatoxin B_1 intoxication, *Cancer Res.*, 35, 2836, 1975.
164. **Kalengayi, M. M. R. and Desmet, V. J.,** Sequential histological and histochemical study of the rat liver during aflatoxin B_1-induced carcinogenesis, *Cancer Res.*, 35, 2845, 1975.
165. **Kalengayi, M. M. R. and Desmet, V. J.,** Liver cell populations and histochemical patterns of adult and fetal type proteins during aflatoxin B_1 hepatocarcinogenesis, in *Primary Liver Tumors*, Remmer, H., Bolt, H. M., Bannasch, P., and Popper, H., Eds., University Park Press, Baltimore, 1978, 467.
166. **Kalengayi, M. M. R. and Desmet, V. J.,** Gamma-glutamyltransferase as oncofetal marker of experimental hepatocarcinogenesis in the rat, *Scand. J. Immunol.*, 8, (Suppl. 8), 547, 1978.
167. **Kalengayi, M. M. R., Ronchi, G., and Desmet, V. J.,** Histochemistry of gamma-glutamyltranspeptidase in rat liver during aflatoxin B_1-induced carcinogenesis, *J. Natl. Cancer Inst.*, 55, 579, 1975.
168. **Karasaki, S.,** Subcellular localization of surface adenosine triphosphatase activity in preneoplastic liver parenchyma, *Cancer Res.*, 32, 1703, 1972.
169. **Karasaki, S.,** Cell proliferation and subcellular localization of alkaline phosphatase activity in rat liver parenchyma during azo dye carcinogenesis, *Cancer Res.*, 35, 482, 1975.

170. **Kitagawa, T.**, Histochemical analysis of hyperplastic lesions and hepatomas of the liver of rats fed 2-fluorenylacetamide, *Gann*, 62, 207, 1971.
171. **Kitagawa, T.**, Sequential phenotypic changes in hyperplastic areas during hepatocarcinogenesis in the rat, *Cancer Res.*, 36, 2534, 1976.
172. **Kitagawa, T. and Pitot, H. C.**, The regulation of serine dehydratase and glucose-6-phosphatase in hyperplastic nodules of rat liver during diethylnitrosamine and N-2-fluorenylacetamide feeding, *Cancer Res.*, 35, 1075, 1975.
173. **Kitagawa, T., Pitot, H. C., Miller, E. C., and Miller, J. A.**, Promotion by dietary phenobarbital of hepatocarcinogenesis by 2-methyl-N,N-dimethyl-4-aminoazobenzene in the rat, *Cancer Res.*, 39, 112, 1979.
174. **Kitagawa, T. and Sugano, H.**, Combination of enzyme histochemistry and radioautography: a new method applied to analysis of hepatocarcinogenesis, *Gann*, 63, 509, 1972.
175. **Kitagawa, T. and Sugano, H.**, Combined enzyme histochemical and radioautographic studies on areas of hyperplasia in the liver of rats fed N-2-fluorenylacetamide, *Cancer Res.*, 33, 2993, 1973.
176. **Kitagawa, T. and Sugano, H.**, Enhancement of azo dye hepatocarcinogenesis with dietary phenobarbital in rats, *Gann*, 68, 255, 1977.
177. **Kitagawa, T. and Sugano, H.**, Enhancing effect of phenobarbital on the development of enzyme-altered islands and hepatocellular carcinomas initiated by 3′-methyl-4-(dimethylamino)azobenzene or diethylnitrosamine, *Gann*, 69, 679, 1978.
178. **Kitagawa, T., Watanabe, R., and Sugano, H.**, Induction of γ-glutamyltranspeptidase activity by dietary phenobarbital in "spontaneous" hepatic tumors of C3H mice, *Gann*, 71, 536, 1980.
179. **Kuhlmann, W. D., Krischan, R., Kunz, W., Guenthner, T. M. and Oesch, F.**, Focal elevation of liver microsomal epoxide hydrolase in early preneoplastic stages and its behavior in the further course of hepatocarcinogenesis, *Biochem. Biophys. Res., Commun.*, 98, 417, 1981.
180. **Kunz, W., Appel, K. E., Rickart, R., Schwarz, M., and Stockle, G.**, Enhancement and inhibition of carcinogenic effectiveness of nitrosamines, in *Primary Liver Tumors*, Remmer, H., Bolt, H. M., Bannasch, P., and Popper, H., Eds., University Park Press, Baltimore, 1978, 261.
181. **Laib, R. J., Stockle, G., Bolt, H. M., and Kunz, W.**, Vinyl chloride and trichloroethylene: comparison of alkylating effects of metabolites and induction of preneoplastic enzyme deficiencies in rat liver, *J. Cancer Res. Clin. Oncol.*, 94, 139, 1979.
182. **Laishes, B. A. and Farber, E.**, Transfer of viable putative preneoplastic hepatocytes to the livers of syngeneic host rats, *J. Natl. Cancer Inst.*, 61, 507, 1978.
183. **Laishes, B. A., Fink, L., and Carr, B. I.**, A liver colony assay for a new hepatocyte phenotype as a step towards purifying new cellular phenotypes that arise during hepatocarcinogenesis, *Ann. N.Y. Acad. Sci.*, 349, 373, 1980.
184. **Laishes, B. A., Ogawa, K., Roberts, E., and Farber, E.**, Gamma-glutamyltranspeptidase: a positive marker for cultured rat liver cells derived from putative premalignant and malignant lesions, *J. Natl. Cancer Inst.*, 60, 1009, 1978.
185. **Laishes, B. A. and Rolfe, P. B.**, Search for endogenous liver colony-forming units in F344 rats given a two-thirds hepatectomy during short-term feeding of 2-acetylaminofluorene, *Cancer Res.*, 41, 1731, 1981.
186. **Lesch, R., Meinhardt, K., and Oehlert, W.**, A histological and autoradiographic study of the induction of tumours in the rat liver by methyl-allyl-nitrosamine, *Z. Krebsforsch.*, 70, 267, 1967.
187. **Lipsky, M. M., Hinton, D. E., Goldblatt, P. J., Klaunig, J. E., and Trump, B. F.**, Iron negative foci and nodules in safrole-exposed mouse liver made siderotic by iron-dextran injection, *Pathol. Res. Pract.*, 164, 178, 1979.
188. **Lipsky, M. M., Hinton, D. E., Klaunig, J. E., Goldblatt, P. J., and Trump, B. F.**, Gamma glutamyl transpeptidase in safrole-induced, presumptive premalignant mouse hepatocytes, *Carcinogenesis*, 1, 151, 1980.
189. **Malkin, A., Kellen, J. A., Kolin, A., Cameron, R., and Farber, E.**, The immunohistochemical detection of chorionic gonadotropin in experimental rat hepatomas, *Scand. J. Immunol.*, 8 (Suppl. 8), 603, 1978.
190. **Malvaldi, G.**, Appearance of iron free hyperplastic hepatocytes following ferric nitrilotriacetate and 2-acetylaminofluorene sequential administration, *Eur. J. Cancer*, 17, 481, 1981.
191. **Narita, T., Watanabe, R., and Kitagawa, T.**, Mechanisms of inhibition by simultaneously administered phenobarbital of 3′-methyl-4-(dimethylamino)azobenzene-induced hepatocarcinogenesis in the rat, *Gann*, 71, 755, 1980.
192. **Novikoff, A. B., Novikoff, P. M., Stockert, R. J., Becker, F. F., Yam, A., Poruchynsky, M. S., Levin, W., and Thomas, P. E.**, Immunocytochemical localization of epoxide hydrase in hyperplastic nodules induced in rat liver by 2-acetylaminofluorene, *Proc. Natl. Acad. Sci. U.S.A.*, 76, 5207, 1979.
193. **Ogawa, K., Kaneko, A., Minase, T., and Onoe, T.**, Persistent changes induced by subcarcinogenic doses of 3′-methyl-4-(dimethylamino)azobenzene in rat liver, *Gann*, 65, 109, 1974.
194. **Ogawa, K., Solt, D. B., and Farber, E.**, Phenotypic diversity as an early property of putative preneoplastic hepatocyte populations in liver carcinogenesis, *Cancer Res.*, 40, 725, 1980.

195. **Ohde, G., Schuppler, J., Schulte-Hermann, R., and Keiger, H.,** Proliferation of rat liver cells in preneoplastic nodules after stimulation of liver growth by xenobiotic inducers, *Arch. Toxicol.*, Suppl. 2, 451, 1979.
196. **Ohmori, T., Watanabe, K., and Williams, G. M.,** Absence of uniform progressive growth of long-term transplants of rat liver neoplastic nodules, *J. Natl. Cancer Inst.*, 65, 485, 1980.
197. **Okita, K., Gruenstein, M., Klaiber, M., and Farber, E.,** Localization of α-fetoprotein by immunofluorescence in hyperplastic nodules during hepatocarcinogenesis induced by 2-acetylaminofluorene, *Cancer Res.*, 34, 2758, 1974.
198. **Okita, K., Kligman, L. H., and Farber, E.,** A new common marker for premalignant and malignant hepatocytes induced in the rat by chemical carcinogens, *J. Natl. Cancer Inst.*, 54, 199, 1975.
199. **Pearson, B. and Defendi, V.,** Histochemical studies of succinic dehydrogenase by means of tetrazolium in rat liver tumors induced by p-dimethylaminoazobenzene, *Cancer Res.*, 15, 593, 1955.
200. **Pitot, H. C.,** The stability of events in the natural history of neoplasia, *Am. J. Pathol.*, 89, 703, 1977.
201. **Pitot, H. C.,** Drugs as promoters of carcinogenesis, *in The Induction of Drug Metabolism*, Estabrook, R. W. and Lindenlaub, E., Eds., Schattauer-Verlag, Stuttgart, 1978, 471.
202. **Pitot, H. C.,** Characteristics of stages of hepatocarcinogenesis, in *Carcinogenesis: Fundamental Mechanisms and Environmental Effects*, Pullman, B., Ts'o, P. O. P., and Gelboin, H., Eds., D. Reidel, Hingham, Maine, 1980, 219.
203. **Pitot, H. C., Barsness, L., and Kitagawa T.,** Stages in the process of hepatocarcinogenesis in rat liver, in *Carcinogenesis, Mechanisms of Tumor Promotion and Cocarcinogenesis*, Vol. 2, Slaga, T. J., Sivak, A., and Boutwell, R. K., Eds., Raven Press, New York, 1978, 433.
204. **Pitot, H. C., Goldsworthy, T., Campbell, H. A., and Poland, A.,** Quantitative evaluation of the promotion by 2,3,7,8-tetrachlorodibenzo-p-dioxin of hepatocarcinogenesis from diethylnitrosamine, *Cancer Res.*, 40, 3616, 1980.
205. **Rabes, H., Hartenstein, R., and Scholze, P.,** Specific stages of cellular response to homeostatic control during diethylnitrosamine-induced liver carcinogenesis, *Experientia*, 26, 1356, 1970.
206. **Rabes, H. M. and Szymkowiak, R.,** Cell kinetics of hepatocytes during the preneoplastic period of diethylnitrosamine-induced liver carcinogenesis, *Cancer Res.*, 39, 1298, 1979.
207. **Ruebner, B. H., Michas, C., Kanayama, R., and Bannasch, P.,** Sequential hepatic histologic and histochemical changes produced by diethylnitrosamine in the rhesus monkey, *J. Natl. Cancer Inst.*, 57, 1261, 1976.
208. **Salmon, W. D. and Copeland, D. H.,** Liver carcinoma and related lesions in chronic choline deficiency, *Ann. N.Y. Acad Sci.*, 57, 664, 1954.
209. **Schauer, A. and Kunze, E.,** Enzyme-histochemical and autoradiographic studies in the course of cancerization of rat liver with diethylnitrosamine, *Z. Krebsforsch.*, 70, 252, 1968.
210. **Scherer, E. and Emmelot, P.,** Kinetics of induction and growth of precancerous liver-cell foci, and liver tumour formation by diethylnitrosamine in the rat, *Eur. J. Cancer*, 11, 689, 1975.
211. **Scherer, E. and Hoffmann, M.,** Probable clonal genesis of cellular islands induced in rat liver by diethylnitrosamine, *Eur. J. Cancer*, 7, 369, 1971.
212. **Schieferstein, G., Pirschel, J., Frank, W., and Friedrich-Freksa, H.,** Quantitative studies on the irreversible loss of two enzyme activities in the rat liver after application of diethylnitrosamine, *Z. Krebsforsch.*, 82, 191, 1974.
213. **Schmitz-Moormann, P., Gedigk, P., and Dharamadhach, A.,** Early histological and histochemical changes during experimental production of liver carcinoma by diethylnitrosamine, *Z. Krebsforsch.*, 77, 9, 1972.
214. **Schor, N. A., Ogawa, K., Lee, G., and Farber, E.,** The use of the D-T diaphorase for the detection of foci of early neoplastic transformation in rat liver, *Cancer Lett.*, 5, 167, 1978.
215. **Sell, S.,** Distribution of alpha-fetoprotein- and albumin-containing cells in the livers of Fischer rats fed four cycles of N-2-fluorenylacetamide, *Cancer Res.*, 38, 3107, 1978.
216. **Sirica, A. E., Barsness, L., Goldsworthy, T., and Pitot, H. C.,** Definition of stages during hepatocarcinogenesis in the rat: potential application to the evaluation of initiating and promoting agents in the environment, *J. Environ. Pathol. Toxicol.*, 2, 21, 1978.
217. **Stratil, P., Dolezalova, V., Nemecek, R., and Simickova, M.,** Relationship between α-fetoprotein positive cells and precancerous lesions in rat liver during 3′-methyl-4-dimethylaminoazobenzene carcinogenesis, *Neoplasma*, 26, 381, 1979.
218. **Takahashi, S., Katayal, S. L., Lombardi, B., and Shinozuka, H.,** Induction of foci of altered hepatocytes by a single injection of azaserine to rats, *Cancer Lett.*, 7, 265, 1979.
219. **Taper, H. S. and Bannasch, P.,** Histochemical correlation between glycogen, nucleic acids, and nucleases in pre-neoplastic and neoplastic lesions of rat liver after short-term administration of N-nitrosomorpholine, *Z. Krebsforsch.*, 87, 53, 1976.
220. **Taper, H. S., Fort, L., and Brucher, J.-M.,** Histochemical activity of alkaline and acid nucleases in the rat liver parenchyma during N-nitrosomorpholine carcinogenesis, *Cancer Res.*, 31, 913, 1971.

221. **Wachstein, M. and Meisel, E.,** Enzymatic histochemistry of ethionine-induced liver cirrhosis and hepatoma, *J. Histochem. Cytochem.*, 7, 189, 1959.
222. **Watanabe, K. and Williams, G. M.,** Enhancement of rat hepatocellular-altered foci by the liver tumor promoter phenobarbital: evidence that foci are precursors of neoplasms and that the promoter acts on carcinogen-induced lesions, *J. Natl. Cancer Inst.*, 61, 1311, 1978.
223. **Weber, A., LeProvost, E., Boisnard-Rissel, M., Berges, J., Schapira, F., and Guillouzo, A.,** Localization of fetal aldolases during early stages of azo-dye hepatocarcinogenesis in rat, *Biochem. Biophys. Res. Commun.*, 92, 591, 1980.
224. **Weiler, E.,** Die Anderung der serologischen Spezifitat von Leberzellen der Ratte wahrend der Cancerogenese durch p-Dimethylaminoazobenzol, *Z. Naturforsch.*, 11b, 31, 1956.
225. **Williams, G. M.,** Functional markers and growth behavior of preneoplastic hepatocytes, *Cancer Res.*, 36, 2540, 1976.
226. **Williams, G. M.,** Enhancement of hyperplastic lesions in the rat liver by the tumor promoter phenobarbital, in *Carcinogenesis, Mechanisms of Tumor Promotion and Cocarcinogenesis*, Vol. 2, Slaga, T. J., Sivak, A., and Boutwell, R. K., Eds., Raven Press, New York, 1978, 449.
227. **Williams, G. M., Hirota, N., and Rice, J. M.,** The resistance of spontaneous mouse hepatocellular neoplasms to iron accumulation during rapid iron loading by parenteral administration and their transplantability, *Am. J. Pathol.*, 94, 65, 1979.
228. **Williams, G. M., Klaiber, M., Parker, S. E., and Farber, E.,** Nature of early appearing, carcinogen-induced liver lesions resistant to iron accumulation, *J. Natl. Cancer Inst.*, 57, 157, 1976.
229. **Williams, G. M., Ohmori, T., Katayama, S., and Rice, J. M.,** Alteration by phenobarbital of membrane-associated enzymes including gamma glutamyl transpeptidase in mouse liver neoplasms, *Carcinogenesis*, 1, 813, 1980.
230. **Williams, G. M., Ohmori, T., and Watanabe, K.,** The persistence and phenotypic stability of transplanted rat liver neoplastic nodules, *Am. J. Pathol.*, 99, 1, 1980.
231. **Williams, G. M. and Watanabe, K.,** Quantitative kinetics of development of N-2-fluorenylacetamide-induced, altered (hyperplastic) hepatocellular foci resistant to iron accumulation and of their reversion or persistence following removal of carcinogen, *J. Natl. Cancer Inst.*, 61, 113, 1978.
232. **Williams, G. M. and Yamamoto, R. S.,** Absence of stainable iron from preneoplastic and neoplastic lesions in rat liver with 8-hydroxyquinoline-induced siderosis, *J. Natl. Cancer Inst.*, 49, 685, 1972.
233. **Yager, J. D. and Yager, R.,** Oral contraceptive steroids as promoters of hepatocarcinogenesis in female Sprague-Dawley rats, *Cancer Res.*, 40, 3680, 1980.
234. **Yamamoto, R. S., Williams, G. M., Frankel, H. H., and Weisburger, J. H.,** 8-Hydroxyquinoline: chronic toxicity and inhibitory effect on the carcinogenicity of N-2-fluorenylacetamide, *Toxicol. Appl. Pharmacol.*, 19, 687, 1971.
235. **Zugibe, F. T., Ed.,**, *Diagnostic Histochemistry*, C. V. Mosby, St. Louis, 1970.
236. **Burstone, M. S., Ed.,** *Enzyme Histochemistry and Its Application in the Study of Neoplasms*, Academic Press, New York, 1962.
237. **Schnitka, T. K. and Seligman, A. M.,** Ultrastructural cytochemistry of enzymes and some applications, in *Methods in Cancer Research*, Vol. 10, Busch, H., Ed., Academic Press, New York, 1973, 37.
238. **Thompson, S. W.,** *Selected Histochemical and Histopathological Methods*, Charles C Thomas, Springfield, Ill., 1966.
239. **Gomori, G.,** Distribution of acid phosphatase in the tissues under normal and pathologic conditions, *Arch. Pathol.*, 32, 189, 1941.
240. **Barka, T. and Anderson, P. J.,** *Histochemistry, Theory, Practice, and Bibliography*, Hoeber Medical Division, Harper & Row, New York, 1963.
241. **Rutenberg, A. M. and Seligman, A. M.,** The histochemical demonstration of acid phosphatase by a post-incubation coupling technique, *J. Histochem. Cytochem.*, 3, 455, 1955.
242. **Wachstein, M.,** Enzymatic histochemistry of the liver, *Gastroenterology*, 37, 525, 1959.
243. **Novikoff, A. B. and Essner, E.,** The liver cell. Some new approaches to its study, *Am. J. Med.*, 29, 102, 1960.
244. **Dixon, M. and Webb, E. C.,** *Enzymes*, 3rd ed., Academic Press, New York, 1979.
245. **Sleyster, E. C. and Knook, D. L.,** Aging and multiple forms of acid phosphatase in isolated rat liver cells, *Mech. Aging Dev.*, 14, 443, 1980.
246. **Wachstein, M. and Meisel, E.,** Histochemistry of hepatic phosphatases at a physiologic pH. With special reference to the demonstration of bile canaliculi, *Am. J. Clin. Pathol.*, 27, 13, 1957.
247. **Novikoff, A. B., Drucker, J., Shin, W.-Y., and Goldfischer, S.,** Further studies of the apparent adenosinetriphosphatase activity of cell membranes in formol-calcium-fixed tissues, *J. Histochem. Cytochem.*, 9, 434, 1961.
248. **Yamaguchi, M.,** Comparison of calcitonin, epinephrine, and glucagon effects on plasma membrane Ca-ATPase activity and calcium content in liver of rats, *Endocrinol. Jpn.*, 27, 273, 1980.

249. **Peterson, R. E., Hamada, N., Yang, K. H., Madhukar, B. V., and Matsumura, F.,** Reversal of 2,3,7,8-tetrachlorodibenzo-p-dioxin-induced depression of ouabain biliary excretion by pregnenolone-16α-carbonitrile and spironolactone in isolated perfused rat livers, *Toxicol. Appl. Pharmacol.*, 50, 407, 1979.
250. **Karasaki, S.,** Ultrastructural and cytochemical studies on hyperbasophilic foci with special reference to the demonstration of cell surface alterations in hepatocarcinogenesis, *Cancer Res.*, 36, 2567, 1976.
251. **Gerber, M. A. and Thung, S. N.,** Enzyme patterns in human hepatocellular carcinoma, *Am. J. Pathol.*, 98, 395, 1980.
252. **Gomori, G.,** *Microscopic Histochemistry. Principles and Practice*, University of Chicago Press, 1952, chap. 8.
253. **Burstone, M. S.,** Histochemical demonstration of phosphatases in frozen sections with naphthol AS-phosphates, *J. Histochem. Cytochem.*, 9, 146, 1961.
254. **Burstone, M. S.,** Histochemical comparison of naphthol AS-phosphates for the demonstration of phosphatases, *J. Natl. Cancer Inst.*, 20, 601, 1958.
255. **Mayahara, H., Hirano, H., Saito, T., and Ogawa, K.,** The new lead citrate method for the ultracytochemical demonstration of activity of non-specific alkaline phosphatase (orthophosphoric monoester phosphohydrolase), *Histochemie*, 11, 88, 1967.
256. **Fishman, W. H.,** Perspectives on alkaline phosphatase isoenzymes, *Am. J. Med.*, 56, 617, 1974.
257. **Gangolli, S. and Wright, M.,** The histochemical demonstration of aniline hydroxylase activity in rat liver, *Histochem. J.*, 3, 107, 1971.
258. **Hayaishi, O., Takikawa, O., Sono, M., and Yoshida, R.,** Enzymatic activation of molecular oxygen, in *Microsomes, Drug Oxidations, and Chemical Carcinogenesis*, Vol. 1, Coon, M. J., Conney, A. H., Estabrook, R. W., Gelboin, H. V., Gillette, J. R., and O'Brien, P. J., Eds., Academic Press, New York, 1980, 1.
259. **Sternberger, L. A.,** *Immunocytochemistry*, 2nd ed., John Wiley & Sons, New York, 1979.
260. **Lin, J.-C., Hiasa, Y., and Farber, E.,** Preneoplastic antigen as a marker for endoplasmic reticulum of putative premalignant hepatocytes during liver carcinogenesis, *Cancer Res.*, 37, 1972, 1977.
261. **Levin, W., Lu, A. Y. H., Thomas, P. E., Ryan, D., Kizer, D. E., and Griffin, M. J.,** Identification of epoxide hydrase as the preneoplastic antigen in rat liver hyperplastic nodules, *Proc. Natl. Acad. Sci. U.S.A.*, 75, 3240, 1978.
262. **Baldwin, R. W.,** Immunology of rat hepatic neoplasia, in *Rat Hepatic Neoplasia*, Newberne, P. M. and Butler, W. H., Eds., MIT Press, Cambridge, 1978, 228.
263. **Novikoff, A. B. and Goldfischer, S.,** Visualization of peroxisomes (microbodies) and mitochondria with diaminobenzidine, *J. Histochem. Cytochem.*, 17, 675, 1969.
264. **Itabashi, M., Mochizuki, Y., and Tsukada, H.,** Peroxisomes in liver tumors of rats induced by 3′-methyl-4-(dimethylamino)-azobenzene, *Gann*, 66, 463, 1975.
265. **Linder, M. C.,** Iron and copper metabolism in cancer, as exemplified by changes in ferritin and ceruloplasmin in rats with transplantable tumors, in *Morris Hepatomas. Mechanisms of Regulation*, Morris, H. P. and Criss, W. E., Eds., Plenum Press, New York, 1978, 643.
266. **Frieden, E.,** Copper and iron metalloproteins, *TIBS*, 1, 273, 1976.
267. **Linder, M., Munro, H. N., and Morris, H. P.,** Rat ferritin isoproteins and their response to iron administration in a series of hepatic tumors and in normal and regenerating liver, *Cancer Res.*, 30, 2231, 1970.
268. **Sell, S.,** Distribution of α-fetoprotein- and albumin-containing cells in the livers of Fischer male rats fed four cycles of N-2-fluorenylacetamide, *Cancer Res.*, 38, 3107, 1978.
269. **Abelev, G. I.,** Cell aspects in study on regulation of alpha-fetoprotein (AFP) synthesis, in *Carcino-Embryonic Proteins*, Vol. 1, Lehmann, F.-G., Ed., Elsevier, Amsterdam, 1979, 99.
270. **Basteris, B.,** Immunofluorescent localization of alpha-fetoprotein and albumin in embryonic fetal and newborn rat, in *Carcino-Embryonic Proteins*, Vol. 2, Lehmann, F.-G., Ed., Elsevier, Amsterdam, 1979, 353.
271. **Sell, S. and Morris, H. P.,** Relationship of rat alpha-fetoprotein to growth rate and chromosome composition of Morris hepatomas, *Cancer Res.*, 34, 1413, 1974.
272. **Wachstein, M. and Meisel, E.,** On the histochemical demonstration of glucose-6-phosphatase, *J. Histochem. Cytochem.*, 4, 592, 1956.
273. **Newsholme, E. A. and Start, C.,** *Regulation in Metabolism*, John Wiley & Sons, London, 1973, chap. 6.
274. **Weber, G. and Cantero, A.,** Glucose-6-phosphatase activity in normal, precancerous, and neoplastic tissues, *Cancer Res.*, 15, 105, 1955.
275. **Hess, R., Scarpelli, D. G., and Pearse, A. G. E.,** The cytochemical localization of oxidative enzymes. II. Pyridine nucleotide-linked dehydrogenases, *J. Biophys. Biochem. Cytol.*, 4, 753, 1958.
276. **Karnovsky, M. J. and Himmelhoch, S. R.,** The use of ethylene diamine tetraacetic acid disodium in the histochemical demonstration of triphosphopyridine nucleotide-linked dehydrogenases, *J. Histochem. Cytochem.*, 9, 203, 1961.

277. **Axelrod, B.,** Other pathways of carbohydrate metabolism, in *Metabolic Pathways,* Vol. 1, 3rd ed., Greenberg, D. M., Ed., Academic Press, New York, 1967, 271.
278. **Pitot, H. C. and Cardelli, J.,** Contribution of the Morris hepatomas to the biochemistry of cancer. Establishment of the phenotypic heterogeneity of neoplasms in vivo, in *Morris Hepatomas. Mechanisms of Regulation,* Morris, H. P. and Criss, W. E., Eds., Plenum Press, New York, 1978, 21.
279. **Hayashi, M., Nakajima, Y., and Fishman, W. H.,** The cytologic demonstration of β-glucuronidase employing naphthol AS-BI glucuronide and hexazonium pararosanilin; a preliminary report, *J. Histochem. Cytochem.,* 12, 293, 1964.
280. **Rutenburg, A. M., Kim, H., Fischbein, J. W., Hanker, J. S., Wasserkrug, H. L., and Seligman, A. M.,** Histochemical and ultrastructural demonstration of γ-glutamyl transpeptidase activity, *J. Histochem. Cytochem.,* 17, 517, 1969.
281. **Vanderlaan, M., Cutter, C., and Dolbeare, F.,** Flow microfluorometric identification of liver cells with elevated gamma-glutamyltranspeptidase activity after carcinogen exposure, *J. Histochem. Cytochem.,* 27, 114, 1979.
282. **Kitagawa, T., Imai, F., and Sato, K.,** Re-elevation of γ-glutamyl transpeptidase activity in periportal hepatocytes of rats with age, *Gann,* 71, 362, 1980.
283. **Fiala, S. and Fiala, E. S.,** Activation by chemical carcinogens of γ-glutamyl transpeptidase in rat and mouse liver, *J. Natl. Cancer Inst.,* 51, 151, 1973.
284. **Tateishi, N., Higashi, T., Nomura, T., Naruse, A., Nakashima, K., Shiozaki, H., and Sakamoto, Y.,** Higher transpeptidation activity and broad acceptor specificity of γ-glutamyltransferases of tumors, *Gann,* 67, 215, 1976.
285. **Tate, S. S., Thompson, G. A., and Meister, A.,** Recent studies on γ-glutamyl transpeptidase, in *Glutathione: Metabolism and Function,* Arias, I. M. and Jakoby, W. B., Eds., Raven Press, New York, 1976, chap. 4.
286. **Prusiner, S., Doak, C. W., and Kirk, G.,** A novel mechanism for group translocation: substrate-product reutilization by γ-glutamyl transpeptidase in peptide and amino acid transport, *J. Cell. Physiol.,* 89, 853, 1976.
287. **Wirth, P. J. and Thorgeirsson, S. S.,** Glutathione synthesis and degradation in fetal and adult rat liver and Novikoff hepatoma, *Cancer Res.,* 38, 2861, 1978.
288. **Curthoys, N. P. and Kuhlenschmidt, T.,** Phosphate-independent glutaminase from rat kidney. Partial purification and identity with γ-glutamyltranspeptidase, *J. Biol. Chem.,* 250, 2099, 1975.
289. **Fiala, S., Fiala, A. E., and Dixon, B.,** γ-Glutamyl transpeptidase in transplantable, chemically induced rat hepatomas and "spontaneous" mouse hepatomas, *J. Natl. Cancer Inst.,* 48, 1393, 1972.
290. **Fiala, S., Mohindru, A., Kettering, W. G., Fiala, A. E., and Morris, H. P.,** Glutathione and gamma glutamyl transpeptidase in rat liver during chemical carcinogenesis, *J. Natl. Cancer Inst.,* 57, 591, 1976.
291. **Taniguchi, N., Tsukada, Y., Mukuo, K., and Hirai, H.,** Effect of hepatocarcinogenic azo dyes on glutathione and related enzymes in rat liver, *Gann,* 65, 381, 1974.
292. **Rabes, H. M., Hartenstein, R., and Ringelmann, W.,** DNA synthesis in rat liver during early stages of azo dye-induced hepatocarcinogenesis, *Cancer Res.,* 32, 83, 1972.
293. **Kottgen, E., Reutter, W., and Gerok, W.,** Induction and superinduction of sialylation of membrane-bound γ-glutamyltransferase during liver regeneration, *Eur. J. Biochem.,* 82, 279, 1978.
294. **DeYoung, L. M., Richards, W. L., Bonzelet, W., Tsai, L. L., and Boutwell, R. K.,** Localization and significance of γ-glutamyltranspeptidase in normal and neoplastic mouse skin, *Cancer Res.,* 38, 3697, 1978.
295. **Sirica, A. E., Richards, W., Tsukada, Y., Sattler, C. A., and Pitot, H. C.,** Fetal phenotypic expression by adult rat hepatocytes on collagen gel/nylon meshes, *Proc. Natl. Acad. Sci. U.S.A.,* 76, 283, 1979.
296. **DeBault, L. E. and Cancilla, P. A.,** γ-Glutamyl transpeptidase in isolated brain endothelial cells: induction by glial cells *in vitro, Science,* 207, 653, 1980.
297. **Fiala, S., Fiala, A. E., Keller, R. W., and Fiala, E. S.,** Gamma glutamyl transpeptidase in colon cancer induced by 1,2-dimethylhydrazine, *Arch. Geschwulstforsch.,* 47, 117, 1977.
298. **Sachdev, G. P., Wen, G., Martin, B., Kishore, G. S., and Fox, O. F.,** Effects of dietary fat and alpha-tocopherol on γ-glutamyl transpeptidase (GGTP) of 7,12-dimethylbenz(a)anthracene (DMBA)-induced mammary carcinomas, *Proc. Am. Assoc. Cancer Res.,* 21, 2, A7, 1980.
299. **Groscurth, P., Fleming, N., and Kistler, G. S.,** The activity and distribution of gamma-glutamyl transpeptidase (γ-GT) in human lung cancers serially transplanted in nude mice, *Histochemistry,* 53, 135, 1977.
300. **Novogrodsky, A., Tate, S. S., and Meister, A.,** Gamma-glutamyl transpeptidase, a lymphoid cell-surface marker: relationship to blastogenesis, differentiation, and neoplasia, *Proc. Natl. Acad. Sci. U.S.A.,* 73, 2414, 1976.
301. **Asghar, K., Reddy, B. G., and Krishna, G.,** Histochemical localization of glutathione in tissues, *J. Histochem. Cytochem.,* 23, 774, 1975.
302. **Meister, A. and Tate, S. S.,** Glutathione and related gamma-glutamyl compounds: biosynthesis and utilization, *Annu. Rev. Biochem.,* 45, 559, 1976.

303. **Sies, H., Wahllander, A., Waydhas, C., Soboll, S., and Haberle, D.,** Functions of intracellular glutathione in hepatic hydroperoxide and drug metabolism and the role of extracellular glutathione, in *Advances in Enzyme Regulation,* Vol. 18, Weber, G., Ed., Pergamon Press, Oxford, 1980, 303.
304. **Flohe, L. and Gunzler, W. A.,** Glutathione-dependent enzymatic oxidoreduction reactions, in *Glutathione: Metabolism and Function,* Arias, I. M. and Jakoby, W. B., Eds., Raven Press, New York, 1976, chap. 2.
305. **Novi, A. M.,** Regression of aflatoxin B_1-induced hepatocellular carcinomas by reduced glutathione, *Science,* 212, 541, 1981.
306. **McManus, J. F. A.,** Histological and histochemical uses of periodic acid, *Stain Technol.,* 23, 99, 1948.
307. **Swigart, R. H., Wagner, C. E., and Atkinson, W. B.,** The preservation of glycogen in fixed tissues and tissue sections, *J. Histochem. Cytochem.,* 8, 74, 1960.
308. **Richards, W. L. and Potter, V. R.,** Scanning microdensitometry of glycogen zonation in the livers of rats adapted to a controlled feeding schedule and to 30, 60, or 90% casein diets, *Am. J. Anat.,* 157, 71, 1980.
309. **Ishikawa, K. and Shimazu, T.,** Daily rhythms of glycogen synthetase and phosphorylase activities in rat liver: influences of food and light, *Life Sci.,* 19, 1873, 1976.
310. **Korsgaard, B. and Wulff, H. R.,** An improved method for the histochemical demonstration of phosphorylase in tissue sections, *Acta Pathol. Microbiol. Scand.,* 70, 236, 1967.
311. **Gomori, G.,** Microtechnical demonstration of iron, a criticism of its methods, *Am. J. Pathol.,* 12, 655, 1936.
312. **Lehy, T., Zeitoun, P., Manchon, P., and Dubrasquet, M.,** Siderose du rat par augmentation du fer alimentaire. Etude histologique et ultrastructurale, *Pathol. Biol.,* 18, 407, 1970.
313. **Daoust, R.,** Modified procedure for the histochemical localization of ribonuclease activity by the substrate film method, *J. Histochem. Cytochem.,* 14, 254, 1966.
314. **Vorbrodt, A.,** Histochemical studies on the intracellular localization of acid deoxyribonuclease, *J. Histochem. Cytochem.,* 9, 647, 1961.
315. **Taper, H. S.,** La detection histochimique de la desoxyribonuclease alcaline, *Ann. Histochim.,* 14, 301, 1968.
316. **Kitagawa, T. and Pitot, H. C.,** Immunohistochemical demonstration of serine dehydratase in rat liver, *Am. J. Pathol.,* 78, 309, 1975.
317. **Potter, V. R.,** Transplantable animal cancer, the primary standard, *Cancer Res.,* 21, 1331, 1961.
318. **Potter, V. R. and Watanabe, M.,** Some biochemical essentials of malignancy: the challenge of diversity, in *Proc. Int. Leukemia-Lymphoma,* Zarafonetis, C. J. D., Ed., Lea & Febiger, Philadelphia, 1968, 33.
319. **Walker, P. R. and Potter, V. R.,** Isozyme studies on adult, regenerating, precancerous and developing liver in relation to findings in hepatomas, in *Advances in Enzyme Regulation,* Vol. 10, Weber, G., Ed., Pergamon Press, New York, 1972, 339.
320. **Weber, G., Kizaki, H., Shiotani, T., Tzeng, D., and Williams, J. C.,** The molecular correlation concept of neoplasia: recent advances and new challenges, in *Morris Hepatomas. Mechanisms of Regulation,* Morris, H. P. and Criss, W. E., Eds., Plenum Press, New York, 1978, 89.
321. **Liebelt, A. G. and Liebelt, R. A.,** Transplantation of tumors, in *Methods in Cancer Research,* Vol. 1, Busch, H., Ed., Academic Press, New York, 1967, chap. 4.
322. **Reuber, M. D.,** Histopathology of transplantable hepatic carcinomas induced by chemical carcinogens in rats, *Gann Monogr.,* 1, 43, 1966.
323. **Morris, H. P. and Meranze, D. R.,** Induction and some characteristics of "minimal deviation" and other transplantable rat hepatomas, in *Special Topics in Carcinogenesis,* Grundmann, E., Ed., Springer-Verlag, New York, 1974, 103.
324. **Reuber, M. D.,** Transplantation studies, in *Mouse Hepatic Neoplasia,* Butler, W. H. and Newberne, P. M., Eds., Elsevier, Amsterdam, 1975, chap. 8, Part A.
325. **Williams, G. M., Klaiber, M., and Farber, E.,** Differences in growth of transplants of liver, liver hyperplastic nodules, and hepatocellular carcinomas in the mammary fat pad, *Am. J. Pathol.,* 89, 379, 1977.
326. **Schaeffer, W. I. and Heintz, N. H.,** A diploid rat liver cell culture. IV. Malignant transformation by aflatoxin B_1, *In Vitro,* 14, 418, 1978.
327. **Heintz, N., Little, B., Bresnick, E., and Schaeffer, W. I.,** Malignant transformation of cultured rat hepatocytes by (+)- and (−)-trans-7,8-dihydro-7,8-dihydroxybenzo(a)pyrene, *Cancer Res.,* 40, 1281, 1980.
328. **Huberman, E., Montesano, R., Drevon, C., Kuroki, T., St. Vincent, L., Pugh, T. D., and Goldfarb, S.,** γ-Glutamyl transpeptidase and malignant transformation of cultured liver cells, *Cancer Res.,* 39, 269, 1979.
329. **San, R. H. C., Shimada, T., Maslansky, C. J., Kreiser, D. M., Laspia, M. F., Rice, J. M., and Williams, G. M.,** Growth characteristics and enzyme activities in a survey of transformation markers in adult rat liver epithelial-like cell cultures, *Cancer Res.,* 39, 4441, 1979.

330. **San, R. H. C., Laspia, M. F., Soiefer, A. I., Maslansky, C. J., Rice, J. M., and Williams, G. M.**, A survey of growth in soft agar and cell surface properties as markers for transformation in adult rat liver epithelial-like cell cultures, *Cancer Res.*, 39, 1026, 1979.
331. **Jirtle, R. L., Biles, C., and Michalopoulos, G.**, Morphologic and histochemical analysis of hepatocytes transplanted into syngeneic hosts, *Am. J. Pathol.*, 101, 115, 1980.
332. **Slifkin, M., Merkow, L. P., Pardo, M., Epstein, S. M., Leighton, J., and Farber, E.**, Growth in vitro of cells from hyperplastic nodules of liver induced by 2-fluorenylacetamide or aflatoxin B_1, *Science*, 167, 285, 1970.
333. **Kitagawa, T., Michalopoulos, G., and Pitot, H. C.**, Unscheduled DNA synthesis in cells from N-2-fluorenylacetamide-induced hyperplastic nodules of rat liver maintained in a primary culture system, *Cancer Res.*, 35, 3682, 1975.
334. **Laishes, B. A., Roberts, E., and Farber, E.**, In vitro measurement of carcinogen-resistant liver cells during hepatocarcinogenesis, *Int. J. Cancer*, 21, 186, 1978.
335. **Williams, G. M.**, The use of liver epithelial cultures for the study of chemical carcinogenesis, *Am. J. Pathol.*, 85, 739, 1976.
336. **Weinstein, I. B., Orenstein, J. M., Gebert, R., Kaighn, M. E., and Stadler, U. C.**, Growth and structural properties of epithelial cell cultures established from normal rat liver and chemically induced hepatomas, *Cancer Res.*, 35, 253, 1975.
337. **Iype, P. T. and Allen, T. D.**, Identification of transformed rat liver epithelial cells in culture, *Cancer Lett.*, 6, 27, 1979.
338. **Carr, B. I. and Laishes, B. A.**, Carcinogen-induced drug resistance in rat hepatocytes, *Cancer Res.*, 41, 1715, 1981.
339. **Shimada, T., Kreiser, D. M., and Williams, G. M.**, Effect of the tumor promoter phenobarbital on membrane-mediated properties of adult rat liver-derived epithelial cells in culture, *In Vitro*, 17, 224, 1981.
340. **Boynton, A. L. and Whitfield, J. F.**, Stimulation of DNA synthesis in calcium-deprived T51B liver cells by the tumor promoters phenobarbital, saccharin, and 12-O-tetradecanoylphorbol-13-acetate, *Cancer Res.*, 40, 4541, 1980.
341. **Swierenga, S. H. H., Whitfield, J. F., Boynton, A. L., MacManus, J. P., Rixon, R. H., Sikorska, M., Tsang, B. K., and Walker, P. R.**, Regulation of proliferation of normal and neoplastic rat liver cells by calcium and cyclic AMP, *Ann. N.Y. Acad. Sci.*, 349, 373, 1980.
342. **Iype, P. T. and Pontzer, C. H.**, Identification of transformed liver cell colonies using concanavalin A attached to agarose beads, *Cancer Res.*, 40, 4663, 1980.
343. **Wanson, J.-C., Bernaert, D., Penasse, W., Mosselmans, R., and Bannasch, P.**, Separation in distinct subpopulations by elutriation of liver cells following exposure of rats to N-nitrosomorpholine, *Cancer Res.*, 40, 459, 1980.
344. **Dolbeare, F., Vanderlaan, M., and Phares, W.**, Alkaline phosphatase and an acid arylamidase as marker enzymes for normal and transformed WI-38 cells, *J. Histochem. Cytochem.*, 28, 419, 1980.
345. **DeGerlache, J., Lans, M., Taper, H., and Roberfroid, M.**, Separate isolation of cells from nodules and surrounding parenchyma of the same precancerous rat liver: biochemical and cytochemical characterization, *Toxicology*, 18, 225, 1980.
346. **Iype, P. T., Turner, S., and Siddiqi, M. S.**, Markers for transformation in rat liver epithelial cells in culture, *Ann. N.Y. Acad. Sci.*, 349, 312, 1980.
347. **Montesano, R., Bannikov, G., Drevon, C., Kuroki, T., Saint Vincent, L., and Tomatis, L.**, Neoplastic transformation of rat liver epithelial cells in culture, *Ann. N.Y. Acad. Sci.*, 349, 323, 1980.
348. **Takano, T., Tatematsu, M., Hasegawa, R., Imaida, K., and Ito, N.**, Dose-response relationship for the promoting effect of phenobarbital on the induction of liver hyperplastic nodules in rats exposed to 2-fluorenylacetamide and carbon tetrachloride, *Gann*, 71, 580, 1980.
349. **Weisburger, J. H., Madison, R. M., Ward, J. M., Viguera, C., and Weisburger, E. K.**, Modification of diethylnitrosamine liver carcinogenesis with phenobarbital but not with immunosuppression, *J. Natl. Cancer Inst.*, 54, 1185, 1975.
350. **Nishizumi, M.**, Enhancement of diethylnitrosamine hepatocarcinogenesis in rats by exposure to polychlorinated biphenyls or phenobarbital, *Cancer Lett.*, 2, 11, 1976.
351. **Nishizumi, M.**, Effect of phenobarbital, dichlorodiphenyltrichloroethane, and polychlorinated biphenyls on diethylnitrosamine-induced hepatocarcinogenesis, *Gann*, 70, 835, 1979.
352. **Uchida, E. and Hirono, I.**, Effect of phenobarbital on induction of liver and lung tumors by dimethylnitrosamine in newborn mice, *Gann*, 70, 639, 1979.
353. **Ito, N., Nakanishi, K., Hagiwara, A., Shibata, M., and Fukushima, S.**, Induction of hyperplastic liver nodules by phenobarbital in rats initiated with N-butyl-N-(4-hydroxybutyl)nitrosamine, *Gann*, 71, 918, 1980.
354. **Kitagawa, T., Hirakawa, T., Ishikawa, T., Nemoto, N., and Takayama, S.**, Induction of hepatocellular carcinoma in rat liver by initial treatment with benzo(a)pyrene after partial hepatectomy and promotion by phenobarbital, *Toxicol. Lett.*, 6, 167, 1980.

355. **Pitot, H. C.,** Drugs as promoters of carcinogenesis, in *The Induction of Drug Metabolism,* Estabrook, R. W. and Lindenlaub, E., Eds., Schattauer-Verlag, Stuttgart, 1979, 471.
356. **Peraino, C., Fry, R. J. M., and Grube, D. D.,** Drug-induced enhancement of hepatic tumorigenesis, in *Carcinogenesis, Mechanisms of Promotion and Cocarcinogenesis,* Vol. 2, Slaga, T. J., Sivak, A., and Boutwell, R. K., Eds., Raven Press, New York, 1978, 421.
357. **Peraino, C., Fry, R. J. M., Staffeldt, E., and Christopher, J. P.,** Enhancing effects of phenobarbitone and butylated hydroxytoluene on 2-acetylaminofluorene-induced hepatic tumorigenesis in the rat, *Food Cosmet. Toxicol.,* 15, 93, 1977.
358. **Reddy, J. K. and Rao, M. S.,** Enhancement by Wy-14,643, a hepatic peroxisome proliferator, of diethylnitrosamine-initiated hepatic tumorigenesis in the rat, *Br. J. Cancer,* 38, 537, 1978.
359. **Ohde, G., Schuppler, J., Schulte-Hermann, R., and Keiger, H.,** Proliferation of rat liver cells in preneoplastic nodules after stimulation of liver growth by xenobiotic inducers, *Arch. Toxicol.,* Suppl. 2, 451, 1979.
360. **Peraino, C., Fry, R. J. M., and Staffeldt, E.,** Enhancement of spontaneous hepatic tumorigenesis in C3H mice by dietary phenobarbital, *J. Natl. Cancer Inst.,* 51, 1349, 1973.
361. **Thorpe, E. and Walker, A. I. T.,** The toxicology of dieldrin (HEOD). II. Comparative long-term oral toxicity studies in mice with dieldrin, DDT, phenobarbitone, β-BHC, and γ-BHC, *Food Cosmet. Toxicol.,* 11, 433, 1973.
362. **Ponomarkov, V., Tomatis, L., and Turusov, V.,** The effect of long-term administration of phenobarbitone in CF-1 mice, *Cancer Lett.,* 1, 165, 1976.
363. **Kitagawa, T., Watanabe, R., and Sugano, H.,** Induction of γ-glutamyl transpeptidase activity by dietary phenobarbital in "spontaneous" hepatic tumors in C3H mice, *Gann,* 71, 536, 1980.
364. **Rossi, L., Ravera, M., Repetti, G., and Santi, L.,** Long-term administration of DDT or phenobarbital-Na in Wistar rats, *Int. J. Cancer,* 19, 179, 1977.
365. **Innes, J. R. M., Ulland, B. M., Valerio, M. G., Petrucelli, L., Fishbein, L., Hart, E. R., Pallotta, A. J., Bates, R. R., Falk, H. L., Gart, J. J., Klein, M., Mitchell, I., and Peters, J.,** Bioassay of pesticides and industrial chemicals for tumorigenicity in mice: a preliminary note, *J. Natl. Cancer Inst.,* 42, 1101, 1969.
366. **Tomatis, L., Turusov, V., Day, N., and Charles, R. T.,** The effect of long-term exposure to DDT on CF-1 mice, *Int. J. Cancer,* 10, 489, 1972.
367. **Turusov, V. S., Day, N. E., Tomatis, L., Gati, E., and Charles, R. T.,** Tumors in CF-1 mice exposed for six consecutive generations to DDT, *J. Natl. Cancer Inst.,* 51, 983, 1973.
368. **Tomatis, L., Partensky, C., and Montesano, R.,** The predictive value of mouse liver tumour induction in carcinogenicity testing. A literature survey, *Int. J. Cancer,* 12, 1, 1973.
369. **Terracini, B., Testa, M. C., Cabral, J. R., and Day, N.,** The effects of long-term feeding of DDT to BALB/c mice, *Int. J. Cancer,* 11, 747, 1973.
370. **Fitzhugh, O. G. and Nelson, A. A.,** The chronic oral toxicity of DDT (2,2-bis(p-chlorophenyl-1,1,1-trichlorethane), *J. Pharmacol. Exp. Ther.,* 89, 18, 1947.
371. **Defchmann, W. B., Keplinger, M., Sala, F., and Glass, E.,** Synergism among oral carcinogens. IV. The simultaneous feeding of four tumorigens to rats, *Toxicol. Appl. Pharmacol.,* 11, 88, 1967.
372. **Sabine, J. R., Horton, B. J., and Wicks, M. B.,** Spontaneous tumors in C3H-A^{vy} and C3H-A^{vy}fB mice: high incidence in the United States and low incidence in Australia, *J. Natl. Cancer Inst.,* 50, 1237, 1973.
373. **Boutwell, R. K.,** Some biological aspects of skin carcinogenesis, *Prog. Exp. Tumor Res.,* 4, 207, 1964.
374. **Grube, D. D., Peraino, C., and Fry, R. J. M.,** The effect of dietary phenobarbital and the induction of skin tumors in hairless mice with 7,12-dimethylbenz(a)anthracene, *J. Invest. Dermatol.,* 64, 258, 1975.
375. **Pollard, M. and Luckert, P. M.,** Promotional effect of sodium barbiturate on intestinal tumors induced in rats by dimethylhydrazine, *J. Natl. Cancer Inst.,* 63, 1089, 1979.
376. **Clemmesen, J., Fuglsang-Frederiksen, V., and Plum, C. M.,** Are anticonvulsants oncogenic?, *Lancet,* 1(7860) 705, 1974.
377. **Schneiderman, M. A.,** Phenobarbitone and liver tumours, *Lancet,* 2(7888), 1085, 1974.
378. **Clemmesen, J. and Hjalgrim-Jensen, S.,** Is phenobarbital carcinogenic. A follow-up of 8087 epileptics, *Ecotoxicol. Environ. Safety,* 1, 457, 1978.
379. **Gold, E., Gordis, L., Tonascia, J., and Szklo, M.,** Increased risk of brain tumors in children exposed to barbiturates, *J. Natl. Cancer Inst.,* 61, 1031, 1978.
380. **Annegers, J. F., Kurland, L. T., and Hauser, W. A.,** Brain tumors in children exposed to barbiturates, *J. Natl. Cancer Inst.,* 63, 3, 1979.
381. **Gold, E. B., Gordis, L., Tonascia, J. A., and Szklo, M.,** Brain tumors in children exposed to barbiturates, *J. Natl. Cancer Inst.,* 63, 3, 1979.
382. **Potter, V. R.,** Initiation and promotion in cancer formation: the importance of studies on intercellular communication, *Yale J. Biol. Med.,* 53, 367, 1980.

383. **Schulte-Hermann, R., Ohde, G., Schuppler, J., and Timmermann-Trosiener, I.,** Enhanced proliferation of putative preneoplastic cells in rat liver following treatment with the tumor promoters phenobarbital, hexachlorocyclohexane, steroid compounds, and nafenopin, *Cancer Res.*, 41, 2556, 1981.
384. **Trosko, J. E., Yotti, L. P., Warren, S. T., Tsushimoto, G., and Chang, C.,** Inhibition of cell-cell communication by tumor promoters, in *Carcinogenesis — A Comprehensive Survey*, Vol. 7, Hecker, E., Fusenig, N. E., Kunz, W., Marks, F., and Thielmann, M. W., Eds., Raven Press, New York, 1982, 565.
385. **Slaga, T. J., Fischer, S. M., Weeks, C. E., and Klein-Szanto, A. J. P.,** Multistage chemical carcinogenesis in mouse skin, in *Biochemistry of Normal and Abnormal Epidermal Differentiation*, Bernstein, I. A. and Seizi, M., Eds., University of Tokyo Press, 1980, 193.
386. **Mondal, S., Brankow, D. W., and Heidelberger, C.,** Two-stage chemical oncogenesis in cultures of C3H/10T1/2 cells, *Cancer Res.*, 36, 2254, 1976.
387. **Peterson, A. R., Mondal, S., Brankow, D. W., Thon, W., and Heidelberger, C.,** Effects of promoters on DNA synthesis in C3H/10T1/2 mouse fibroblasts, *Cancer Res.*, 37, 3223, 1977.
388. **Kennedy, A. R. and Little, J. B.,** Investigation of the mechanism for enhancement of radiation transformation in vitro by 12-O-tetradecanoylphorbol-13-acetate, *Carcinogenesis*, 1, 1039, 1980.
389. **Colburn, N. H.,** Tumor promoter produces anchorage independence in mouse epidermal cells by an induction mechanism, *Carcinogenesis*, 1, 951, 1980.
390. **Scherer, E. and Emmelot, P.,** Kinetics of induction and growth of precancerous liver-cell foci, and liver tumour formation by diethylnitrosamine in the rat, *Eur. J. Cancer*, 11, 689, 1975.
391. **Peraino, C., Richards, W. L., and Stevens, F. J.,** unpublished data.

Chapter 2

PROMOTION OF HEPATIC NEOPLASIA BY GONADAL STEROIDS

James D. Yager, Jr.

TABLE OF CONTENTS

I. INTRODUCTION

A. Synthetic Steroids and Hepatic Neoplasia in Humans

In a recent review, Lipsett[1] discussed the role of hormones, with emphasis on estrogens and androgens, in the causes of human cancer. Estrogens or their synthetic analogues such as diethylstilbestrol, ethinylestradiol, and others have been associated with cancer in various human tissues whose growth is under hormonal control. Specific examples are the association of postmenopausal estrogen therapy with endometrial cancer and the occurrence of clear cell adenocarcinoma of the vagina in young women exposed to diethylstibestrol in utero.

The earliest reports of an association between treatment with gonadal steroids and hepatic neoplasia came from observations made on patients being treated for Fanconi's anemia by androgenic hormones.[2,3] Other reports also appeared confirming the relationship between androgen treatment and hepatic neoplasia.[4] The 1972 paper by Horvath et al.[5] described the first case of hepatoma associated with the use of oral contraceptive steroids. This was followed in 1973 by the paper of Baum et al.[6] describing the occurrence of liver adenomas in seven patients with a common history of oral contraceptive use. This latter paper focused attention on the possible association between ingestion of synthetic steroids and hepatic neoplasia. Subsequently, numerous reports have indicated that liver adenomas and, less frequently, hepatocellular carcinomas may appear in women using oral contraceptives.[1,4,7-16] To date, the results of two case-control studies[7,13] and a national survey[11] have been published. The case-control study of Rooks et al.[13] concerned the association of hepatocellular adenoma with oral contraceptive use in 79 female patients and in 220 age- and neighborhood-matched controls. Among other things, these investigators concluded that: (1) risk of hepatocellular adenoma increases with increased duration of oral contraceptive use and (2) the risk is positively correlated with the hormonal potency of the oral contraceptive preparation used. In the U.S., the risk of developing hepatic neoplasms is low, the annual incidence of hepatocellular neoplasms for non- or short-term-users of oral contraceptives being about 1.0 and 1.3/million in women 16 to 30 and 31 to 44 years of age, respectively.[13] Rooks et al.[13] estimate the risk of long-term users of low potency oral contraceptives to increase to an incidence of 3.4/100,000. While this represents a substantial increase in risk for developing hepatocellular neoplasia, the actual risk is still relatively small.[9]

Two synthetic estrogens, ethinylestradiol and mestranol, and a number of synthetic progestins are used in oral contraceptives in the U.S.[17] While the study of Edmonson et al.[7] indicated that the synthetic estrogen mestranol was more frequently used by patients who developed hepatocellular adenoma, Rooks et al.[13] were unable to determine which estrogenic component posed the greater risk. Nor were they able to distinguish whether the increased risk was associated with the estrogenic or progestin component of the oral contraceptives. Additional studies are needed to define more clearly the role of these hormone analogues in hepatic neoplasia. In addition, it should be noted that in some instances, the hepatic adenomas regress upon cessation of steroid treatment.[4,18] Thus, at least up to a point, the adenomas are dependent upon the continuous presence of the hormones.

B. Carcinogenicity of Synthetic Steroids in Experimental Animals

Experimental studies on the role of sex hormones in hepatocarcinogenesis were stimulated by the early observations of sex differences in tumor incidence in strains of rats fed certain hepatocarcinogens.[19] Such studies demonstrated the potential cocarcinogenic effects of hormones in liver. A considerable amount of work on the carcinogenicity of oral contraceptive steroids was carried out during the evaluation of the safety of these drugs.[20,21] In general, these studies indicated that prolonged feeding of high doses of various natural and synthetic sex steroids (estrogens and progestins) caused generally small but significant increases in benign and malignant tumors in different organs of rats and mice. With regard to liver neoplasms, synthetic estrogens and progestins caused small but significant increases in benign hepatocellular adenomas in rats and mice of both sexes.[20-24] Schardein et al.[22] fed male and female Sprague-Dawley rats a diet containing a mixture of 98% norethinodrone acetate and 2% ethinylestradiol at levels approximately 10 and 100 times the human dose. Livers were analyzed for the presence of regenerative nodules, hepatocellular adenomas, and hepatomas. Regenerative nodules were distinguished in standard hematoxylin- and eosin-stained histological sections as hyperplastic areas forming distinct nodules which caused compression of surrounding parenchyma. Hepatocytes within different nodules ranged in their cytological appearance from well-organized, normal looking to disordered, hypertrophied, vacuolated cells. No hepatocellular carcinomas were detected in the 104-week experimental period. Hyperplastic nodules were detected in 13% (13/100) and 10% (10/100) of the animals in the low and high dose groups, respectively; controls had an incidence of 2% (4/200). Hepatocellular adenomas were not detected in controls (0/200) and were present in 3% (3/100) and 4% (4/100) of the animals fed the low and high doses of these synthetic contraceptive steroids, respectively.

However, it should be pointed out that in this[22] and other studies of Schardein[23,24] the overall total tumor incidence in all organs together was not increased in the treated animals. Schuppler and Gunzel[21] recently reviewed data on liver tumors in rats and mice fed steroid hormones in long-term carcinogenicity studies where the hormones were fed at levels up to 200 to 400 and even, in some cases, 6250 times the human contraceptive dose. Taking into account the spontaneous rate of liver tumors, sex, and strain differences, they found various sex steroids, including norethynodrel, norethisterone, and a combination of these two plus mestranol caused an increase in hepatocellular adenomas in rats and/or mice. They came to the conclusion that the evidence suggesting that steroidal hormones are able to initiate hepatocarcinogenesis is weak. They went on to speculate that a promoting effect of these hormones was a possibility based on their ability to stimulate liver growth.[21]

Reinterpreting their statements, we could propose that sex steroids are not complete carcinogens for liver. Rather, they may be cocarcinogenic and/or promoters of hepatocarcinogenesis initiated by other environmental, chemical, or physical agents (see below). Recently, Higashi et al.[25] reported the results of a study involving daily intubation of 0.075 mg ethinylestradiol and 6 mg of norethindrone (doses this author estimates to be 1000 or more times the human contraceptive dose) to female Wistar rats for 1 year. Hyperplastic nodules appeared in 18/18 rats and a hepatocellular carcinoma in only 1 of 18. Control animals did not develop any such lesions. This further emphasizes the weak complete hepatocarcinogenicity of such synthetic sex steroid hormones.

II. MECHANISMS OF CARCINOGENESIS IN LIVER

A. Two-Stage Carcinogenesis in Liver

It is now widely recognized that carcinogenesis is a multistage process. At least two stages, initiation and promotion, can be distinguished experimentally. Initiation can be caused by exposure to a subcarcinogenic dose of an initiating agent. Initiation is considered to be a persistent, if not irreversible, event possibly caused by mutation in somatic cells. For the most part, initiators can be shown to be mutagens in various test systems. Promotion, on the other hand, represents a process that is, at least to a point, reversible. It involves chronic treatment with a chemical agent that ultimately enhances tumor incidence and number. Promoters are not mutagenic and are thought to act through epigenetic mechanisms.

The processes of initiation and promotion have been experimentally demonstrated in various tissues and organs including skin,[26] pancreas,[27] colon,[28] mammary gland,[29] and liver.[30] Peraino et al.[31] presented the first definitive evidence that hepatocarcinogenesis consists of at least two separable stages. Initiation was caused by feeding rats a diet containing a low level (0.02%) 2-acetylaminofluorene (AAF) for 18 days. Next the AAF-initiated animals were fed a diet containing 0.05% phenobarbital for a prolonged period. Significant increases in both tumor incidence and number were seen in livers of animals treated with both agents compared to animals fed AAF or phenobarbital alone. More recent studies have resulted in the development of improved protocols for detection of and distinction between initiating and promoting agents for liver.[30] Initiation can be accomplished by single dose treatment with a carcinogen administered 24 hr after surgical partial hepatectomy, a time when hepatocyte DNA synthesis is maximal and has an apparent cocarcinogenic effect.[32] Subsequent feeding of liver tumor promoters results in enhanced tumor formation.[30]

Previous studies have clearly documented the fact that distinct populations of hepatocytes representing focal and nodular hyperplastic lesions develop before hepatocellular carcinomas.[30,33] More recently, histochemical techniques have been employed to reveal the presence of enzyme-altered foci of hepatocytes. Generally, the histochemical procedures used take advantage of the fact that many populations of altered hepatocytes representing putative preneoplastic foci express some fetal-like phenotypic properties such as ATPase deficiency, glucose-6-phosphatase deficiency, and the presence of gamma glutamyl transpeptidase (GGT).[30,33] Of the markers, the appearance of GGT positive foci is the most widely used to detect and quantitate putative preneoplastic foci in livers of animals being treated with actual or suspected initiators, promoters, or complete hepatocarcinogens.

B. Gonadal Steroids: Promoters, Initiators, or Complete Hepatocarcinogens?

Results from studies on the effects of gonadal steroids on various biological systems suggest that they might behave as promoters of hepatocarcinogenesis. Complete carcinogens must, of course, be able to initiate and promote in their target tissues. As indicated above, the process of initiation involves irreversible effects on cells and is currently thought to involve mutation. Most, if not all, initiators and complete carcinogens are mutagenic. Several studies have been carried out to determine the mutagenicity of various natural and synthetic sex steroid hormones. Lang and Redmann[34] recently reported the results of mutagenicity studies using the Ames Salmonella/microsome mutagenicity test. Certain sex steroids, natural and synthetic, estrogens and progestins, were tested with several Salmonella strains using microsomes from uninduced mouse liver and from rat liver induced by Aroclor® 1254. Neither ethinylestradiol, norethynodrel, nor any other steroid tested, demonstrated mutagenicity in this assay. Mestranol (3-*O*-methylethinylestradiol) was not tested, but presumably would also have been negative.

A very recent report by Drevon et al.[35] described the results of mutagenicity studies on four estrogens (diethylstilbesterol, ethinylestradiol, estradiol-17β, and estrone) using an hepatocyte-mediated mutagenicity assay in V-79 cells. Except for ethinylestradiol, the toxicity of the estrogens for the V-79 cells was reduced by the presence of isolated hepatocytes. However, none of the estrogens enhanced the mutation frequency in the V-79 cells as determined by the appearance of resistance to 8-azaguanine or ouabain. This was true whether or not the hepatocytes were obtained from Aroclor®-treated rats.

A study was also carried out to determine whether mestranol and norethindrone, separately and in combination, had any effects on bone marrow chromosomes in rats.[36] In this study, norethindrone was fed to rats at doses of 5 and 7 mg/100 g body weight and mestranol at 2, 3, 5, and 10 mg/100 g body weight, doses far in excess of the effective human contraceptive dose. The animals were sacrificed at 8, 16, 24, and 48 hr after treatment and their bone marrow cells were fixed for study of chromosome aberrations. No chromosomal aberrations of any kind were found, and there was no evidence of increased ploidy or changes in chromosome number. While these results suggest that these two steroids do not exert effects on chromosomes, the study lacked a positive control rendering the negative results more difficult to interpret.

An additional in vivo study has been performed to determine whether ethinylestradiol or estrone bind covalently to rat liver DNA.[37] The radioactive estrogens were given to rats and binding to DNA determined 8 hr later. Binding to DNA was detected, but at a level about 10,000 times lower than that for a typical hepatocarcinogen such as aflatoxin B_1 or dimethylnitrosamine.

The results of the mutagenicity and chromosome studies discussed above suggested that the gonadal steroids would not be efficient initiators or complete carcinogens and that they would probably act as either cocarcinogens and/or promoters. Two other observations suggest that their potency as promoters should be evaluated. First, as described above, their weak ability to induce hepatocellular adenomas when fed in very high dose together with their known liver growth stimulating potential suggested that they might be acting as promoters.[21] In addition, several cases have been reported in which hepatocellular adenomas regressed after women stopped ingesting the oral contraceptive preparations they were using at the time of diagnosis.[4,18] This suggests that, as with promoters in general, their neoplastic effects are, at least up to a point, reversible. These observations prompted studies on the promoting potential of oral contraceptive steroids.

1. Gonadal Steroids as Promoters

To date, only three papers have appeared reporting the results of studies clearly indicating that synthetic gonadal steroids can promote hepatic neoplasia. Taper[38] carried out a study designed to determine the effect of two synthetic estrogens, estradiol-17-phenylpropionate and estradiol benzoate, on hepatocarcinogenesis initiated by *N*-nitrosomorpholine (NNM). In this study, ovariectomized female Wistar rats were divided into four treatment groups: (1) NNM alone, (2) NNM accompanied by a single dose of estrogen at the time of the first NNM treatment; (3) NNM followed by estrogen treatment once every 3 weeks; and (4) no NNM but treatment with estrogen as in (3). The initiating agent, NNM, was given at 2.6 mg/100 g body weight in aqueous solution by intragastric intubation five times weekly for 3 weeks. The estrogens were given in combination, the source being the long-term drug Dimenforman Prolongatum. This preparation contains 10 mg estradiol-17-phenylpropionate and 2.5 mg estradiol benzoate in 1 mℓ. Animals receiving chronic estrogen treatment were injected i.m. at 3-week intervals at a total dose per injection of 645 μg/100 g of body weight. Animals were killed 300 days after beginning carcinogen treatment and their livers examined grossly for tumors by slicing into 5 mm slices. Hematoxylin- and eosin-stained histological sections were prepared and examined in detail.

Table 1 shows the results of the macroscopic observations. NNM followed by chronic estrogen treatment (Group 3) caused a 3.5-fold increase in the total number of macroscopic hepatic tumors and a 3.5-fold increase in the number of tumors per rat compared to the controls receiving only NNM. Estrogen treatment alone (Group 4) had no tumorigenic effect. Simultaneous treatment with NNM and a single estrogen injection (Group 2) appeared to cause a small reduction in the total number of tumors. Table 2 shows the results of the microscopic evaluations of the livers of these rats. In this evaluation, foci were small lesions that did not show disruption of liver architecture. Nodules, on the other hand, were larger lesions involving several lobules and showing disruption of normal architecture. The number of foci detected in the livers of NNM-treated rats was too great to count, so in Table 2 the numbers for this class of lesions reflect the number of animals in which foci were found. Nodules and carcinomas were able to be counted, and these numbers in Table 2 reflect the total number of such lesions in rats of each group.

The data in Table 2 show that differences occurred in the type of foci found in livers from rats in different treatment groups. However, attention should be focused on the incidence of basophilic foci which, according to the report of Squire and Levitt,[39] seem to have the greatest significance with regard to the development of neoplasms. Of 31 animals in Group

Table 1
MACROSCOPIC OBSERVATION OF LIVERS OF TREATED RATS

			Number of liver tumors					
Group[a]	Number of rats	Liver weight per 100 g body weight (mean ± SD)	<1 mm	1—5 mm	5—10 mm	>10 mm	All sizes	Number of tumors per rat
1	31	3.09 ± 1.55	32	0	0	4	36	1.1
2	21	2.64 ± 0.29	7	9	1	2	19	0.9
3	31	4.32 ± 1.80	61	39	10	9	119	3.8
4	27	3.41 ± 0.83	0	0	0	0	0	0.0

[a] Group 1: NNM only; Group 2: NNM plus a single estrogen injection at the time of the first NNM treatment; Group 3: NNM followed by estrogen treatment once every 3 weeks; Group 4: chronic estrogen treatment alone as in Group 3.

Adapted from Taper, H. S., *Cancer*, 42, 462, 1978. With permission.

Table 2
MICROSCOPIC EVALUATION OF RESULTS

	Experimental Group			
	I	II	III	IV
Number of rats	31	21	31	27
Total number of rats with foci nodules and liver tumors	25/31	19/21	29/31	0/27
Liver foci[a]				
Clear cell	23	15	10	0
Eosinophilic	14	14	18	0
Mixed	3	1	5	0
Basophilic	2	0	19	0
Liver nodules				
Clear cell	4	4	0	0
Eosinophilic	5	4	9	0
Mixed	2	1	8	0
Basophilic	0	0	6	0
Total	11	9	23	0
Heptatocellular carcinomas (degree of differentiation)				
High	0	1	5	0
Moderate	1	0	3	0
Poor	0	0	1	0
Glandulo-papillary	2	1	0	0
Total	3	2	9	0
Other malignant liver tumors	1	0	1	0
Tumors in other organs[b]				
Benign	2	1	11	0
Malignant	0	0	4	0

[a] For liver foci the numbers indicate the amounts of rats bearing each particular type of these lesions. Other numbers indicate the exact amount of liver nodules and other tumors microscopically detected in each experimental group.

Table 2 (continued)
MICROSCOPIC EVALUATION OF RESULTS

[b] Benign tumors. Group I: clear cell and one basophilic kidney adenoma; Group II: one basophilic kidney adenoma; Group III: two eosinophilic, eight basophilic kidney adenomas, one mammary fibroadenoma. Malignant tumors. Group III: two myeloblastic leukemias, one mammary adenocarcinoma, one malignant Wilms' tumor.

From Taper, H. S., *Cancer*, 42, 462, 1978. With permission.

3 (NNM followed by chronic estrogen treatment), 19 had basophilic foci compared to 2 of 31 in the Group 1 controls (NNM alone). The number of liver nodules and the total number of hepatocellular carcinomas were also substantially increased, twofold and threefold, respectively, in the animals initiated by NNM and subsequently treated with estrogens once every 3 weeks. Chronic estrogen administration following NNM treatment also increased the incidence of benign and malignant tumors in other organs (Table 2).

The estrogen dose used in these studies, while given as an injection of 645 μg/100 g of body weight once every 3 weeks, averaged to be 30 μg/100 g of body weight per day.[38] While not extraordinarily high, this average daily estrogen dose is higher than the level of ethinylestradiol alone (0.8 μg/100 g/day) fed in the carcinogenicity study of Schardein[23] and higher than the level of mestranol alone (2.5 μg/100 g/day) fed in the promotion study of Yager and Yager.[40] However, it is comparable to the dose used when Schardein et al.[22] fed animals a combination of 98% nonethindrone acetate:2% ethinylestradiol (37 μg/100 g/day) in another carcinogenicity study. The results obtained by Taper[38] employing an initiation/promotion protocol strongly suggest that chronic treatment of NNM initiated animals with estradiol-17-phenylpropionate plus estradiol benzoate enhances the incidence of hepatic neoplasia. Thus, estrogen treatment according to this protocol promotes carcinogen-initiated hepatocarcinogenesis.

The second study on promotion of hepatic neoplasia by synthetic gonadal steroids was carried out in our laboratory.[40] Table 3 shows the protocol used to determine whether mestranol (M), norethynodrel (N), or M + N could promote the appearance of diethylnitrosamine (DEN)-initiated hepatic neoplasia. Female Sprague-Dawley rats, adapted to a basal control diet,[40] were subjected to a surgical partial hepatectomy at 7 weeks of age, 158 ± 12 g of body weight. The animals were intubated with DEN (5 mg/kg of body weight) 24 hr later. After another 24 hr, the animals were transferred to diets containing the various test compounds at the doses indicated in Table 3. There were 15 animals per group and 5 per group were killed after 16 weeks, 10 per group after 40 weeks. The dose levels of M and N were approximately 10 to 15 times the human dose as calculated for a 50 kg woman ingesting the oral contraceptive, Enovid E®.[17,40] The phenobarbital (PB) groups were included as positive controls since the previous work of Peraino et al.[31] indicated that it is a promoter of hepatocarcinogenesis.

Figure 1 shows the body weights of the animals in the different treatment groups over the course of the experiment. It is apparent that the animals ingesting a diet containing the synthetic steroids, particularly mestranol, had reduced body weights throughout the treatment period. Food consumption data[64] indicated that the steroid-fed animals did not ingest less diet. Thus, the steroid-treated animals appear to have a decreased capacity for food utilization, an effect also seen by Schardein.[23] Table 4 shows the liver weights per 100 g of body weight for animals in the different treatment groups. No significant differences were detected at 4 months. At 9 months, liver weights per 100 g of body weight in the groups receiving phenobarbital, M, N, and M + N were significantly greater than control.

Table 3
PROMOTION PROTOCOL

1. Rats — female Sprague-Dawley
2. Protocol
3. Treatment Groups[a]/dosing (mg/kg/day)
   - DEN → mestranol (M), 0.02—0.03
   - DEN → norethynodrel (N), 0.5—0.75
   - DEN → phenobarbital (P), 19.4—27.4 (0.05% in diet)
   - DEN → M + N
   - DEN → control (basal diet)
   - H_2O → M + N
   - H_2O → P

[a] There were 15 rats per group. Five per group were killed after 16 weeks and 10 after 40 weeks.

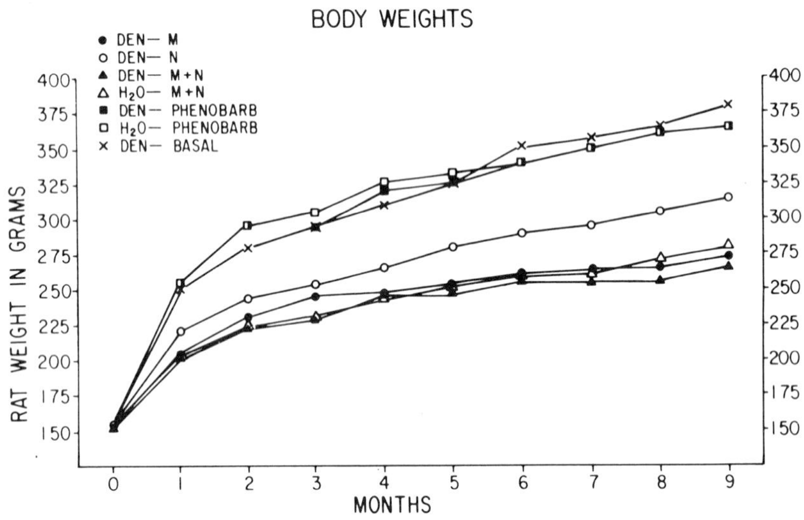

FIGURE 1. Monthly body weight curves for the seven groups of animals over the course of the experiment. (From Yager, J. D., Jr. and Yager, R., *Cancer Res.*, 40, 3680, 1980. With permission.)

Table 4
LIVER WEIGHT PER 100 g OF BODY WEIGHT OF ANIMALS FED DIET CONTAINING ORAL CONTRACEPTIVE STEROIDS

	Liver weight per 100 g body weight	
Treatment	**4 Month kill**	**9 Month kill**
DEN → M	3.45 ± 0.35[a]	3.27 ± 0.30[b,c]
DEN → N	3.08 ± 0.19	3.11 ± 0.38[b,c]
DEN → M + N	3.06 ± 0.22	3.38 ± 0.42[b]
H_2O → M + N	3.25 ± 0.21	3.68 ± 0.25[b]
DEN → PB	3.19 ± 0.18	3.23 ± 0.45[b,d]

Table 4 (continued)
LIVER WEIGHT PER 100 g OF BODY WEIGHT OF ANIMALS FED DIET CONTAINING ORAL CONTRACEPTIVE STEROIDS

	Liver weight per 100 g body weight	
Treatment	4 Month kill	9 Month kill
$H_2O \rightarrow$ PB	3.54 ± 0.81	3.28 ± 0.36[b,c]
DEN → basal	2.88 ± 0.42	2.59 ± 0.14[c]

[a] Mean ± SD, 5 rats per group at 4 months; 10 rats per group at 9 months.
[b] Significantly greater than DEN → basal, $p < 0.001$.
[c] Significantly less than $H_2O \rightarrow M + N$, $p < 0.01$.
[d] Significantly less than $H_2O \rightarrow M + N$, $p < 0.05$.

From Yager, J. D., Jr. and Yager, R., *Cancer Res.*, 40, 3680, 1980. With permission.

The number of GGT foci per square centimeter of liver are shown in Figure 2[40] and the significance of the differences in GGT foci per square centimeter among selected groups are indicated in Table 5. Focusing on the 9-month data, the results clearly show that M and M + N significantly enhance the appearance of GGT foci in DEN initiated animals. The number of foci in the groups DEN → M, DEN → M + N, and DEN → PB were comparable. This is especially interesting since the level of mestranol in the diet was approximately 1/1000 that of PB (Table 3). Thus, on a weight basis, the steroids may be considerably more potent promoters than PB. Another interesting observation can be made from the results shown in Figure 2. At 9 months, the number of foci in the $H_2O \rightarrow M + N$ group was significantly greater than DEN → Basal and $H_2O \rightarrow$ PB groups. Table 6 shows the incidence and number of hepatocellular lesions at 9 months as detected in histological sections stained with hematoxylin and eosin. As in the study of Taper,[38] the types of foci differ among the treatment groups. However, the incidence of basophilic foci is considerably elevated in the animals in groups DEN → M and DEN → M + N. The low incidence of more advanced lesions at this time most likely reflects the low initiating dose of DEN together with the fact that the carcinogen was given by intubation.

The results obtained with norethynodrel are less clear than with mestranol or M + N together. The number of GGT foci at 9 months was not significantly greater than in the $H_2O \rightarrow M + N$ control group, but was significantly less than the DEN → M group. In addition, no increase in basophilic foci was seen. Additional studies are necessary to define the promoting potential of norethynodrel. However, if it is a promoter, it has less potency than mestranol and it is likely that the results seen in animals ingesting M + N are due to M.

Assuming that the GGT foci and basophilic foci represent putative preneoplastic lesions and are correlated with the number of hepatocellular carcinomas that would ultimately arise, the results shown above suggest that mestranol is a promoter of hepatocarcinogenesis. When compared to phenobarbital on the basis of effective doses, mestranol appears to be quite potent. Furthermore, the number of foci was slightly but significantly increased in animals only treated with M + N alone. This suggests that M, N, or the combination either may have weak complete carcinogenic activity or, more likely, may be a reflection of mestranol's potent promoting potential acting on a spontaneous incidence of initiation.

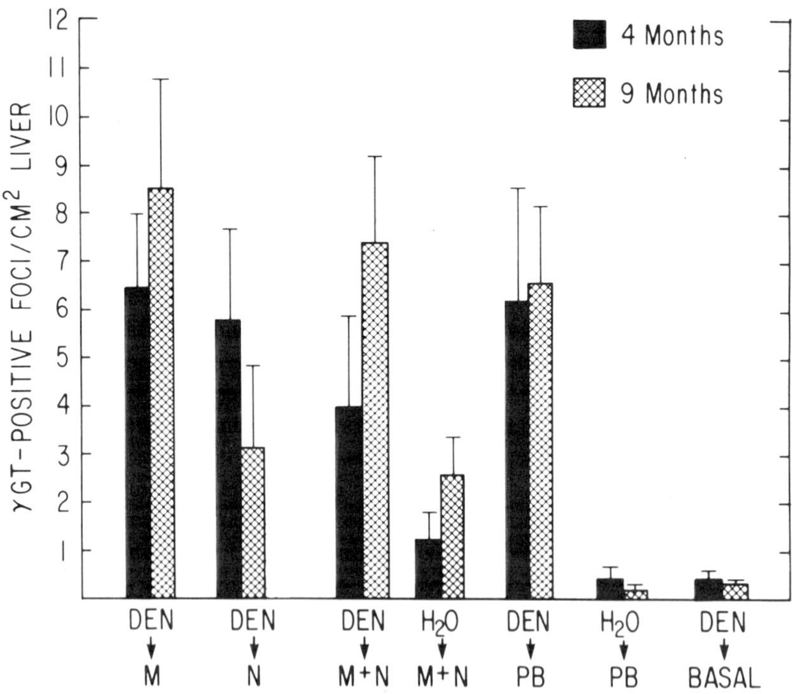

FIGURE 2. GGT foci per square centimeter in livers of animals from the seven treatment groups. Columns, mean; bars, SE. (From Yager, J. D., Jr. and Yager, R., *Cancer Res.*, 40, 3680, 1980. With permission.)

Table 5
SIGNIFICANCE OF DIFFERENCES IN GGT FOCI PER SQUARE CENTIMETER LIVER AMONG SELECTED EXPERIMENTAL GROUPS

	p for selected group comparisons[a]			
	H_2O ——→ M + N		DEN ——→ basal	
Group	(4 months)	(9 months)	(4 months)	(9 months)
DEN → M	<0.05	<0.01	<0.01	<0.001
DEN → N	NS[b]	NS	<0.05	NS
DEN → M + N	NS	<0.05	NS	<0.001
DEN → PB	<0.05	NS	<0.01	<0.001
H_2O → M + N			NS	<0.001

Note: The rank sum test was used to determine these levels of significance. However, realizing the problems associated with making multiple individual comparisons between groups, we also conducted a Newman-Keuls analysis of variance. This test confirmed the significance of the differences indicated with at least $p < 0.05$.

[a] See Figure 2 for the actual numbers of GGT foci per square centimeter liver in all experimental groups.

[b] NS, not significant; $p > 0.05$.

From Yager, J. D., Jr. and Yager, R., *Cancer Res.*, 40, 3680, 1980. With permission.

Table 6
INCIDENCE AND NUMBER OF HEPATOCELLULAR LESIONS DETECTED BY HISTOPATHOLOGICAL EVALUATION

	Foci					
Groups	Clear cell	Eosinophilic (ground glass)	Basophilic	Mixed	Neoplastic nodules	Hepatocellular carcinomas
DEN → M	10[a] (2.4)[b]	2 (2.5)	7 (2.0)	9 (5.4)	0	0
DEN → N	5 (1.6)	2 (3.0)	1 (1.0)	6 (2.3)	0	1 (1.0)
DEN → M + N	9 (2.3)	2 (1.5)	6 (1.8)	8 (5.0)	3 (1.0)	0
DEN → PB	0	4 (1.8)	2 (1.0)	4 (2.3)	0	0
H_2O → M + N	3 (2.3)	2 (1.0)	2 (1.5)	10 (3.9)	0	0
H_2O → PB	0	1 (1.0)	0	2 (1.0)	0	0
DEN → basal	0	0	1 (1.0)	4 (2.0)	0	0

Note: All sections were taken from one lobe of the liver and stained with H & E. Each group had ten animals.

[a] Numbers of animals in group with at least one lesion.
[b] Numbers in parentheses, lesions per lesion-bearing rat.

From Yager, J. D., Jr. and Yager, R., *Cancer Res.*, 40, 3680, 1980. With permission.

An additional observation that may ultimately bear on mechanisms should be described. In analyzing the frozen sections stained for GGT activity, it was evident that some treatments had caused the appearance of diffuse GGT-positive staining in a pattern that radiated from the portal areas. No distinct cellular alterations were observed in hematoxylin- and eosin-stained sections from the same rat. Upon decoding the slides after counting the foci, it was determined that the diffuse GGT staining was detected only in animals fed a diet containing mestranol. No diffuse staining was seen in rats fed a diet containing norethynodrel alone, phenobarbital, or control diet. Determination of GGT in liver homogenates confirmed this finding. GGT activity was significantly elevated in livers of animals ingesting mestranol.[40] A general increase in liver GGT activity has previously been found to be associated with intrahepatic cholestasis in the absence of ductal cell proliferation.[41] Thus, mestranol may produce a mild cholestatic response which may be a significant component of its mechanism(s) of promotion (see below).

The most recent report of promotion of hepatocarcinogenesis by a synthetic estrogen was by Cameron et al.[42] They found that feeding ethinylestradiol at 10 ppm to male Fischer 344 rats treated 2 weeks previously with DEN, promoted the appearance of GGT positive foci and hyperplastic nodules. From the results of their study, Cameron et al.[42] concluded that ethinylestradiol is a moderately strong promoter of preneoplastic liver lesions.

2. *Gonadal Steroids as Initiators*

As discussed above, the process of initiation is thought to involve mutation in somatic cells and most initiating agents can be shown to be mutagenic in one or more mutagenicity assays. However, it is not at all clear whether initiation must involve mutation. In fact it is likely that, at least in some instances, cell transformation can be caused by nonmutational, epigenetic mechanisms. Teratomas most likely represent neoplasms that have arisen through such a mechanism. The synthetic steroids have not been demonstrated to be mutagenic. However, in experimental systems, chronic treatment with such steroids causes a low but significant increase in incidence of various types of neoplasms including GGT foci (Figure 2), hepatocellular adenomas,[22] and carcinomas.[25] Thus, the question arises as to whether these agents have weak initiating potential, and that this, together with their ability to promote, makes them complete carcinogens or whether the tumors that arise are due to their promoting potential working on a low level of spontaneous initiation.

a. Initiation Potential of Mestranol

We devised an experimental protocol, similar to that shown in Table 3, to determine whether mestranol had detectable initiating potential.[43] Rats were intubated with mestranol 24 hr following partial hepatectomy. After 24 hr had passed, the animals were transferred to a diet containing 0.05% phenobarbital to promote any hepatocytes that might have been initiated by the mestranol treatment. The animals were killed 4 months later and the number of GGT foci determined. The results indicated that the mestranol treatment did not cause a significant increase in the number of such foci.[43] Thus, mestranol does not exhibit significant initiating potential as detectable by this type of protocol.

b. Hepatogenotoxicity of Gonadal Steroids

The detection of DNA repair synthesis in rat hepatocytes in primary culture appears to be a useful test for detection of the genotoxic potential of various suspect chemical agents.[44-46] We have been unable to detect the induction of repair synthesis by any natural or synthetic gonadal steroids in cultured rat hepatocytes obtained from either male or female rats.[43] Thus, these compounds, including mestranol and ethinylestradiol, do not exhibit genotoxic properties in hepatocytes as detectable using this in vitro assay.

The negative results obtained in the several different types of tests designed to detect mutagenic or genotoxic effects of synthetic gonadal steroids suggest that they lack the ability to initiate the process of carcinogenesis through mechanisms involving somatic cell mutations. However, in a recent pilot study, we found that mestranol caused a small (1.5-fold) but significant increase in sister chromatid exchange frequency in CHO cells.[65] This effect was dependent on the presence of liver microsomes. Additional studies are under way to critically evaluate this potentially interesting preliminary observation.

III. POSSIBLE MECHANISMS OF PROMOTION BY GONADAL STEROIDS

Much is known about the numerous biochemical and cellular effects of promoters, particularly phobol esters.[47] However, it is not clear which of their known effects are critical to their promoting properties.

In liver, phenobarbital, a known promoter of hepatocarcinogenesis, has numerous biochemical and cellular effects on hepatocytes. These effects include induction of hyperplasia and hypertrophy, both of which involve major changes in gene expression.[30,31,48] The mammalian liver has been demonstrated to contain estrogen receptors that most likely mediate the numerous changes in liver function caused by estrogens.[49] Eisenfeld et al.[49] postulate that perhaps many of the side effects of oral contraceptive steroids might be mediated via the normal estrogen receptor mechanism. Pitot and Sirica[30] have urged that the relationship between the effects of promoting agents and their interaction with specific receptors be investigated more extensively, not only in liver but in other organ systems as well. Thus, it is important to determine whether promotion by the synthetic gonadal steroids[38,40,42] is due to the hormonal effects of the estrogenic components as mediated through estrogen receptors. Use of estrogens of varying potencies and antiestrogenic compounds may prove to be of some value. In this regard, it is interesting that norethynodrel, a progestin with weak estrogenic activity, did not appear to be as potent a promoter as mestranol.[40]

Synthetic estrogens have been reported to stimulate cell proliferation in rat liver.[31,50] This response could be a result of anabolic biochemical and cellular effects of these agents on hepatocytes. On the other hand, the stimulation of hepatocyte proliferation may reflect regenerative hyperplasia resulting from toxic effects of synthetic steroids. It has been well documented that these agents, particularly synthetic estrogens, impair bile secretion resulting in mild cholestasis.[41,51] This toxic effect on the hepatocytes is associated with decreased mixed function oxidase activity,[51-54] changes in bile composition particularly characterized by increased cholesterol content,[55,56] alterations in liver GGT,[41,57] alterations in hepatocyte membranes including inhibition of Na^+, K^+ATPase activity,[58,59] and changes in membrane lipid structure and function perhaps due to increased cholesterol content and decreased fluidity.[59] Cytologically, hepatocytes in ethinylestradiol-treated rats are seen to be swollen and rounded up resulting in gaps between cells that are occupied by microvilli.[50] These latter types of membranous changes also appear in regenerating liver and may be a manifestation of the increased cell proliferation in livers of synthetic estrogen-treated rats.[50]

Determination of the extent to which the cholestatic response and its associated biochemical and cellular changes are important in promotion in the liver by the synthetic gonadal steroids requires investigation. Several compounds such as *S*-adenosyl-L-methionine[55] have been shown to reverse at least some of these changes. Thus, the ability of these compounds to inhibit promotion by mestranol or ethinylestradiol should be investigated. It should also be noted that cholestasis and at least some of the associated changes listed above are not essential components of the general process of promotion in liver since they are not all caused by phenobarbital and, in fact, in some cases can even be reversed by phenobarbital treatment.[52,56] However, this does not necessarily mean that they are not essential for promotion by the synthetic estrogens.

Numerous studies have demonstrated that tumor promoters have dramatic effects on cell membranes.[47] Recently several laboratories have reported that tumor promoters can decrease communication between cells as detected using in vitro cell culture systems.[60,61] If promoters have such effects in vivo, the consequences could include decreases in the intercellular exchange of growth regulator molecules. This could allow latent "initiated" cells to begin growth to give a population or clone of cells at greater risk for incurring additional changes leading to the neoplastic state.[62] In view of the fact that the synthetic estrogens appear to have many effects on membranes, we have carried out pilot studies on the effects of several synthetic gonadal steroids on metabolic cooperation in V-79 cells.[60] The results of these preliminary studies were positive. Both mestranol and norethynodrel (a progestin with estrogenic activity) decreased metabolic cooperation in this system.[66] More detailed studies are now required to test further the role of cell-cell communication in promotion by synthetic gonadal steroids and other promoters of liver[63] and other tissues.

IV. CONCLUSIONS

Synthetic gonadal steroids have been shown to be involved in the etiology of benign hepatocellular adenomas and carcinomas in women who have been ingesting oral contraceptive steroids for prolonged periods of time. Experimental studies have indicated that these agents are not mutagenic nor highly genotoxic. However, three separate animal studies have shown these types of compounds, especially the estrogens, to be promoters of hepatocarcinogenesis.

Synthetic gonadal and anabolic steroids have numerous biochemical and cellular effects on liver cells. It is not known which of these effects are essential to their promoting potential, and additional studies will be required to determine the mechanism(s) responsible for this extremely undesirable side effect.

ACKNOWLEDGMENTS

I wish to thank Dr. J. Zurlo for critical review of this manuscript. The research conducted in my laboratory was supported by grant CA 23916 and the actual experimental work was conducted while I was in the Department of Pathology at the Dartmouth Medical School. I wish to thank Drs. Longnecker and Roebuck for their support and advice during the course of these studies and D. Fifield, R. Fifield, M. Swan, and S. Ball for their valuable technical assistance.

REFERENCES

1. **Lipsett, M. B.,** Interaction of drugs, hormones, and nutrition in the causes of cancer, *Cancer,* 43, 1967, 1979.
2. **Recant, L. and Lacy, P.,** Fanconi's anemia and hepatic cirrhosis, *Am. J. Med.,* 39, 464, 1965.
3. **Bernstein, M. S., Hunter, R. L., and Yachnin, S.,** Hepatoma and peliosis hepatis developing in a patient with Fanconi's anemia, *N. Engl. J. Med.,* 284, 1135, 1971.
4. **Sherlock, S.,** Hepatic tumors and sex hormones, in *Primary Liver Tumors,* Remmer, H., Bolt, H. M., Bannasch, P., and Popper, H., Eds., University Park Press, Baltimore, 1978, 201.
5. **Horvath, E., Kovacs, K., and Ross, R. C.,** Ultrastructural findings in a well differentiated hepatoma, *Digestion,* 7, 74, 1972.
6. **Baum, J. K., Holtz, F., Bookstein, J. J., and Klein, E. W.,** Possible association between benign hepatomas and oral contraceptives, *Lancet,* 2, 926, 1973.
7. **Edmondson, H. A., Henderson, B., and Benton, B.,** Liver-cell adenomas associated with use of oral contraceptives, *N. Engl. J. Med.,* 294, 470, 1976.
8. **Gindhart, T. D.,** Liver tumors and oral contraceptives: pathology and pathogenesis, *Ann. Clin. Lab. Sci.,* 8, 443, 1978.
9. **Goldfarb, S.,** Sex hormones and hepatic neoplasia, *Cancer Res.,* 36, 2584, 1978.
10. **Christopherson, W. M. and Mays, E. T.,** Relation of steroids to liver oncogenesis, *J. Toxicol. Environ. Health,* 5, 207, 1979.
11. **Nissen, E. D., Kent, D. R., and Nissen, S. E.,** Role of oral contraceptive agents in the pathogenesis of liver tumors, *J. Toxicol. Environ. Health,* 5, 231, 1979.
12. **Vana, J., Murphy, G. P., Aronoff, B. L., and Baker, H. W.,** Survey of primary liver tumors and oral contraceptive use, *J. Toxicol. Environ. Health,* 5, 255, 1979.
13. **Rooks, J. B., Ory, H. W., Ishak, K. G., Strauss, L. T., Greenspan, J. R., Paganini, A., and Tayler, C. W., Jr.,** Epidemiology of hepatocellular adenoma: the role of oral contraceptive use, *JAMA,* 242, 644, 1979.
14. **Neuberger, J., Nunnerly, H. B., Davis, M., Portmann, B., Laws, J. W., and Williams, R.,** Oral contraceptive-associated liver tumors: occurrence of malignancy and difficulties in diagnosis, *Lancet,* 1, 273, 1980.
15. **Monroe, P. S., Riddell, R. H., Siegler, M., and Baker, A. L.,** Hepatic angiosarcoma: possible relationship to long-term oral contraceptive ingestion, *JAMA,* 246, 64, 1981.
16. **Thung, S. N. and Gerber, M.,** Precursor stage of hepatocellular neoplasm following long-term exposure to orally administered contraceptives, *Hum. Pathol.,* 12, 472, 1981.
17. **Hatcher, R. A., Stewart, G. K., Stewart, F., Guest, F., Stewart, D. W., and Jones, S. A.,** Combined oral contraceptives, in *Contraceptive Technology 1980—1981,* rev. ed., Irvington Publishers, New York, 1980, 26.
18. **Edmondson, H. A., Reynolds, T. B., Henderson, B., and Benton, B.,** Regression of liver cell adenomas associated with oral contraceptives, *Ann. Intern. Med.,* 86, 180, 1977.
19. **Firminger, H. J. and Reuber, M. D.,** Influence of adrenocortical, androgenic and anabolic hormones on the development of carcinoma and cirrhosis of the liver in A × C rats fed N-2-fluorenyldiacetamide, *J. Natl. Cancer Inst.,* 27, 559, 1961.
20. IARC Monograph, *Evaluation of Carcinogenic Risk of Chemicals to Man,* Vol. 6, International Agency for Research on Cancer, Lyons, 1974.
21. **Schuppler, J. and Gunzel, P.,** Liver tumors and steroid hormones in rats and mice, *Arch. Toxicol.,* Suppl. 2, 181, 1979.

22. **Schardein, J. L., Kaump, D. H., Woosley, E. T., and Jellema, M. M.,** Long-term toxicologic and tumorigenesis studies on an oral contraceptive agent in albino rats, *Toxicol. Appl. Pharmacol.*, 16, 10, 1970.
23. **Schardein, J. L.,** Studies of the components of an oral contraceptive agent in albino rats. I. Estrogenic component, *J. Toxicol. Environ. Health*, 6, 885, 1980.
24. **Schardein, J. L.,** Studies of the components of an oral contraceptive agent in albino rats. II. Progestogenic component and comparison of effects of the components and the combined agent, *J. Toxicol. Environ. Health*, 6, 895, 1980.
25. **Higashi, S., Tomita, T., Mizumoto, R., and Nakakuki, K.,** Development of hepatoma in rats following oral administration of synthetic estrogen and progestogen, *Gann*, 71, 576, 1980.
26. **Boutwell, R. K.,** The function and mechanism of promoters of carcinogenesis, *CRC Crit. Rev. Toxicol.*, 2, 419, 1974.
27. **Roebuck, B. D., Yager, J. D., Jr., Longnecker, D. S., and Wilpone, S. A.,** Promotion by unsaturated fat of azaserine-induced pancreatic carcinogenesis in the rat, *Cancer Res.*, 41, 3961, 1981.
28. **Reddy, B. S., Narisawa, T., Maronpot, R., Weisburger, J. H., and Wynder, E. L.,** Animal models for the study of dietary factors and cancer of the large bowel, *Cancer Res.*, 35, 3421, 1975.
29. **Carroll, K. K.,** Lipids and carcinogenesis, *J. Environ. Pathol. Toxicol.*, 3, 253, 1980.
30. **Pitot, H. C. and Sirica, A. E.,** The stages of initiation and promotion in hepatocarcinogenesis, *Biochim. Biophys. Acta*, 605, 191, 1980.
31. **Peraino, C., Fry, R. J. M., Staffeldt, E., and Kisieleski, W. E.,** Effects of varying exposure to phenobarbital on its enhancement of 2-acetylaminofluorene-induced hepatic tumorigenesis in the rat, *Cancer Res.*, 33, 2701, 1973.
32. **Cayama, E., Tsuda, H., Sarma, D. S. R., and Farber, E.,** Initiation of chemical carcinogenesis requires cell proliferation, *Nature (London)*, 275, 60, 1978.
33. **Farber, E.,** The sequential analysis of liver cancer induction, *Biochim. Biophys. Acta*, 605, 149, 1980.
34. **Lang, R. and Redmann, U.,** Non-mutagenicity of some sex hormones in the Ames salmonella/microsome mutagenicity test, *Mutat. Res.*, 67, 361, 1979.
35. **Drevon, C., Piccoli, C., and Montesano, R.,** Mutagenicity assays of estrogenic hormones in mammalian cells, *Mutat. Res.*, 89, 83, 1981.
36. **Ansari, S. R. and Adhami, U. M.,** Effect of antifertility drugs (norethindrone and mestranol) on the bone marrow chromosomes of albino rat (*Rattus-norvegicus*), *Indian J. Hered.*, 9, 7, 1977.
37. **Jaggi, W., Lutz, W. K., and Schlatter, C.,** Covalent binding of ethinylestradiol and estrone to rat liver DNA in vivo, *Chem. Biol. Interact.*, 23, 13, 1978.
38. **Taper, H. S.,** The effect of estradiol-17-phenylpropionate and estradiol benzoate on N-nitrosomorpholine-induced liver carcinogenesis in ovariectomized female rats, *Cancer*, 42, 462, 1978.
39. **Squire, R. A. and Levitt, M. H.,** Report of a workshop on classification of specific hepatocellular lesions in rats, *Cancer Res.*, 35, 3214, 1975.
40. **Yager, J. D., Jr. and Yager, R.,** Oral contraceptive steroids as promoters of hepatocarcinogenesis in female Sprague-Dawley rats, *Cancer Res.*, 40, 3680, 1980.
41. **Ronchi, G. and Desmet, V. J.,** Histochemical study of gamma glutamyl transpeptidase (GGT) in experimental intrahepatic and extrahepatic cholestasis, *Beitr. Pathol. Bd.*, 150, 316, 1973.
42. **Cameron, R., Imaida, K., and Ito, N.,** Promotive effects of ethinylestradiol in hepatocarcinogenesis initiated by diethylnitrosamine in male rats, *Gann*, 72, 339, 1981.
43. **Yager, J. D., Jr. and Fifield, D. S., Jr.,** Lack of hepatogenotoxicity of oral contraceptive steroids, *Carcinogenesis*, 3, 625, 1982.
44. **Williams, G. W.,** Detection of chemical carcinogens by unscheduled DNA synthesis in rat liver primary cell cultures, *Cancer Res.*, 37, 1845, 1977.
45. **Yager, J. D., Jr. and Miller, J. A., Jr.,** DNA repair in primary cultures of rat hepatocytes, *Cancer Res.*, 38, 4385, 1978.
46. **Probst, G. S., McMahon, R. E., Hill, L. E., Thompson, C. Z., Epp, J. K., and Neal, S. B.,** Chemically-induced unscheduled DNA synthesis in primary rat hepatocyte cultures. A comparison with bacterial mutagenicity using 218 compounds, *Environ. Mut.*, 3, 11, 1981.
47. **Slaga, T. J., Sivak, A., and Boutwell, R., Eds.,** Mechanisms of tumor promotion, in *Carcinogenesis, A Comprehensive Survey*, Vol. 2, Raven Press, New York, 1978.
48. **Shenoy, S. T. and Peraino, C.,** Changes in liver composition in phenobarbital-induced hepatomegaly, *Exp. Mol. Pathol.*, 27, 134, 1977.
49. **Eisenfeld, A. J., Aten, R. F., and Weinberger, M. J.,** Commentary: oral contraceptives — possible mediation of side effects via an estrogen receptor in liver, *Biochem. Pharmacol.*, 27, 2571, 1978.
50. **Cole, F. M. and Sweeney, G. D.,** Changes in rat hepatocyte plasma membranes caused by synthetic estrogens, *Lab. Invest.*, 42, 225, 1980.
51. **Roberts, R. J. and Plaa, G. L.,** Effect of norethandrolone, acetohexamide, and enovid on α-naphthisothiocyanate-induced hyperbilirubinemia and cholestasis, *Biochem. Pharmacol.*, 15, 333, 1966.

52. **Mackinnon, A. M. and Simon, F.,** Pharmacological reversal of cholestasis-associated decrease in hepatic cytochrome P-450, *Biochem. Pharmacol.*, 24, 748, 1975.
53. **Mackinnon, A. M., Sutherland, E., and Simon, F. R.,** Qualitative alteration in hepatic microsomal cytochrome P-450 apoproteins associated with bile duct ligation, and the administration of ethinyl estradiol, phenobarbital and 3-methylcholanthrene, *Biochem. Pharmacol.*, 27, 29, 1978.
54. **Sweeney, G. D. and Cole, F. M.,** Effects of ethinyl estradiol on liver microsomal mixed function oxygenase activity in male rats, *Lab. Invest.*, 42, 231, 1980.
55. **Stramentinoli, G., DiPadova, C., Gualano, M., Rovagnati, P., and Galli-Kienle, M.,** Ethinylestradiol-induced impairment of bile secretion in the rat: protective effects of S-adenosyl-L-methionine and its implication in estrogen metabolism, *Gastroenterology*, 80, 154, 1981.
56. **Davis, R. A. and Kern, F.,** Effects of ethinyl estradiol and phenobarbital on bile acid synthesis and biliary bile acid and cholesterol excretion, *Gastroenterology*, 70, 1130, 1976.
57. **Tazi, A., Galteau, M. M., and Siest, G.,** Effect of imipramine on hepatic gamma-glutamyltransferase in female rats. Interaction with contraceptives, *Biochem. Pharmacol.*, 29, 2874, 1980.
58. **Heikel, T. A. J. and Lathe, G. H.,** The effect of 17α-ethinyl-substituted steroids on adenosine triphosphatases of rat liver plasma membrne, *Biochem. J.*, 118, 187, 1970.
59. **Davis, R. A., Kern, F., Jr., Showalter, R., Sutherland, E., Sinensky, M., and Simon, F. R.,** Alterations of hepatic Na^+, K^+-ATPase and bile flow by estrogen. Effects on liver surface membrane lipid structure and function, *Proc. Natl. Acad. Sci. U.S.A.*, 75, 4130, 1978.
60. **Yotti, L. P., Chang, C. C., and Trosko, J. E.,** Elimination of metabolic cooperation in Chinese hamster cells by tumor promoters, *Science*, 206, 1089, 1980.
61. **Murray, A. W. and Fitzgerald, D. J.,** Tumor promoters inhibit metabolic cooperation in cocultures of epidermal and 3T3 cells, *Biochem. Biophys. Res. Commun.*, 91, 395, 1979.
62. **Potter, V. R.,** Initiation and promotion in cancer formation: the importance of studies on intercellular communication, *Yale, J. Biol. Med.*, 53, 367, 1980.
63. **Williams, G. M., Telang, S., and Tong, C.,** Inhibition of intercellular communication between liver cells by the liver tumor promoter 1,1,1-trichloro-2,2-bis(p-chlorophenyl)ethane, *Cancer Lett.*, 11, 339, 1981.
64. **Yager, J. D., Jr. and Yager, R.,** unpublished observations.
65. **Galloway, S. and Yager, J. D., Jr.,** unpublished observations.
66. **Trosko, J. E. and Yager, J. D., Jr.,** unpublished observations.

Chapter 3

ENHANCEMENT OF TUMOR FORMATION IN MOUSE LUNG*,**

H. P. Witschi

TABLE OF CONTENTS

** Research sponsored by the Office of Health and Environmental Research, U.S. Department of Energy, under contract W-7405-eng-26 with the Union Carbide Corporation.

I. INTRODUCTION

In 1977 Witschi et al. reported that it was possible to enhance development of mouse lung tumors with the common food additive butylated hydroxytoluene (BHT). Two different mouse strains, Swiss-Webster and A/J, were treated with a single dose of urethan (ethyl carbamate). One week later, half of the urethan-treated animals were injected once a week with 300 mg BHT per kilogram dissolved in corn oil; the other half received corn oil alone. Mice were killed 10 weeks (A/J) or 14 weeks (Swiss-Webster) after urethan treatments. Significantly more tumors were visible on the surface of the lung of animals treated with BHT compared with controls. In mice not exposed to urethan, BHT had no effect.[1]

These observations seemed to indicate that some of the factors involved in two-stage carcinogenesis play a role in the development of not only epithelial tumors in mouse skin, but also tumors originating from pulmonary epithelial cells. Further work showed that indeed, BHT had many properties of a promoting agent in mouse lung.[2] Not all observations made to date fulfill the strict criteria usually applied to two-stage carcinogenesis in mouse skin. Nevertheless, we feel that the information available strongly supports the view that the mouse lung tumor-BHT system can be taken as a valid example of two-stage carcinogenesis.

II. BACKGROUND

The rationale for testing BHT as a possible promoting agent for lung tumors in mice was as follows. In 1974 the bulk of available evidence suggested that practically all promoting agents were chemicals capable of eliciting gene activation and cell proliferation in mouse skin.[3] It was also assumed that most, if not all, lung tumors in mice originated from Type II alveolar cells.[4] When it was discovered that administration of BHT produced extensive Type II cell proliferation in mouse lung,[5] it was, therefore, a logical step to examine whether lung tumor formation could be enhanced by repeatedly inducing Type II cell proliferation.

A. Mechanisms of Action of Promoting Agents

Information on mechanisms of action of promoting agents has been and continues to be greatly refined. Many promoters produce cell proliferation in their target tissue, although not all agents capable of doing so act as promoting agents.[3] These aspects are dealt with elsewhere in this series.[6]

B. Lung Tumors in Mice

Lung tumors are among the more common spontaneously occurring neoplasms. However, their spontaneous incidence depends on strain and age. Up to 70% of Strain A mice at the age of 2 years may have one or several tumors per lung. Swiss-Webster is another strain in which lung tumors develop spontaneously with high incidence. In other strains, such as C57BL or C3H, only a few animals (5 to 15%) will develop tumors.[4] The tumors can be classified into epithelial tumors (often called alveologenic carcinoma), adenoma, Type II cell tumor, Type A tumor, Type B tumor, and bronchioalveolar tumors (or some other term). Epithelial tumors appear as circumscribed white nodules which are frequently located directly beneath the pleura. They are easily identified with the naked eye or under a dissecting microscope. Under the light microscope the tumors form an adenomatous pattern with closely packed columns of cuboidal or columnar cells; they are devoid of a capsule and infiltrate and compress the surrounding pulmonary tissues.[4] Other tumors, such as squamous cell carcinomas or vascular tumors, are very rare in untreated mice.[7]

There is still some question as to the cell type of origin for epithelial lung tumors. Initially they were classified under the light microscope into two groups described as alveolar and bronchiolar, thus implying a different cellular origin.[8] However, early electron microscopic studies showed that the tumor cells contained lamellar bodies, a characteristic feature of Type II alveolar epithelial cells.[9] Isolated individual cells from urethan-induced tumors were found to synthesize surfactant and respond to steroids.[10-12] This gave further support to the view that lung tumors in mice were derived from Type II alveolar cells. In contrast, some newer observations suggest that lung tumors may have different cells of origin. When pregnant Swiss-Webster mice were treated with ethylnitrosourea on the 16th day of gestation and their offspring were killed when 1 to 3 months old, it was found that all animals had multiple lung adenomas (average 35). Of 149 tumors examined, 86 were defined as bronchiolar tumors, derived from the nonciliated bronchiolar cells (the so-called Clara cells), and 61 were classified as alveolar tumors derived from Type II cells.[13] The two tumor types could be distinguished by light microscopy with comparative ease. Type II cell tumors consisted of continuous bands of uniform cuboidal cells lining alveolar septa and filling alveolar spaces. Occasionally the cells formed tubular patterns resembling fetal lung tissue. Clara cell or bronchiolar cell tumors consisted of columnar epithelial cells arranged in a tubular or papillary pattern. Electron microscopy confirmed that the tumors had two distinctly different cells of origin, Type II alveolar cells and Clara cells. Under the scanning electron microscope, alveolar cell tumors had a smooth surface, whereas Clara cell tumors were characterized by a rough surface with numerous microvilli.[14]

We recently examined more than 100 tumors from Strain A/J or from Swiss-Webster mice treated with a single dose of urethan (1000 mg/kg).[83] The criteria used to distinguish Type II alveolar cell tumors from Clara cell tumors in paraffin sections were those described by Kauffman et al.[13] In A/J mice, 70% of all tumors could be classified as having originated from Type II alveolar cells, whereas in Swiss-Webster mice only 20% could be identified as Type II cell tumors. The remaining 80% showed morphologic features characteristic of Clara cell tumors. These observations need confirmation by more detailed electron microscopy studies and need to be extended to other mouse strains. They point out, however, that the apparently conflicting data on the cells of origin of mouse lung tumors may be due to the fact that different observers used different mouse strains.

In mouse strains with a high spontaneous incidence of lung tumors, the administration of many chemical and physical agents will produce within a few months a substantial increase in both tumor incidence (expressed as number of tumor-bearing animals) and tumor multiplicity (expressed as number of tumors per lung).[4] The chemical which has been most widely used to produce lung tumors in susceptible mouse strains is urethan. As early as 2 to 3 months following a single injection of urethan, white round nodules appear on the surface of the lung. The number of visible tumors is proportional to the dose of urethan given. In Strain A mice, 1 mg of urethan usually produces one tumor per lung, whereas in Swiss-Webster mice the same dose produces about 0.5 tumor per lung. Other strains develop substantially fewer tumors after urethan administration.[2,4]

Tumor multiplicity is most conveniently determined by counting the macroscopically visible surface nodules. It has been maintained from time to time that this procedure might underestimate the actual number of tumors, since tumors originating deep in the lung parenchyma might not be counted on the lung surface. In an early histologic study it was found, however, that new tumor foci are formed only during the first 2 months following a single injection of urethan. After this time, no new foci are formed which will eventually grow into macroscopic, recognizable tumors, and from approximately 4 months after urethan administration the number of tumors apparent on the surface reaches a plateau.[15] This early observation was recently corroborated. In A/J mice treated with urethan, the number of surface tumors was counted at 2 to 10 months after urethan. Each lung was cleared[16] and the number of tumors was recounted. Practically a 1:1 relationship between surface tumors and tumors visible in cleared lungs was found, regardless of number of tumors per lung or of time after urethan treatment (Figure 1). It can thus be concluded that surface counting of tumors accurately reflects the total number of tumors per lung visible to the naked eye.

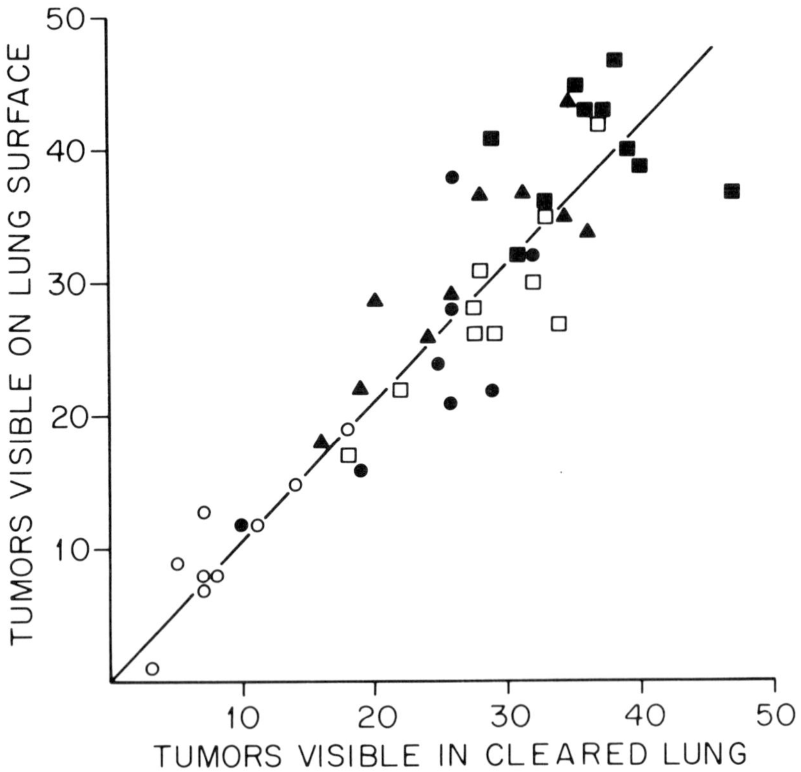

FIGURE 1. Male A/J mice were injected i.p. with 1000 mg urethan per kilogram and killed 2 (○), 4 (●), 6 (□), 8 (■), or 10 (▲) months later. For each lung, the number of tumors was counted first on the lung surface and then again in the cleared[16] lungs.

C. Effects of BHT on Normal Mouse Lung

In 1972 it was reported that the antioxidant BHT would product acute lung damage in mice. A few days after a single dose of BHT (400 mg/kg), lung lesions indicative of a proliferative change in the alveolar epithelium were found. The histopathological changes resolved 1 week after BHT treatment. No damage was found in other tissues.[17] Initially, it was thought that BHT would simply produce cell hyperplasia in mouse lung.[6,18] Combined morphologic-biochemical studies showed that the effects of BHT were somewhat more complex. Within the first 24 hr after injection, BHT produces extensive and diffuse necrosis of Type I alveolar cells. This is followed 2 to 4 days later by proliferation and division of Type II alveolar cells. Eventually Type II cells differentiate into Type I alveolar cells, and within 6 to 8 days after BHT treatment an essentially normal looking alveolar epithelium is restored and only a few areas of fibrosis may persist. Proliferation of alveolar interstitial cells and capillary endothelial cells reaches a peak 5 and 6 days after BHT injection, respectively[19,20] (Table 1).

BHT-induced proliferation of Type II alveolar cells is therefore a secondary event which follows initial injury to the Type I epithelial cells. The morphologic observations, together with data on accumulation and on disappearance of BHT in the lung,[21] seem to preclude a direct action of BHT on Type II alveolar cells. BHT has been shown to produce lung injury in several mouse strains, followed by extensive cell proliferation.[22,23] The morphologic and biochemical events associated with BHT-induced lung damage and following Type II alveolar cell proliferation have been reproduced in several laboratories.[24-28] Interestingly, BHT seems to produce lung damage only in mice, but not in other rodents such as the rat or the hamster.[26,29,30]

Table 1
CELL PROLIFERATION IN MOUSE LUNG FOLLOWING I.P. INJECTION OF 400 MG BHT/KG

Days after BHT injection	No. of cells labeled/10,000 lung cells[a]		
	Epithelial	Interstitial	Endothelial
1	14	15	11
2	261	99	54
3	330	132	48
4	182	248	83
5	162	348	35
6	41	105	156
7	70	164	137
8	40	92	50
9	18	58	15

[a] Data calculated from labeling index and differential cell count; original data by Adamson et al.[20]

III. ENHANCEMENT OF URETHAN-INDUCED LUNG TUMOR FORMATION BY BHT

A. Temporal Relationships

BHT enhances lung tumor formation only if it is given to mice after the administration of an initiating dose of urethan. In Swiss-Webster mice injected i.p. with 1000 mg of urethan per kilogram, an average of four tumors per lung was found 14 weeks later. Treatment of the animals with a total of 13 weekly injections of 300 mg BHT per kilogram, beginning 1 week after urethan treatment, produced an average of 13 tumors per lung. In mice of the same strain and from the same source, the procedure was reversed. Animals were given 13 weekly injections of 300 mg BHT per kilogram; controls received corn oil. All animals were given 1000 mg of urethan per kilogram 1 week after the last BHT injection. Both BHT-treated animals and controls had an average of three to four tumors per lung 14 weeks later.[2] The same observation was made in an experiment in which BHT was administered in the diet. A/J mice were given 500 mg of urethan per kilogram, and instead of receiving weekly BHT injections, the animals were offered (for a 24-hr period once a week for 8 consecutive weeks) a diet containing 0.75% BHT. Tumors were counted 4 months after urethan treatment. The animals given BHT had twice as many tumors as the controls. In the same experiment another group of mice were fed a BHT diet continuously for 2 weeks. These animals were injected with 1000 mg of urethan per kilogram, and the BHT diet was replaced by an ordinary laboratory diet without any BHT added. The animals exposed to BHT prior to urethan injection had the same average number of tumors per lung as the controls 14 weeks later.[31]

Thus, in two different experiments and by two different routes of exposure, it was found that BHT enhances tumor formation in mouse lung only if the treatment is begun 1 week after urethan treatment, whereas it has no effect if it is given before urethan treatment. The data allow exclusion of the possibility that BHT enhances tumor formation by altering the metabolism of urethan. BHT is a known inducer of hepatic mixed-function oxidases,[32] and as such might conceivably affect metabolic activation or deactivation of urethan to a proximate carcinogen. However, pretreatment with BHT does not influence tumor incidence or multiplicity. Since urethan is usually completely excreted from an experimental animal within 24 hr,[33] it is also unlikely that BHT, given for the first time 1 week after urethan treatment, will influence its metabolism.

It was also found that delay of BHT administration until 6 weeks after urethan treatment enhanced tumor formation.[2] In a recent experiment Swiss-Webster mice were given 1000 mg of urethan per kilogram, urethan and BHT treatments (300 mg/kg for a total of 4 weekly injections) were begun 1, 4, 7, 10, 13, or 19 weeks later. The time allowed for tumor expression between the first BHT injection and the time the animals were killed was 15 to 16 weeks; thus animals were killed 16, 19, 22, 25, 28, or 35 weeks after urethan injection.[34] In BHT-treated animals the number of tumors per lung was always higher than in controls (Figure 2). BHT thus effectively enhances tumor development even if the beginning of treatment is delayed until 5 months after administration of the initiating agent.

In summary, BHT enhances tumor formation in urethan-initiated mouse lung if it is given up to several months after the carcinogen, but not if exposure to BHT precedes exposure to urethan. BHT thus meets one important criterion commonly attributed to promoting agents. The next question to be addressed is whether BHT alone has tumorigenic action.

B. Effects of BHT Alone

BHT is a common food additive and at present still is on the list of GRAS substances. Its toxicity has been extensively evaluated in several species in long-term feeding studies. The general consensus is that there is no evidence that BHT might be a carcinogen in rodents. When BHT was tested in an assay specifically designed to measure lung tumor formation in mice, it had no effect.[35] It is of interest that BHT in two long-term feeding studies has been found to produce a slight increase in the incidence of so-called spontaneous lung tumors.[36,37] The data are, however, inconclusive. In one study the number of animals examined and some other shortcomings in experimental design precluded the drawing of firm conclusions.[36] In the second study it was found that lung tumor incidence and multiplicity in female mice fed BHT were significantly higher in the low-dose group, but not in the higher-dose group. Increased incidence of lung tumors in female mice could therefore not be associated unequivocally with the administration of BHT. No increased tumor incidence and tumor multiplicity were found in the male mice tested. It was concluded that under the conditions of this bioassay BHT would not produce tumors.[37] Thus, several animal studies designed to evaluate the carcinogenic potential of BHT gave negative results. In our own experiments we did not obtain evidence that BHT would enhance tumor incidence or tumor multiplicity in animals not exposed to urethan. BHT thus fulfills a second criterion for a promoting agent: it seems not to have tumorigenic activity per se.

C. Route of BHT Exposure

Experiments with radiolabeled BHT in mice have shown that the kinetics of uptake into an elimination of BHT or its metabolites from mouse lung are comparable regardless of whether BHT is injected i.p. or administered orally.[38] Given by either route BHT produces a similar degree of lung damage. Thus, BHT reaches its target following absorption from the peritoneal cavity or from the gastrointestinal tract.

It was therefore not unexpected to find that BHT would enhance tumor promotion following i.p. injection[2] as well as following gastric intubation[38] or ingestion in the diet[31] (Table 2). The data show that BHT enhances tumor formation in mouse lung regardless of route of administration. Although this finding is not of particular interest to mechanistic studies, it might nevertheless raise some concern with regard to the continued use of BHT as a food additive.

D. Dose-Response Relationships: Urethan

The dose-response to urethan was studied in one experiment with Swiss-Webster mice[2] (Figure 3). Four different doses of urethan were used, and animals were given 13 weekly injections of BHT. When animals were killed 14 weeks after urethan treatment, it was found

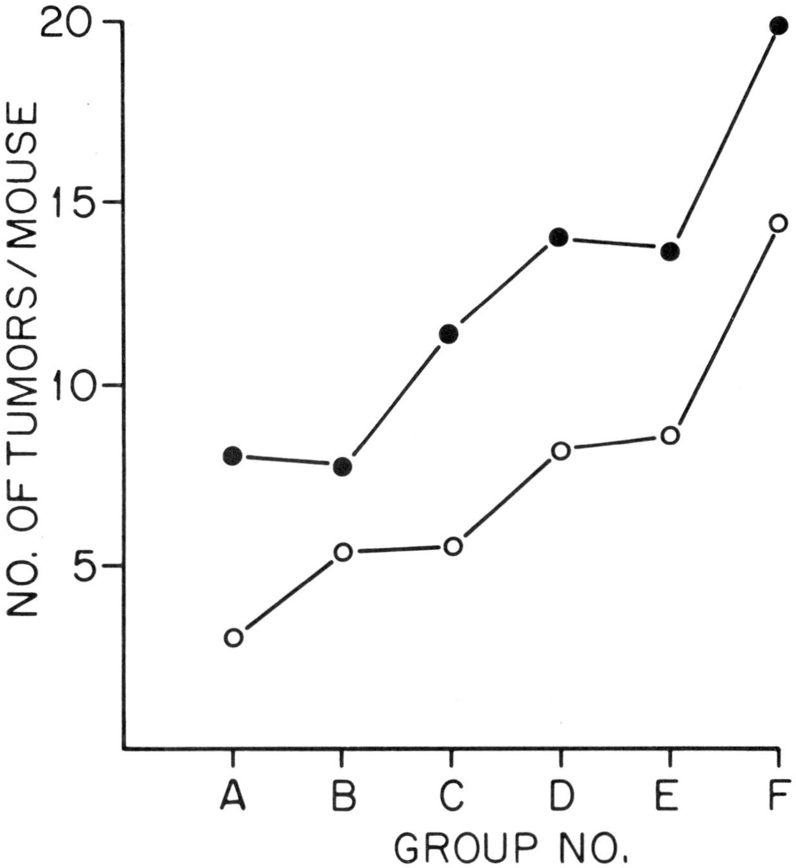

FIGURE 2. Swiss-Webster mice were injected with 1000 mg urethan per kilogram and received i.p. either 300 mg BHT/kg (●) or corn oil (○). The following treatment schedules were used. Group A: BHT once a week in weeks 1 to 4 after urethan treatment; killed 16 weeks after urethan treatment. Group B: BHT in weeks 4 to 7; killed at 19 weeks. Group C: BHT in weeks 7 to 10; killed at 22 weeks. Group D: BHT in weeks 10 to 13; killed at 25 weeks. Group E: BHT in weeks 13 to 16; killed at 28 weeks. Group F: BHT in weeks 19 to 22; killed at 35 weeks. (Data redrawn from Witschi, H. P. and Kehrer, J. P., *J. Am. Coll. Toxicol.*, 1, 171, 1982. With permission.

that the BHT treatment significantly enhanced tumor formation in animals given 100 to 1000 mg of urethan per kilogram. However, with the lowest dose of urethan used (50 mg/kg), no significant increase in tumor multiplicity was found, nor was there an increased tumor incidence. The percentage of tumor-bearing animals treated with 50 mg of urethan per kilogram plus BHT was not significantly different from the percentage of tumor-bearing mice treated with corn oil. More recently we found that 0.75% BHT in the diet enhanced significantly the number of tumors in animals injected with 1000 mg of urethan per kilogram, but was without effect in mice given 50, 25, or 5 mg of urethan per kilogram.[84] So far it has not been possible to produce enhanced tumor formation or development with low doses of urethan. BHT does not fulfill one criterion to be considered of importance for promoting agents — the capability to enhance tumor formation following administration of subcarcinogenic doses of an initiating agent.

E. Dose-Response Relationships: BHT

The effects of various doses of BHT upon lung tumor development were studied in Swiss-

Table 2
ENHANCEMENT OF LUNG TUMOR FORMATION BY DIFFERENT ROUTES OF ADMINISTRATION OF BHT

Initial dose of urethan (mg/kg)	Strain	Treatment	No. of tumors/mouse 14—16 weeks after urethan (± SE)	Ref.
1000	Swiss-Webster	300 mg BHT/kg i.p., 13 weekly injections	12.6 ± 1.8 (24)[a]	2
		Oil, i.p.	3.7 ± 0.5 (26)	
1000	Swiss-Webster	300 mg BHT/kg by stomach tube, once a week for 13 weeks	14.7 ± 2.8 (23)	38
		Oil, stomach tube	5.5 ± 1.2 (22)	
500	A/J	0.75% BHT in diet continuously for 8 weeks	12.4 ± 1.3 (24)	31
		Control diet	8.0 ± 0.9 (26)	

[a] Number of animals in parentheses.

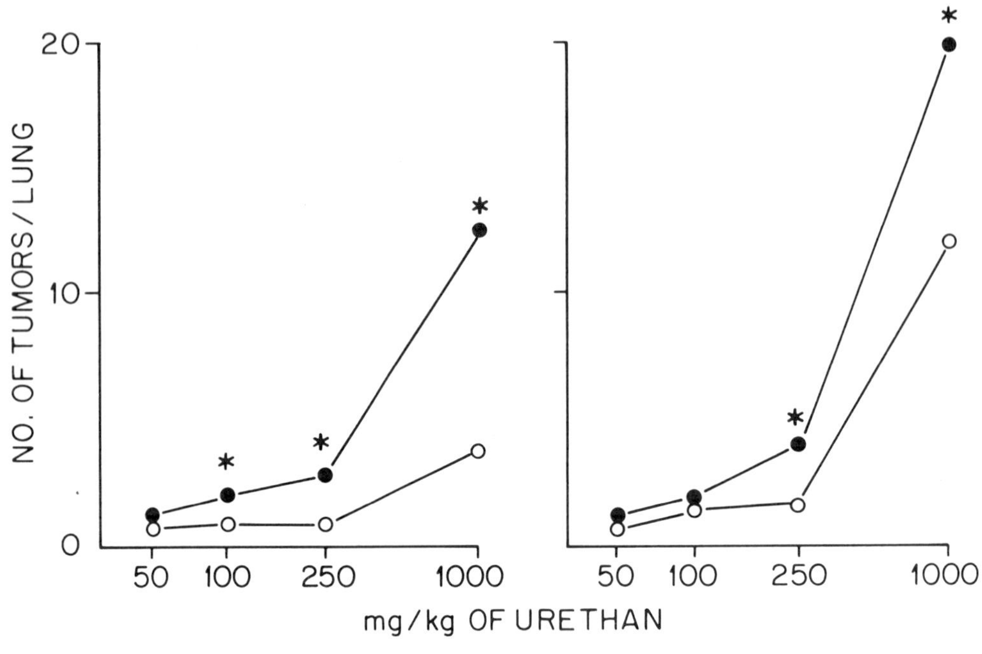

FIGURE 3. Dose response to urethan. Swiss-Webster mice were injected with 50 to 1000 mg of urethan per kilogram and given a total of 13 weekly BHT injections (●). Control animals received urethan and corn oil (○). Animals were killed 14 weeks (left panel) or 24 weeks (right panel) after urethan treatment. (Data redrawn from Witschi, H. P. and Lock, S., *Toxicol. Appl. Pharmacol.*, 50, 391, 1979. With permission.)

Webster mice treated with 1000 mg of urethan per kilogram and given 6 weekly injections of 300, 200, 100, or 50 mg BHT per kilogram.[34] The lowest dose of BHT (50 mg/kg) was as effective in enhancing tumor response as the highest dose (300 mg/kg). An absence of a dose-response to BHT was also noted in studies in which the antioxidant was given to animals in the diet.[31] In one experiment, A/J mice were treated with 500 mg of urethan per kilogram and had continuous access to food containing BHT for 8 weeks. Cumulative BHT intake per mouse was calculated to be 868 mg. An average of 12.5 tumors per lung was found, compared with 8 tumors per lung in animals on a control diet. The same strain of mice treated with 500 mg of urethan per kilogram was exposed once a week for a 24-hr period to BHT in the food for 8 consecutive weeks. The cumulative BHT intake was 126 mg per mouse. In BHT-treated animals, 10.3 tumors per lung were found in the treated animals at the end of the experiments compared with an average of 5 tumors per lung in controls.

It must be concluded that there is so far no indication of a dose-response to BHT. The lowest dose of BHT needed to enhance urethan-induced lung tumors in mice has yet to be determined, and BHT is effective over a 100-fold dose range (Figure 4). There is one important proviso to this conclusion, however: 6 weekly injections of 50 mg/kg BHT amount to a cumulative dose of 300 mg BHT per kilogram. This regimen significantly enhances tumor formation.[34] However, it was also found that one or two injections of 300 mg BHT per kilogram do not enhance tumor development. The minimum number of injections required is four.[2] Since two injections of 300 mg/kg of BHT amount to a cumulative dose of 600 mg/kg, it is obvious that repeated or continuous exposure to BHT for more than 2 weeks is necessary to influence tumor development.

F. Effects of BHT in Resistant Mouse Strains

Although BHT has been found to enhance reproducibly tumor development in Swiss-Webster and A/J mice, it has no effect in strains with a low spontaneous incidence of lung tumors. In BALB/c, C57BL, and C3H mice treated with urethan followed by 13 injections of BHT, BHT has been found to produce cell proliferation in lung comparable to that seen in Swiss-Webster and A/J mice.[22] However, lung tumor formation was not enhanced by BHT.[2]

IV. EFFECTS OF DIFFERENT INITIATORS AND PROMOTERS IN MOUSE LUNG

A. Effects of BHT Following Treatment with Different Initiators

There is only a limited data base available to document that BHT enhances tumor formation in animals initiated by other carcinogens. In a feeding study some evidence suggested that BHT enhances lung tumor formation in animals pretreated with diethylnitrosamine; the data are not clear-cut.[39] In Swiss-Webster mice given dimethylnitrosamine or 3-methylcholanthrene, treatment with BHT had no effect,[34] whereas in A/J mice given the same carcinogen, BHT did enhance tumor formation.[40] The reasons for this conflicting observation are not clear at present. In A/J mice the tumor response to 3-methylcholanthrene was very good, with animals developing an average of 4 tumors per lung. In Swiss-Webster mice only 0.4 tumor per lung developed with the same dose of 3-methylcholanthrene. Failure of BHT to have an effect in Swiss-Webster mice might have been due to too small a number of initiating events. In analogy to what was found with 50 mg urethan per kilogram, BHT might not be effective in this situation. However, the same reasoning cannot be applied to the data obtained with dimethylnitrosamine. In Swiss-Webster mice 10 mg dimethylnitrosamine per kilogram produced an average of 2.5 tumors per lung and BHT failed to enhance tumor development. In A/J mice, 7 mg dimethylnitrosamine per kilogram produced 0.8 tumors per lung and BHT had a significant effect. Further studies are needed to establish unambiguously whether BHT is as effective as a promoting agent for other chemical carcinogens as it is for urethan.

B. Enhancement of Lung Tumor Development by Agents Other Than BHT

BHT is not the only agent which may promote lung tumors in mice. The systemic

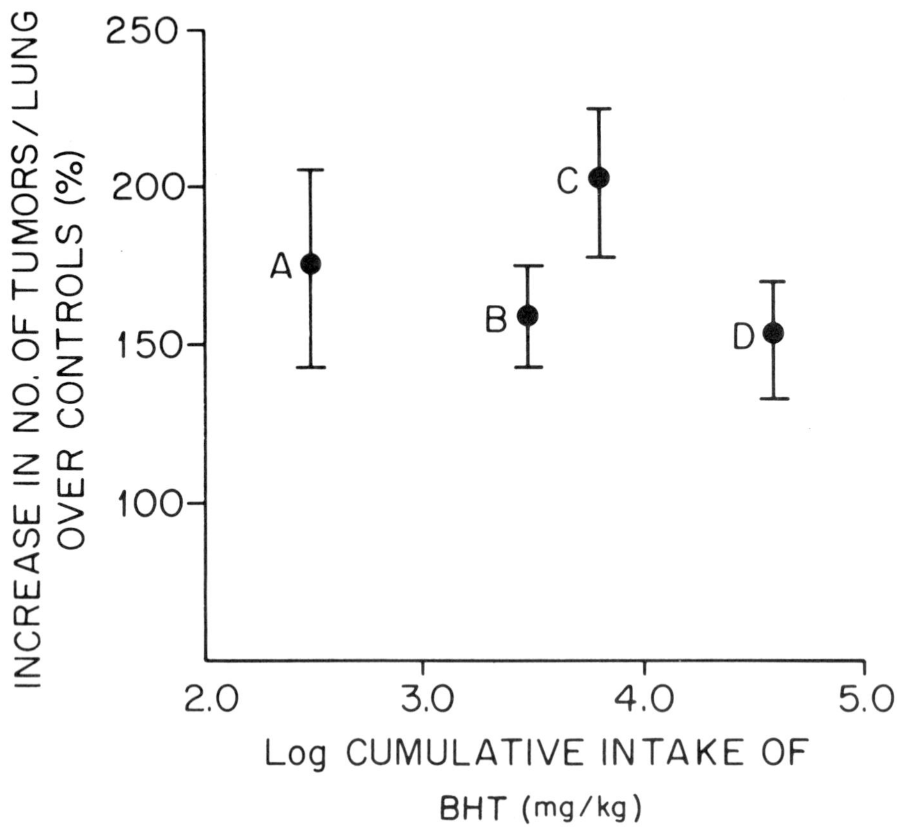

FIGURE 4. Dose response to BHT. Data are calculated as percentage increase in lung tumors in animals treated with BHT compared with corresponding controls. Group A: Swiss-Webster mice, 1000 mg of urethan per kilogram, 6 weekly injections of 50 mg BHT per kilogram. Groups B to D: A/J mice, 500 mg urethan per kilogram i.p. Group B: 8 weekly injections of 300 mg BHT per kilogram. Group C: exposed for 24 hr once a week for 8 consecutive weeks to 0.75% BHT in food. Group D: exposed continuously for 8 weeks to 0.75% BHT in food. All animals were killed 4 months after urethan treatment. (Group A data redrawn from Witschi, H. P. and Kehrer, J. P., *J. Am. Coll. Toxicol.*, 1, 171, 1982. Group B to D redrawn from Witschi, H. P., *Toxicology*, 21, 95, 1981. With permission.)

promoting ability of phorbol was tested in AKR mice.[41] Repeated injections in adult mice did not produce lung tumors. Dimethylnitrosamine, injected into newborn or 10-day-old animals, produced only a few tumors. However, when dimethylnitrosamine was injected at birth, subsequent treatment with phorbol increased both tumor incidence and multiplicity. When dimethylnitrosamine administration was delayed until 10 days after birth, no promoting effect of phorbol was observed. It was concluded that phorbol might act as a systemic promoter in lung, among other tissues, provided the initiating stimulus was given early after birth. Additional evidence has now become available that phorbol or its active compound 12-*O*-tetradecanoylphorbol-13-acetate has systemic promoting ability.[42] The effects on mouse lung tumors appear not to have been evaluated further in a systemic way.

Saccharin was initially considered to be a carcinogen, but it is now thought to be a promoting agent.[43] Commercial saccharin preparations (but not pure saccharin) were given daily at 1 g/kg by stomach tube to Strain A mice. The mice were injected with 100 or 1000 mg of urethan per kilogram 1 week later. Saccharin treatment was continued daily, five times a week, for another 16 weeks. When the animals were killed, it was found that all those treated with the higher dose of urethan and saccharin preparation had a significantly increased tumor multiplicity (2 to 4 times above control values).[44] Together with evidence on the effects of saccharin in other systems,[45] the data strongly suggest that saccharin acts as a promoting agent. Unfortunately, the experiment is somewhat inconclusive, inasmuch as saccharin treatment was initiated before urethan administration. This experimental design does not allow exclusion of a cocarcinogenic effect of saccharin. It is hoped that data will become available on lung tumor development in animals given saccharin only after urethan treatment. This could be important for the evaluation of the promoting potential of saccharin and could also provide a stimulus for studies that would establish whether the mouse lung tumor assay may be used to detect not only initiators, but also promoting agents.

Of even more practical importance would be to study the possible role of inhaled agents on the development of lung tumors. Tumor promotion appears to be an important and general mechanism in respiratory carcinogenesis in several animal models and possibly even in humans.[45] Determination of whether a toxic inhalant also promotes tumor formation in mouse lung seems to have been done with one agent only, diesel exhaust. The number of tumors found in animals injected with urethan and subsequently exposed to diesel exhaust was slightly higher than the number of tumors in mice injected with urethan and exposed to air only.[47] However, the low number of tumors found in any group precluded definitive conclusions. The data are preliminary; nevertheless, they indicate that lung tumor formation in mice might be enhanced not only by bloodborne agents, but also by inhalants.

Finally, it is interesting to contemplate whether any inhalant capable of stimulating Type II alveolar proliferation in mouse lung might enhance adenoma development. One agent known to produce Type II cell proliferation is oxygen.[48] Some early work, although not designed as initiation-promotion studies, nevertheless indicated that oxygen might enhance tumor development. Strain A mice injected with a single dose of dibenz[*a,h*]anthracene and exposed immediately thereafter for 2 days to 100% oxygen developed significantly more tumors than animals treated with dibenz[*a,h*]anthracene and kept in air.[49] Similar observations were made when Strain A mice were given 1000 mg of urethan per kilogram and placed for 2 days into 70% O_2; with lower doses of urethan, no effect of oxygen was found.[50] In mice born within 24 hr after their mothers received urethan, those born and kept in an atmosphere of 100% oxygen for 24 hr had significantly more tumors at 6 months of age than animals not exposed to oxygen.[51] However, in experiments with adult A/J mice designed as initiation-promotion studies, no effect of 100% oxygen on tumor development was found.[34] Furthermore, not only hyperoxia, but also hypoxia, increases tumor multiplicity after urethan injection.[51,52] Oxygen may thus enhance tumor formation by altering blood flow to the lung or possibly by altering the metabolism of the administered carcinogens rather than by producing increased turnover of Type II alveolar cells.

V. MECHANISMS OF ACTION

A. Toxicity of BHT

BHT is a widely used food additive and as such was subject to numerous toxicity studies.[53] In both acute and long-term animal studies, it has few overt toxic effects; lung damage in mice[17,19] and hemorrhagic death in rats[54,55] appear to be the only serious manifestation of toxicity in experimental animals. Induction of hepatic mixed-function oxidases by BHT has not been considered to be an undesirable effect,[56] although it gave rise to some concern in an evaluation of the continued use of BHT as a food additive.[36] Overall, the available data on the toxicity of BHT seem not to raise undue concern.[53]

Biotransformation of BHT by mixed-function oxidases may play a role in producing untoward effects in liver and lung. A specific BHT-binding protein has been found in rat liver.[57] Rat liver microsomal preparations are capable of forming in vitro several metabolites of BHT.[58] These studies suggest that there are highly reactive metabolites which might bind to cellular macromolecules. In vivo binding of BHT to macromolecules from several tissues has been found in rats.[59] One ring-oxygenated metabolite, BHT-OOH, has recently been synthesized and found to be ten times more toxic in mice than the parent compound.[60] However, the same compound does not produce acute lung damage.[61] Nevertheless, it now appears to be reasonably well established, contrary to what had been thought,[21] that BHT needs to be metabolically activated in order to produce acute lung injury.[29] The first evidence for this was provided in experiments which showed that cedar wood beddings protected mice against BHT.[23] Animals placed on cedar shavings before or even a few hours after BHT injection failed to develop lung damage. Protective effects were also observed with some known constituents of cedar terpenes. This observation was confirmed and extended.[29] Treatment of mice with inhibitors of mixed-function oxidases such as SKF 525A (2-diethylaminoethyl-2,2-diphenylvalerate hydrochloride), colbaltous chloride, and piperonyl butoxide protects against BHT induced lung damage, if compounds are given before or even a few hours after BHT. This protective effect is most likely explained by destruction of pulmonary cytochrome HP 450 by cobaltous chloride or piperonyl butoxide or by competition between SKF 525A and BHT at its target site, thus precluding formation of toxic metabolites. Further evidence that BHT needs metabolic activation was provided by the finding that BHT binds covalently to mouse pulmonary macromolecules. In rats, which do not develop lung damage after BHT treatment, less covalently bound material is found in the lung.

Some data available show that, in vitro, BHT is cytotoxic and may cause swelling and lysis of cells and depress metabolic activities such as RNA and protein synthesis.[62-65] In phytohemagglutinin-stimulated lymphocytes, a mixture of BHT and Tween®-80 produces a marked uncoiling of chromosomes as well as extensive cell membrane damage.[66,67] BHT perturbs artificial membrane systems[68] and inactivates lipid-containing mammalian and bacterial viruses.[69] It is thought that by this mechanism BHT protects chicken against infection with Newcastle virus,[70] and it remains to be established whether the life-lengthening effect of BHT in BALB/c mice[71] is related to a similar chemotherapeutic effect.

In conclusion, several observations suggest that BHT, in order to produce lung damage in mice, needs metabolic activation to a more toxic metabolite. However, BHT may also interfere with structural and functional integrity of biological membranes. How exactly these mechanisms relate to the pathogenesis of lung cell necrosis and enhancement of tumor formation remains to be established.

B. Mechanisms of Lung Tumor Promotion by BHT

Originally it was thought that BHT would enhance lung tumor development because it produces Type II alveolar cell proliferation in lung. This hypothesis was strengthened when it was found that butylated hydroxyanisole (BHA) and ethoxyquin fail to stimulate Type II cell division[1] and do not enhance lung tumor development in urethan-treated mice.[34] However, the bulk of available evidence now strongly suggests that proliferation of Type II alveolar cells is not a key element in lung tumor development.

It was initially thought that each weekly injection of BHT would be followed by a burst of cell proliferation in lung. Newer data show that this is not so. For reasons not yet understood, maximum cell proliferation in lung is seen after the first BHT injection only (Figure 5). After the second BHT injection, the increase in pulmonary labeling indexes is markedly reduced. A slight rebound is seen after the fourth injection, but then the animals become resistant to further BHT injections. Continuous bursts of cell proliferation are thus not a feature of repeated BHT injections.

In mice treated with SKF 525A, BHT injections are not followed by cell proliferation in the lung.[29] When animals were initiated with urethan and then repeatedly given BHT, preceded by a dose of SKF 525A known to prevent cell proliferation, the same number of tumors was found as in animals given BHT without SKF 525A. In both groups (BHT plus

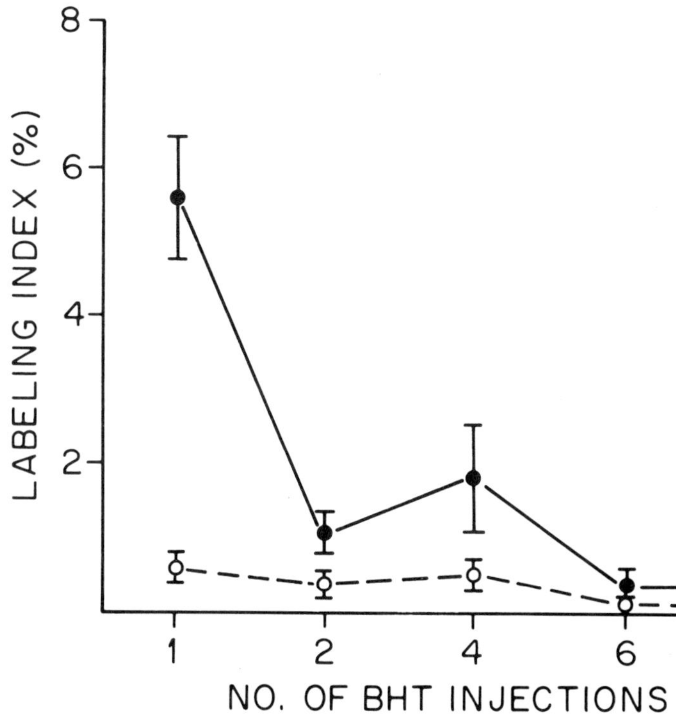

FIGURE 5. Labeling index in lungs of mice following repeated injections of BHT. Male A/J mice were injected with 1000 mg of urethan per kilogram and, beginning 1 week later, received weekly injections of 300 mg BHT per kilogram. Labeling indexes were determined with a 90-min pulse of (^{3}H)thymidine 3 days after 1, 2, 4, 6, or 8 injections. (Details of measuring labeling index are given by Adamson, et al.[20]; original and unpublished data.)

SKF 525A or BHT alone), tumor multiplicity was significantly greater than in animals given urethan and corn oil.[34] Thus, BHT enhances tumor formation whether or not it produces cell proliferation in lung. This was also found in experiments in which a dose of BHT (50 mg/kg), too small to produce measurable cell division, produced a similar number of lung tumors as did a large dose of BHT.[34]

On the other hand, agents which cause cell proliferation in mouse lung do not enhance tumor formation. If mice are exposed for 3 days to 100% oxygen and then removed into air, a burst of cell proliferation in lung similar to the one produced with BHT follows. Repeated exposure to oxygen after urethan treatment does not enhance tumor formation in lung.[34] Cell proliferation in lung can also be caused by i.p. injection of methylcyclopentadienyl manganese tricarbonyl (MMT); no enhancement of tumor development was seen in mice treated with urethan and this compound.[40] There exists, thus, a clear discrepancy between cell proliferation in lung and tumor promotion. Our observations do not allow us to exclude the possibility that repeated BHT treatment might produce a selective proliferation of initiated cells even in the absence of overall detectable proliferation. On the other hand, production of overall cell proliferation in lung by agents other than BHT is clearly without any effect. This suggests that the effect of BHT on lung tumor development could be rather specific.

The possibility that the antioxidant properties of BHT are related to its tumor-enhancing effects needs to be considered. At the moment this seems unlikely, since other antioxidants such as butylated hydroxyanisole, vitamin E, and ethoxyquin do not promote tumor formation in mouse lung.[34,40] The mechanism of action of BHT remains so far unknown. Molecular mechanisms believed to be involved in the promotion of skin tumors in mice have, of course, been extensively investigated.[72] No such studies have been done in mouse lung.

C. Does BHT Produce More Tumors or Only Accelerate Tumor Growth?

All quantitative data on the effect of BHT were obtained by counting surface tumors. It cannot be said whether BHT treatment indeed increases the number of tumors formed or simply accelerates tumor growth so that they become visible earlier on the lung surface.

Two sets of data suggest that BHT indeed increases the number of tumors formed. When comparing the number of tumors visible on the lung surface against the total number of tumors visible in cleared lungs, we found a 1:1 relationship[31] (Figure 1). Thus, surface counting reflects accurately the total number of tumors visible to the naked eye. More tumors seen after BHT treatment may be interpreted to mean that more tumors were formed. It was also possible to enhance tumor formation if BHT was given for the first time not at 1 week after urethan treatment, but after 10 to 19 weeks.[34] It had been claimed earlier that, following a single injection of urethan, new microscopically visible tumor foci develop only within the first 2 months, but not later.[15] Since it was possible to enhance tumor formation with BHT treatment begun 10 weeks or later after urethan treatment, the conclusion might be drawn that BHT, indeed, somehow enhances the formation of new tumors rather than accelerating the growth of already formed foci which are visible only under the microscope.

On the other hand, it was found that the difference between tumor multiplicity in BHT-treated animals and in controls was greater 4 months after urethan treatment than it was 6 months after urethan treatment.[2] As time progresses, the difference diminishes even further.[84] These data must be interpreted to mean that BHT accelerates tumor growth.

In most experiments the initiating dose of urethan given produced a 90 to 100% tumor incidence in both control and BHT-treated animals. This, of course, does not allow evaluation of possible effects of BHT on tumor incidence. In animals treated with other initiators, with lower doses of urethan, or with no carcinogen at all, a significantly increased number of tumor-bearing animals was occasionally, but not regularly found in animals treated with BHT.[31,34] In conclusion, while it is certain that BHT does increase the number of tumors per lung, it is not yet clear whether this is caused by accelerated tumor growth or by increased formation of tumors. Furthermore, it has not been established yet whether after BHT treatment more animals develop tumors than would without BHT treatment. More studies are needed to determine whether BHT indeed produces more tumors or acts to accelerate growth of preformed tumors.

D. Anticarcinogenesis Action of BHT

A discussion of the lung tumor-enhancing properties of BHT would not be complete without mentioning that in other experimental systems BHT has been found to have the opposite effect. Addition of BHT to a diet containing benzo[*a*]pyrene,[73] or prefeeding mice with BHT prior to administration of dimethylhydrazine[74] or diethylnitrosamine[75] significantly reduced the incidence of tumors in the gastrointestinal tract. BHT also inhibited tumorigenesis in mouse skin[76] and in rat mammary glands.[73] BHT can thus protect against chemical carcinogenesis, as do several other antioxidants.[77]

The observations that BHT may protect against or enhance tumor formation are not necessarily mutually exclusive. In all experiments in which a protective effect of BHT was found, BHT was administered prior to or concomitantly with the carcinogen. BHT is a good inducer of mixed-function oxidases in liver and probably also in other tissues.[32,56] It may thus shift pathways of metabolism towards more efficient detoxification of a chemical.[78] It may, however, act differently once cells have been initiated by a carcinogen. This is best exemplified by comparing two studies which examined the effects of BHT on 2-acetylaminofluorene-induced carcinogenesis in rat liver. In animals prefed with BHT, protection was found.[79] In another study acetylaminofluorene was given first, followed by administration of BHT in the diet. BHT substantially enhanced tumor formation.[80] The temporal sequence of exposure to a carcinogen and BHT may therefore be crucial in determining the biological response. Furthermore, the observations by Peraino et al.[80] show that BHT has promoting capabilities in organs other than mouse lung. Recent studies with an in vitro system support this view.[81]

VI. CONCLUSIONS

There is now good experimental evidence to show that several elements of two-stage carcinogenesis apply to the development of lung tumors in mice. At least three agents which have been identified as promoters in skin, urinary bladder, and liver will also enhance tumor formation in lung: phorbol,[41] saccharin,[44] and BHT.[1,2,82]

The most extensive observations on enhancement of lung tumor formation have been made with BHT. It fulfills most criteria of a typical promoting agent. BHT is effective only if animals are treated after exposure to an initiating agent, but not if they are treated beforehand.[2] Administration of BHT can be delayed up to 5 months after urethan treatment and still enhance tumor formation.[34] BHT enhances lung tumor formation regardless of its route of administration (i.p. injection,[2] gavage,[38] or ingestion in the diet[31]). The lowest dose of BHT required to produce an effect has not yet been determined. Finally, in at least one mouse strain, BHT also enhances tumor formation in animals treated with 3-methylcholanthrene or diethylnitrosamine.[40,84]

On the other hand, no evidence is available yet to show that BHT would enhance tumor development in animals treated with subcarcinogenic doses of an initiating compound. Nor has it been possible to produce more tumors with BHT in mouse strains which respond poorly to urethan.[3] The question has not been resolved whether BHT accelerates growth of preformed tumors only or whether it induces the formation of more tumors. BHT does not fulfill all the criteria usually set for promoters in the skin tumor model. Nevertheless, we think that the data on the effects of BHT on mouse lung tumor development have broadened the concept of two-stage carcinogenesis. Evidence for initiation-promotion is now available for such epithelial tissues as liver, colon, stomach, urinary bladder, and mammary gland. No promoting agent in any of these systems fulfills strictly all criteria usually reserved for skin promoters. This may make it necessary to adopt less rigid criteria as to what constitutes a "true" two-stage carcinogenesis system. Two-stage carcinogenesis is an important concept. Much information can be gained from it in discovering general principles underlying the biological response to multichemical exposure. Two-stage carcinogenesis is an excellent example to study and to document the role of chemical interactions when exposure to two or more agents is separated in time.

The mechanism of action of BHT in the mouse lung tumor model is not clear. The original hypothesis was that BHT enhanced tumor formation by repeatedly pushing the target cells for urethan into mitosis.[1] Newer data make this assumption rather unlikely.[34,40] Unfortunately, the mouse tumor system has several drawbacks which make mechanistic studies difficult. In the classical skin tumor system, kinetic data on time of appearance of tumors, increase in number of tumors with time, and biological characteristics of tumors may be obtained by continuous observation of the animals. To obtain similar data on lung tumors, animals would have to be killed serially; this would be economically prohibitive. Even in highly inbred and highly susceptible mouse strains, a substantial variation in the incidence of tumors is found after treatment with urethan. A large number of experimental animals are required to demonstrate a significant difference in tumor multiplicity between controls and BHT-treated animals, since in all experiments done so far, the difference in tumor multiplicity between controls and treated animals was usually only two- to threefold. Studies of the effect of BHT at a mechanistic level will not be easily accomplished. The lung is a very heterogeneous tissue composed of over 40 different cell types, and studies on isolated cell populations present technical difficulties. Moreover, the cells of origin of lung tumors in mice are not known with certainty yet and may be different in various strains.

A last consideration of enhancement of lung tumor formation in mice by BHT and other compounds relies on a more practical aspect, carcinogenesis testing. The mouse skin system has been refined so that it is possible to assay for complete carcinogens, initiators, cocarcinogens, promoters, and even copromoters. The mouse lung tumor system so far has been used only as a screening assay for complete carcinogens.[4] Its use as such may be expanded by including BHT as a possible promoting agent. This seems feasible by incorporating BHT in the diet. Evidence, although limited, is also available to show that the lung tumor system detects promoting agents other than BHT. The potential use of the lung tumor system as a screening test for promoters needs to be evaluated further.

REFERENCES

1. **Witschi, H. P., Williamson, D., and Lock, S.,** Enhancement of urethan tumorigenesis in mouse lung by butylated hydroxytoluene, *J. Natl. Cancer Inst.*, 58, 301, 1979.
2. **Witschi, H. P. and Lock, S.,** Enhancement of adenoma formation in mouse lung by butylated hydroxytoluene, *Toxicol. Appl. Pharmacol.*, 50, 391, 1979.
3. **Boutwell, R. K.,** The function and mechanism of promoters of carcinogenesis, *CRC Crit. Rev. Toxicol.*, 2, 419, 1974.
4. **Shimkin, M. B. and Stoner, G. D.,** Lung tumors in mice: application to carcinogenesis bioassay, *Adv. Cancer Res.*, 21, 1, 1975.
5. **Witschi, H. P. and Côté, M. G.,** Biochemical pathology of lung damage produced by chemicals, *Fed. Proc.*, 35, 89, 1976.
6. **Slaga, T. J., Ed.,** *Mechanisms of Tumor Promotion*, Vols. I—III, CRC Press, Boca Raton, Fla., in press.
7. **Fry, R. J. M. and Witschi, H. P.,** Lung tumors in mice, in *Carcinogenicity, Mutagenicity and Other Short Term Tests*, Douglas, J. F., Ed., Humana Press, Clifton, N.J., in press.
8. **Amaral-Mendes, J. J.,** Histopathology of primary lung tumors in the mouse, *J. Pathol.*, 97, 415, 1969.
9. **Brooks, R. E.,** Pulmonary adenomas of strain A mice: an electron microscopic study, *J. Natl. Cancer Inst.*, 41, 719, 1968.
10. **Snyder, C., Malone, B., Nettesheim, P., and Snyder, F.,** Urethan-induced pulmonary adenomas as a tool for the study of surfactant biosynthesis, *Cancer Res.*, 33, 2437, 1973.
11. **Adamson, I. Y. R. and Klass, D. J.,** Effects of prednisolone on the differentiation of mouse lung adenomas in culture, *Cancer Res.*, 36, 1669, 1976.
12. **Stoner, G. D., Kikkawa, Y., Kniazeff, A. J., Miyai, K., and Wagner, R. M.,** Clonal isolation of epithelial cells from mouse lung adenoma, *Cancer Res.*, 35, 2177, 1975.
13. **Kauffman, S. L., Alexander, L., and Sass, L.,** Histologic and ultrastructural features of the Clara cell adenoma of the mouse lung, *Lab. Invest.*, 40, 708, 1979.
14. **Sato, K. and Kauffman, S. L.,** A scanning electron microscopic study of the type II and Clara cell adenoma of the mouse lung, *Lab. Invest.*, 43, 28, 1980.
15. **Shimkin, M. B. and Polissar, M. J.,** Some quantitative observations on the induction and growth of primary pulmonary tumors in strain A mice receiving urethan, *J. Natl. Cancer Inst.*, 16, 75, 1955.
16. **Yuhas, J. M.,** Radiotherapy of experimental lung tumors in the presence and absence of a radioprotective drug, S-2-(3-aminopropylamino)ethylphosphorthioic acid (WR-2721), *J. Natl. Cancer Inst.*, 50, 69, 1973.
17. **Marino, A. A. and Mitchell, J. T.,** Lung damage in mice following intraperitoneal injection of butylated hydroxytoluene, *Proc. Soc. Exp. Biol. Med.*, 140, 122, 1972.
18. **Witschi, H. P. and Saheb, W.,** Stimulation of DNA synthesis in mouse lung following intraperitoneal injection of butylated hydroxytoluene, *Proc. Soc. Exp. Biol. Med.*, 147, 690, 1974.
19. **Hirai, K. I., Witschi, H. P., and Côté, M. G.,** Electron microscopy of butylated hydroxytoluene-induced lung damage in mice, *Exp. Mol. Pathol.*, 27, 295, 1977.
20. **Adamson, I. Y. R., Bowden, D. H., Côté, M. G., and Witschi, H. P.,** Lung injury induced by butylated hydroxytoluene. Cytodynamic and biochemical studies in mice, *Lab. Invest.*, 36, 26, 1977.

21. **Williamson, D., Esterez, P., and Witschi, H. P.,** Studies on the pathogenesis of butylated hydroxytoluene-induced lung damage in mice, *Toxicol. Appl. Pharmacol.*, 43, 577, 1978.
22. **Witschi, H. P., Kacew, S., Tsang, B., and Williamson, D.,** Biochemical parameters of BHT-induced cell growth in mouse lung, *Chem. Biol. Interact.*, 12, 29, 1976.
23. **Malkinson, A. M.,** Prevention of butylated-hydroxytoluene-induced lung damage in mice by cedar terpene administration, *Toxicol. Appl. Pharmacol.*, 49, 551, 1979.
24. **Smith, L. J., Kaplan, H. B., and Brody, J. S.,** Response of normal and beige mouse alveolar type 2 cells to lung injury, *Am. Rev. Respir. Dis.*, 122, 942, 1980.
25. **Smith, L. J. and Brody, J. S.,** Influence of corticosteroids on mouse alveolar type 2 cell response to acute lung injury, *Am. Rev. Respir. Dis.*, 123, 459, 1981.
26. **Larsen, J. C. and Tarding, F.,** Stimulation of DNA synthesis in mouse and rat lung following administration of butylated hydroxytoluene, *Arch. Toxicol.*, Suppl. 1, 147, 1978.
27. **Omaye, S. T., Reddy, K. A., and Cross, C. E.,** Effect of butylated hydroxytoluene and other antioxidants on mouse lung metabolism, *J. Toxicol. Environ. Health*, 3, 829, 1977.
28. **Kuo, J. F., Brackett, N. L., Stubbs, J. W., Shoji, M., and Helfman, D.,** Involvement of cyclic nucleotide systems in enlarged mice lungs produced by butylated hydroxytoluene, *Biochem. Pharmacol.*, 27, 1671, 1978.
29. **Kehrer, J. P. and Witschi, H. P.,** Effects of drug metabolism inhibitors on butylated hydroxytoluene-induced pulmonary toxicity in mice, *Toxicol. Appl. Pharmacol.*, 53, 333, 1980.
30. **Saccone, G. T. P. and Pariza, M. W.,** Effects of dietary butylated hydroxytoluene and phenobarbital on the activities of ornithine decarboxylase and thymidine kinase in rat liver and lung, *Cancer Lett.*, 5, 145, 1978.
31. **Witschi, H. P.,** Enhancement of tumor formation in mouse lung by dietary butylated hydroxytoluene, *Toxicology*, 21, 95, 1981.
32. **Gilbert, D. and Golberg, L.,** BHT-oxidase. A liver microsomal enzyme induced by the treatment of rats with butylated hydroxytoluene, *Food Cosmet. Toxicol.*, 5, 481, 1967.
33. **Mirvish, S.,** The carcinogenic action and metabolism of urethan and *N*-hydroxyurethan, *Adv. Cancer Res.*, 11, 1, 1968.
34. **Witschi, H. P. and Kehrer, J. P.,** Adenoma development in mouse lung following treatment with possible promoting agents, *J. Am. Coll. Toxicol.*, 1, 171, 1982.
35. **Stoner, G. D., Shimkin, M. B., Kniazeff, A. J., Weisburger, J. H., and Weisburger, E. K.,** Test for carcinogenicity of food additives and chemotherapeutic agents by the pulmonary tumor response in strain A mice, *Cancer Res.*, 33, 3069, 1973.
36. *Fed. Reg.*, 42, 27603, 1977.
37. National Cancer Institute, Bioassay of butylated hydroxytoluene (BHT) for possible carcinogenicity, in Carcinogenesis, Tech. Rep., Ser. No. 150, 1979 (CAS No. 128-37-0, NCI-CG-TR-150), U.S. Department of Health, Education and Welfare, Washington, D.C., 1979.
38. **Witschi, H. P. and Lock, S.,** Toxicity of butylated hydroxytoluene in mouse following oral administration, *Toxicology*, 9, 132, 1978.
39. **Clapp, N. K., Tyndall, R. L., Cumming, R. B., and Otten, J. A.,** Effects of butylated hydroxytoluene alone or with diethylnitrosamine in mice, *Food Cosmet. Toxicol.*, 12, 367, 1974.
40. **Witschi, H. P., Hakkinen, P. J., and Kehrer, J. P.,** Modification of lung tumor development in A/J mice, *Toxicology*, 21, 37, 1981.
41. **Armuth, V. and Berenblum, I.,** Systemic promoting action of phorbol in liver and lung carcinogenesis in AKR mice, *Cancer Res.*, 32, 2259, 1972.
42. **Goerttler, K., Loehrke, H., Schweizer, J., and Hesse, B.,** Systemic two-stage carcinogenesis in the epithelium of the forestomach of mice using 7,12-dimethylbenz(*a*)anthracene as initiator and the phorbol ester 12-*0*-tetradecanoylphorbol-13-acetate as promoter, *Cancer Res.*, 39, 1293, 1979.
43. **Hicks, R. M., Chowaniec, J., and Wakefield, J. St. J.,** Experimental induction of bladder tumors by a two stage system, in *Carcinogenesis — A Comprehensive Survey*, Vol. 2, Slaga, T. J., Sivak, A., and Boutwell, R., Eds., Raven Press, New York, 1978, 475.
44. **Theiss, J. C., Arnold, L. J., and Shimkin, M. B.,** Effect of commercial saccharin preparations on urethan-induced lung tumorigenesis in strain A mice, *Cancer Res.*, 40, 4322, 1980.
45. **Cohen, S. S.,** Tumor promotion in bladder carcinogenesis, in *Mechanisms of Tumor Promotion*, Vol. 2, Slaga, T. J., Ed., CRC Press, Boca Raton, Fla., 1983, chap. 6.
46. **Steele, V. E., Klein-Szanto, A. J. P., and Nettesheim, P.,** Tumor promotion in respiratory carcinogenesis, in *Mechanisms of Tumor Promotion*, Vol. 2, Slaga, T. J., Ed., CRC Press, Boca Raton, Fla., 1983, chap. 4.
47. National Research Council, Health Effects of Exposure to Diesel Exhaust, Report of the Health Effects Panel of the Diesel Impact Study Committee, National Academy of Sciences, Washington, D.C., 1981, 87.

48. **Adamson, I. Y. R. and Bowden, D. H.,** The type 2 cell as progenitor of alveolar epithelial regeneration: a cytodynamic study in mice after exposure to oxygen, *Lab. Invest.*, 30, 35, 1974.
49. **Heston, W. E. and Pratt, A. W.,** Effect of concentration of oxygen on occurrence of pulmonary tumors in strain A mice, *J. Natl. Cancer Inst.*, 22, 707, 1959.
50. **DiPaolo, J. A.,** Influence of altered atmospheric oxygen on urethan-induced pulmonary tumors in mice, *J. Natl. Cancer Inst.*, 23, 535, 1959.
51. **DiPaolo, J. A.,** Effects of oxygen concentration on carcinogenesis induced by transplacental exposure to urethan, *Cancer Res.*, 22, 299, 1962.
52. **Mori-Chavez, P.,** Lung tumors induced at high altitude by urethan (ethyl carbamate) in strain A mice, *J. Natl. Cancer Inst.*, 29, 945, 1962.
53. **Daniel, J. W.,** The safety of antioxidants — fact or fallacy, in *Impact of Toxicology on Food Processing*, Ayres, J. C. and Kirschman, J. C., Eds., AVI Publishing, Westport, Conn., 1981.
54. **Takahashi, O. and Hiraga, K.,** Dose-response of hemorrhagic death by dietary butylated hydroxytoluene (BHT) in male rats, *Toxicol. Appl. Pharmacol.*, 43, 399, 1978.
55. **Suzuki, H., Hakao, T., and Haraja, K.,** Vitamin K deficiency in male rats fed diets containing butylated hydroxytoluene (BHT), *Toxicol. Appl. Pharmacol.*, 50, 261, 1979.
56. **Gilbert, D. and Golberg, L.,** Liver response tests, liver enlargement and stimulation of microsomal producing enzyme activity, *Food Cosmet. Toxicol.*, 3, 417, 1965.
57. **Scully, M. F., Bray, P. J., and Nievel, J. G.,** Early interaction of radioactive butylated hydroxytoluene with protein factors of varying stability in rat liver, related to the onset of sequential biochemical changes leading to the induction of drug-metabolizing enzymes and liver enlargement, *Biochem. Soc. Trans.*, 4, 526, 1976.
58. **Shaw, Y. S. and Chen, C.,** Ring hydroxylation of di-*t*-butylhydroxytoluene by rat liver microsomal preparations, *Biochem. J.*, 128, 1285, 1972.
59. **Nakagawa, H., Hiraja, K., and Suga, T.,** Biological fate of butylated hydroxytoluene (BHT); binding in vivo of BHT to macromolecules of rat liver, *Chem. Pharm. Bull. (Tokyo)*, 27, 442, 1979.
60. **Yamamoto, K., Tajima, K., and Miyatami, T.,** The acute toxicity of butylated hydroxytoluene and its metabolites in mice, *Toxicol. Lett.*, 6, 173, 1980.
61. **Hakkinen, P. J. and Witschi, H. P.,** unpublished observations, 1980.
62. **Surak, G. J., Bradley, R. L., Branen, A. L., Ribelin, W. E., and Shrago, E.,** Effects of butylated hydroxytoluene on *Tetrahymena pyriformis Food Cosmet. Toxicol.*, 14, 541, 1971.
63. **Epstein, S. S., Saporoschetz, I. B., and Hutner, S. H.,** Toxicity of antioxidants to *Tetrahymena pyriformis J. Protozool.*, 14, 238, 1967.
64. **Milner, S. M.,** Effects of the food additive butylated hydroxytoluene on monolayer cultures of primate cells, *Nature (London)*, 216, 557, 1967.
65. **Leslie, S. W., Gad, S. C., and Acosta, D.,** Cytotoxicity of butylated hydroxytoluene and butylated hydroxyanisole in cultured heart cells, *Toxicology*, 10, 281, 1978.
66. **Sciorra, L. J., Maier, R., Thompson, S., and Kaufmann, B. H.,** An analysis of the uncoiling effect of a BHT-Tween 80/absolute ethanol mixture on Velban® arrested human metaphase cells, *Cytologia*, 41, 63, 1976.
67. **Sciorra, L. J., Kaufmann, B. N., and Maier, R.,** The effects of butylated hydroxytoluene on the cell cycle and chromosome morphology of phytohaemagglutinin-stimulated leucocyte cultures, *Food Cosmet. Toxicol.*, 12, 33, 1974.
68. **Eletr, S., Williams, M. A., Watkins, T., and Keith, A. D.,** Perturbations of the dynamics of lipid alkyl chains in membrane systems: effect on the activity of membrane-bound enzymes, *Biochim. Biophys. Acta*, 339, 190, 1974.
69. **Snipes, W., Person, S., Keith, A., and Cupp, J.,** Butylated hydroxytoluene inactivates lipid-containing viruses, *Science*, 188, 64, 1975.
70. **Brogh, M., Jr.,** Butylated hydroxytoluene protects chickens exposed to Newcastle disease virus, *Science*, 197, 1291, 1977.
71. **Clapp, N. K., Satterfield, L. C., and Bowles, N. D.,** Effect of the antioxidant butylated hydroxytoluene (BHT) on mortality in BALB/c mice, *J. Gerontol.*, 34, 497, 1979.
72. **Slaga, T. J., Sivak, A., and Boutwell, R. K.,** *Carcinogenesis — A Comprehensive Survey*, Vol. 2, Raven Press, New York, 1978.
73. **Wattenberg, W.,** Inhibition of carcinogenesis and toxic effects of polycyclic hydrocarbons by phenolic antioxidants and ethoxyquin, *J. Natl. Cancer Inst.*, 48, 1425, 1972.
74. **Clapp, N. K., Bowles, N. D., Satterfield, L. C., and Klima, W. C.,** Selective protective effect of butylated hydroxytoluene against 1,2-dimethylhydrazine carcinogenesis in BALB/c mice, *J. Natl. Cancer Inst.*, 63, 1081, 1979.
75. **Clapp, N. K., Tyndall, R. L., Klima, W. C., and Bowles, N. D.,** Selective sex-related modification of diethylnitrosamine-induced carcinogenesis in BALB/c mice by concomitant administration of butylated hydroxytoluene, *J. Natl. Cancer Inst.*, 61, 177, 1978.

76. **Slaga, T. J. and Bracken, W. M.,** The effects of antioxidants on skin tumor initiation and aryl hydrocarbon hydroxylase, *Cancer Res.*, 37, 1631, 1977.
77. **Wattenberg, L. W.,** Inhibition of chemical carcinogenesis, *J. Natl. Cancer Inst.*, 60, 11, 1978.
78. **Grantham, P. H., Weisburger, J. H., and Weisburger, E. K.,** Effect of the antioxidant butylated hydroxytoluene (BHT) on the metabolism of the carcinogens *N*-2-fluorenylacetamide and *N*-hydroxy-*N*-2-fluorenylacetamide, *Food Cosmet. Toxicol.*, 11, 209, 1973.
79. **Ulland, B. W., Weisburger, J. N., Yamamato, R. S., and Weisburger, E. K.,** Antioxidants and carcinogenesis: butylated hydroxytoluene, but not diphenyl-*p*-phenylenediamine, inhibits cancer induction by *N*-2-fluorenylacetamide and by *N*-hydroxy-*N*-2-fluorenylacetamide in rats, *Food Cosmet. Toxicol.*, 11, 199, 1973.
80. **Peraino, C., Fry, R. J., Staffeldt, E., and Christopher, P.,** Enhancing effects of phenobarbital and butylated hydroxytoluene on 2-acetylaminofluorene-induced hepatic tumorigenesis in the rat, *Food Cosmet. Toxicol.*, 15, 93, 1977.
81. **Trosko, J. E., Yotti, L. P., Warren, S. T., Tushimoto, G., and Chang, C.,** Inhibition of cell-cell communication by tumor promoters, in *Carcinogenesis — A Comprehensive Survey*, Vol. 7, Hecker, E., Fusenig, N. E., Kunz, W., Marks, F., and Thielmann, H. W., Eds., Raven Press, New York, 1982, 565.
82. **Bojān, F., Nagy, A., and Herman, K.,** Effect of butylated hydroxytoluene and paraquat on urethan tumorigenesis in mouse lung, *Bull. Environ. Contam. Toxicol.*, 20, 573, 1978.
83. **Haschek, W. M. and Witschi, H. P.,** unpublished observations.
84. **Witschi, H. P., and Morse, C. C.,** Enhancement of lung tumor formation in mice by dietary butylated hydroxytoluene: dose-time relationships and cell kinetics, *J. Natl. Cancer Inst.*, in press.

Chapter 4

TUMOR PROMOTION IN RESPIRATORY TRACT CARCINOGENESIS

Vernon E. Steele and Paul Nettesheim

TABLE OF CONTENTS

I. INTRODUCTION

The respiratory tract is an organ system which is exposed to a great variety of environmental pollutants. These pollutants are complex mixtures and contain chemicals which, according to classical definitions, can be grouped into initiators (and carcinogens), promoters, and cocarcinogens.[1-5] The basic definitions of an initiator and a promoter do not need to be restated in this chapter, but the term promoter as opposed to cocarcinogen needs to be defined for the purpose of this presentation. A promoter enhances tumor induction synergistically when given after an initiator;[6] a cocarcinogen does so when given simultaneously with the initiator. Obviously this is a simplistic, operational definition. Various cocarcinogenic effects in respiratory carcinogenesis have been reviewed and will not be dealt with here.[7-9]

What evidence is there for tumor promotion in human lung carcinogenesis? There is no direct proof that it occurs based on human data, since the tumor enhancement observed in certain situations (see below) could very well be all due to cocarcinogenic mechanisms. Because of this, animal and cell culture models have been designed to delineate the cocarcinogenic and promotion processes. Human epidemiological studies will almost certainly not allow the detection of promotional effects as defined by animal model systems in the laboratory. We can only look for more than additive effects of environmental agents in humans, and then examine them more closely in animal model systems. In this chapter, we will review: (1) human lung cancer studies in which synergistic effects of two types of exposures occur, and where reasons exist to suspect that the synergism may be due to promotion, and (2) animal and tissue culture systems model systems which have been used to examine tumor promotion and its possible mechanisms.

II. ENHANCEMENT OF RESPIRATORY TRACT TUMORS IN HUMANS

A. Asbestos Exposure and Tobacco Smoke

In the late 1960s epidemiologists studied the causes of death of asbestos workers over a 20-year period and concluded that cigarette smoking increased their risk of dying from bronchogenic carcinomas by 8-fold over that of nonsmoking asbestos workers, and 92-fold over that of nonsmoking nonasbestos workers.[10-12] In a more recent and larger study, the mortality ratio of asbestos workers with a history of smoking to asbestos workers who did not smoke regularly was 7:1.[13] The mortality ratio decreased with decreasing number of cigarettes smoked per day and with increasing numbers of years since cessation of smoking. The question which arose during this study was whether exposure to asbestos dust and cigarette smoking act independently or synergistically in causing death from lung cancer. In smoking asbestos workers, the lung cancer death rate was 602 per 100,000 man years or 590 lung cancer deaths above the background rate of nonsmoking, nonasbestos workers (Table 1). If one adds the death rates of nonsmoking asbestos workers (111) and of smoking nonasbestos workers (47), the figure is 158 lung cancer deaths per 100,000 man years. This is the calculated lung cancer death rate if asbestos and smoking effects were strictly additive and if no synergism were to exist. The difference of 432 lung cancer deaths (590 deaths minus 158 deaths) is due to the synergism of asbestos and cigarette smoke exposure which may very well be promotional in nature (see below).

A similar study of male and female asbestos workers in London examined their smoking histories and deaths from lung cancer.[14] The lung cancer death rate in women also suggested synergistic or multiplicative interactions between asbestos and tobacco smoke. However, this greater than additive effect was not seen in males. This may be because of the low number (6%) of nonsmokers in the male group. Overall, the findings existing to date strongly support the synergistic interaction of asbestos and cigarette smoking in induction of lung cancer.

Table 1
LUNG CANCER DEATH RATES IN ASBESTOS AND NONASBESTOS WORKERS WHO ARE SMOKERS OR NONSMOKERS

Lung Cancer

Asbestos worker	Cigarette smoker	Death rate[a]	Excess deaths	Relative risk[b]
No	No	11.3	0	1.0
Yes	No	58.4	+47.1	5.2
No	Yes	122.6	+111.3	10.9
Yes	Yes	601.6	+590.3	53.2

[a] Rate per 100,000 man years.

[b] Represents each death rate divided by the rate for nonasbestos nonsmoker controls.

Modified from Hammond, E. C., Selikoff, I. J., and Seidman, H.

B. Uranium Ore Dust and Tobacco Smoke

An excess respiratory cancer rate has also been found in underground uranium miners who smoke cigarettes.[15] Of the 62 lung cancer deaths, 52 were in excess of the incidence found in the general population. Both smoking and nonsmoking uranium miners had respiratory cancer rates which were higher than that of nonuranium miners. Among white uranium miners, 60 lung cancer deaths were observed for smokers, contrasted with 2 for nonsmokers. This excess of 58 deaths is far above that expected if the effects were simply additive, i.e., 2 plus 15 cancer deaths due to mining and smoking, respectively. When the data from uranium miners are compared to data from hard rock miners, an excess cancer death rate is apparent that also strongly suggests synergism between radiation and cigarette smoke.

A separate study of uranium miners in Uranium City, North Saskatchewan, Canada has revealed a significantly higher incidence of abnormal sputum cytology for smokers who are miners compared to nonmining smokers.[16] Abnormal sputum cytology consisted of moderate and marked atypical cells and cancer cells (classifications which have been previously described[17]). Such cells suggest different stages in a progression to invasive carcinoma.[18] The probability of smoking miners having abnormal sputum cytology was 1.7 times higher than expected if the effects of mining and smoking were simply additive.

C. Nickel and Asbestos Exposure

In an early study, the distribution of respiratory cancer in nickel workers did not appear to correlate with exposure to nickel alone, but rather correlated with "total dust" in mining areas and smelters.[19] The excess risk of developing lung and nasal sinus cancers seemed to be found only in nickel mining-refining employees, not in nickel metal working employees.

Recently it has been found that in nickel ore samples from mines where smelter workers suffer from unusually high incidences of respiratory cancers, the nickel ore is heavily contaminated with crysotile asbestos.[20] Dust control previously instituted in smelters has sharply reduced the incidence of cancer among workers. It is likely that the combination of nickel and asbestos is responsible for the unusually high lung cancer rate, and that this represents another case of synergistic interaction of two agents in human respiratory cancer.

From these data on human studies it is difficult to judge what the mechanism underlying the above-additive cancer rates is, and whether or not tumor promotion is involved in any of these situations. In the cases involving asbestos, a promotional mechanism may seem likely since asbestos by itself is not known to induce bronchogenic carcinoma in humans. However, it is equally possible that asbestos acts as a cocarcinogen by adsorbing carcinogens and acting as a "carrier" for it, as discussed in the following text.

III. ANIMAL MODELS OF TWO-STAGE CARCINOGENESIS

Since humans are potentially exposed to a multitude of carcinogens and promoting agents, the interacting, or promoting effects of these agents are difficult if not impossible to separate and investigate. Therefore, we must rely on animal models with controllable exposures to delineate these processes in order to develop an understanding of the contributions of various agents to the overall process of carcinogenesis. Several current model systems used to study multistage carcinogenesis in the respiratory system will be discussed.

A. Asbestos and Carcinogen Exposure

Epidemiological evidence as reviewed above shows that asbestos workers who also smoke heavily have a much higher incidence of pulmonary cancer than workers exposed to either agent alone. Since carcinogenic polyaromatic hydrocarbons (PAH) are known to be present in cigarette smoke, several investigators have used these agents in combination with asbestos to establish animal models to study the synergism between the two agents.[21-23] Both Miller et al.[21] and Pylev and Shabad[22] showed that intratracheal injections of asbestos and benzo(a)pyrene combined into rats or hamsters enhanced the lung tumor yield over either agent instilled alone four- to sixfold (Table 2). In another study, Mossman and Craighead[23] showed that 3-methylcholanthrene adsorbed to asbestos has an enhanced tumorigenicity in exposed tracheal explants compared to either agent alone. From these experiments it can be concluded that the animal models can mimic at least some of the synergistic effects between PAHs and asbestos observed in humans.

Several possible mechanisms have been discussed to explain the tumor enhancing effect of asbestos fibers.

1. Adsorption of carcinogens to asbestos fibers may play an important role in any cocarcinogenic effect of the fibers. Harrington and Smith[24] showed that different kinds of asbestos adsorb benzo(a)pyrene to different degrees. In their studies, chrysotile was the most effective adsorbent and amosite was the least effective.
2. Particulates may increase the retention of carcinogens in the airways. Shabad et al.[25] found that India ink particles increased the retention of benzo(a)pyrene (B(a)P) in the lungs of rats after intratracheal injection.
3. Particles may greatly increase the local concentration of a carcinogen in lung tissue.
4. Asbestos fibers may also facilitate uptake of carcinogens into the cells since fibers readily penetrate the epithelial lining.[23] Cellular uptake of polycyclic hydrocarbons is also facilitated by the capacity of asbestos to disperse BP in a monomeric state on its surface and thus increase solubilization on the aqueous phase of the cell.[26]
5. Trace elements associated with asbestos have been shown by Thomson and co-workers[27] to affect the ability of cells to metabolize carcinogens. Such an effect could increase the formation of and prolong the existence of ultimate carcinogenic metabolites.
6. Asbestos fibers alone could act as a direct promoting stimulus. Mossman et al.[28] have shown that asbestos induces several promotion-related enzymes such as ornithine decarboxylase and $Na^+ - K^+$ + ATPase activity in hamster trachea and suggest that asbestos might act as a tumor promoter.

Table 2
INDUCTION OF LUNG CANCER IN RATS BY INTRATRACHEAL INJECTION OF ASBESTOS AND BENZO(A)PYRENE

Treatment	No. animals	No. tumor bearing animals	%
Asbestos (3 × 2 mg)	49	0	0
Benzo(a)pyrene (1 × 5 mg)	19	0	0
Asbestos (1 × 2 mg) + benzopyrene (1 × 5 mg)	11	6	54.5

Modified from Pylev, L. N. and Shabad, L. M.[22]

The first true two-stage carcinogenesis study, in which carcinogen and asbestos were administered sequentially, used the heterotopic tracheal transplant system.[29] Tracheas, transplanted subcutaneously onto the backs of syngeneic hosts, were exposed to 7,12-dimethylbenz(a)anthracene (DMBA) for 4 weeks. At the end of 4 weeks, asbestos was introduced into the tracheas at one tenth the carcinogenic dose. At 29 months the experiment was terminated. The results are shown in Table 3. In the four groups receiving both asbestos and DMBA, grossly invasive carcinomas arose, while only one of the four groups exposed to DMBA only developed tumors (namely the 100 μg DMBA group). This enhancement was by a mechanism not involving the adsorptive properties of the fibers. An explanation for this type of promoting influence is suggested by several studies which show that mucociliary epithelium when exposed to asbestos, either in whole animals or in culture, undergoes extensive necrosis and subsequent regenerative hyperplasia.[30,31] Topping et al.[30] showed that asbestos exposure alone had toxic and severely irritant effects in rat tracheal epithelium. The acute changes were marked: epithelial hyperplasia, hypersecretion, and submucosal inflammation. Manifestations of chronic changes included focal squamous metaplasias, epithelial erosions, and a low incidence of carcinomas. We conclude that the tumor enhancing effect of asbestos fibers has two components: promotional activity and carcinogen carrier function.

B. Radioisotopes and Chemical Carcinogenesis

The carcinogenicity of radionuclides for lung tissue is well documented and was recently reviewed.[32] Several factors synergistically enhance polonium-210-induced lung cancer in animal models.[33] In one such study, hamsters were given intratracheal instillations of ^{210}Po and B(a)P simultaneously or sequentially at low levels.[34] Administration of the two agents simultaneously led to an additive effect, but no clear evidence of any synergistic interaction was observed (Table 4). In contrast, sequential administration led to a greater than fourfold enhancement over either agent given alone. These data suggest that agents present in cigarette smoke might act synergistically with radon daughters to enhance the formation of lung tumors in uranium miners. However, since both agents are carcinogens, it is difficult to determine whether one is observing promotional or syncarcinogenic effects. Other factors present in cigarette smoke or in the uranium mines could act as the promoting stimulus to cells initiated by either ^{210}Po or B(a)P.

C. Chemical Carcinogens and Tumor Promoters

The experiments discussed in the preceding section do not offer unequivocal proof that tumor promotion is a phenomenon occurring in the respiratory tract. One might be studying syncarcinogenesis since all the agents involved are carcinogenic. Therefore, experiments

Table 3
CARCINOMA INCIDENCE IN TRACHEAS EXPOSED TO DMBA AND SUBSEQUENTLY TO ASBESTOS

DMBA (μg)	Asbestos (μg)	No. Tracheas with carcinomas[a] / No. tracheas exposed (%)
0	200	0/40 (0)
12.5	0	1/36 (3)
12.5	200	1/40 (3)
25	0	0/38 (0)
25	200	9/40 (23)
50	0	0/34 (0)
50	200	6/40 (15)
100	0	7/38 (18)
100	200	9/40 (23)

[a] Includes invasive and noninvasive carcinomas.

Modified from Topping, D. C. and Nettesheim, P.[29]

Table 4
INTERACTION BETWEEN POLONIUM POLONIUM-210 AND BENZO(A)PYRENE IN HAMSTER LUNGS

Exposure	No. animals with lung tumors / No. animals at risk	%
Experiment A		
^{210}Po (15 weeks)	19/165	11.5
B(a)P (15 weeks)	5/66	7.6
^{210}Po + B(a)P (given simultaneously for 15 weeks)	33/147	22.4
Experiment B		
^{210}Po (single dose)	1/139	0.7
B(a)P (7 weeks)	*[a]	<4.0
^{210}Po followed sequentially by B(a)P (7 weeks)	23/135	17.0

[a] *Data not shown.

Modified from McGrandy, R. B., Kennedy, A. R., Terzaghi, M., and Little, J. B.[34]

with the classical initiator DMBA and promoter 12-*O*-tetradecanoylphorbol-13-acetate (TPA) were needed to determine whether two-stage carcinogenesis can occur in respiratory tract mucosa. Using the heterotopic transplant model, it was shown[35-37] that exposures to low doses of DMBA followed by the tumor promoter TPA resulted in a greatly increased tumor yield compared to DMBA alone. Table 5 shows the results of two independent studies. In the first study the tumor incidence was more than tripled when TPA was administered following DMBA exposure. In the second study, using a lower initiating DMBA dose, a sevenfold enhancement was observed. In addition, tumors developed much earlier in the tracheas exposed to DMBA and TPA than in tracheas exposed to DMBA only.

Systemic initiation-promotion of lung parenchyma as opposed to trachea-bronchial mucosa has also been demonstrated.[38-41] These studies are presented in Chapter 3 of this volume.

IV. IN VITRO MODELS OF TWO-STAGE CARCINOGENESIS

The study of mechanisms of two or multiple stage carcinogenesis at the cellular and biochemical level requires availability of well-defined culture systems. The development of such systems occurred in essentially three steps: (1) the establishment of organ and cell culture techniques for long-term maintenance of airway epithelium, (2) the demonstration of neoplastic transformation in the in vitro system, and (3) the demonstration of initiation-promotion.

Of the various tracheal culture systems reported in the literature,[42-45] the organ culture-cell culture has been the most successful in terms of neoplastic transformation.[46-48] Tracheal pieces are placed in organ culture under conditions which support maintenance of differentiated epithelium.[42] During this time, the cultures are exposed to the carcinogen. After the end of exposure, the tracheal explants are transferred to a new culture dish and are maintained in an enriched medium which maximizes epithelial outgrowth onto the bottom of the dish (Figure 1). Every 10 to 14 days, the explants are transferred to a new dish. In that way, multiple epithelial outgrowth cultures are established (usually ten outgrowth cultures from each explant), which are considered to be primary cultures. These epithelial cell cultures that are derived from carcinogen-exposed tracheal organ cultures are then examined over subsequent weeks for appearance of various phenotypic changes and the development of neoplastic cell populations.

The most significant changes which develop in cultures derived from carcinogen exposed explants are (1) escape from senescence of primary cultures, (2) appearance of atypical foci (Figure 2), (3) "immortalization", i.e., primary cultures are subculturable and become permanent cell lines, (4) acquisition of anchorage independence of growth, and (5) neoplastic transformation as measured by in vivo tumorigenicity (Table 6). Of these changes, only escape from senescence and appearance of atypical foci require explanation. Primary cultures derived from normal or sham-exposed tracheal explants will continue to proliferate and expand for 2 to 3 weeks after the removal of the explant; however, after that time proliferation ceases and most cultures "senesce" and finally die. In contrast, many of the carcinogen-exposed cultures continue to expand slowly until foci composed of highly proliferative small cells with high nuclear-to-cytoplasmic ratios appear (atypical foci) that grow rapidly and take over the culture. The third phase, subculturability (and immortalization), only occurs when atypical foci develop and reach a certain size.

The key observation made in the transformation studies is that preceding the appearance of neoplastic cells, a change occurs in the cultures which is characterized by escape from "senescence" and immortalization. It is this change which makes it possible to select for the "carcinogen altered" cells that are at an increased risk to become neoplastically transformed.

After it had been learned that neoplastic transformation could be achieved in the explant outgrowth cultures, the same system was used to study two-stage carcinogenesis using *N*-methyl-*N'*-nitro-*N*-nitrosoguanidine (MNNG) and TPA as initiator and promoter, respectively.[50] Concentrations of TPA likely to be effective in such experiments were established in initial studies measuring stimulation of DNA synthesis in tracheal organ cultures by TPA.[48]

In the initiation-promotion studies, tracheal organ cultures were exposed on days 3 and 6 to MNNG and then on days 9, 15, 21, and 27 of culture to TPA (1-hr exposures). Three events were scored: (1) appearance of morphologically altered cells, (2) establishment of

Table 5
TUMOR PROMOTION IN RAT TRACHEAL TRANSPLANTS USING DMBA AS THE INITIATOR AND TPA AS THE PROMOTER

DMBA (μg/pellet)	TPA (μg/pellet)	No. of tracheas at risk	No. of tracheas with carcinomas	%
Experiment 1[a]				
200	100	22	16	73
200	0[b]	20	4	20
0[b]	100	20	0	0
Experiment 2[c]				
100	100	56	19	34
100	0[b]	38	2	5
100	—[d]	26	1	4

[a] Modified from Topping, D. C. and Nettesheim, P.[35]
[b] Blank pellets devoid of DMBA and TPA.
[c] Modified from Klein-Szanto, A. J. P. and Nettesheim, P.[37]
[d] No pellet inserted.

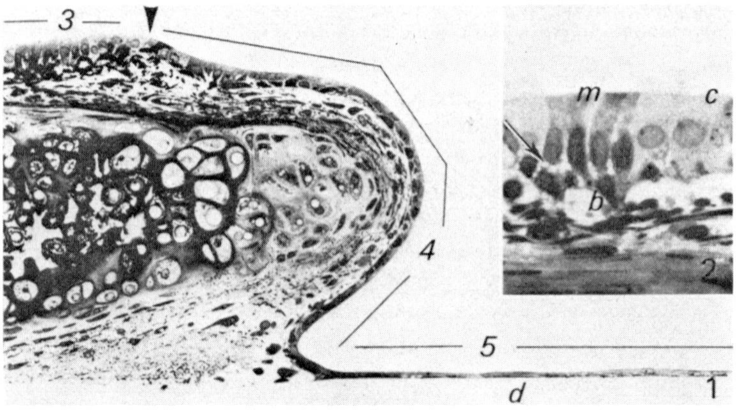

FIGURE 1. Cross section of tracheal explant in outgrowth culture (4 days old). The epithelium extends from the lumenal surface (3) over the cut edge of the explant (4) and onto the culture dish (5) (Magnification × 270). Inset: differentiated cells on the explant. Normal ciliated (c), mucus (m), and basal (b) are observed. Arrow indicates broadened intercellular spaces (Magnification × 1000). (From Heckman, C. A., Marchok, A. C., and Nettesheim, P.[49])

cell line cultures and (3) development of oncogenicity. The MNNG concentration used in these studies was extremely low namely, 0.1 ng/mℓ. Exposure to MNNG alone, TPA alone, and the combination of MNNG and TPA resulted in induction of roughly the same number of cell lines per explant (control cultures yielded none). The first significant difference noted between the treated groups was that in the cultures exposed to both MNNG and TPA, foci

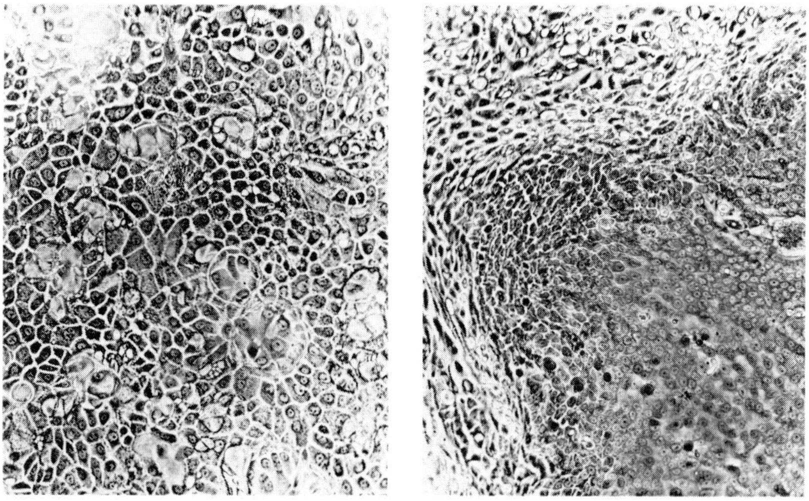

a b

FIGURE 2. (a) Primary tracheal epithelial cell culture from unexposed explant. (b) Focal area of intense mitotic activity and morphologically altered cells (Magnification × 80). (From Steele, V. E., Marchok, A. C., and Nettesheim, P., *Mechanisms of Tumor Promotion and Co-carcinogenesis*, Slaga, T. J., Boutwell, R. K., and Sivak, A., Eds., Raven Press, New York, 291. With permission.)

Table 6
DEVELOPMENT OF ONCOGENICITY IN CELL CULTURES DERIVED FROM CARCINOGEN-TREATED EXPLANTS

	No. of explants[a] producing		
MNNG (μg/mℓ)	Long-term primary cell culture[b]	Cell line culture[c]	Tumorigenic cell line[d]
0	6	0	0
0.001	9	7	5
1.0	10	8	6
10.0	10	10	9

[a] Ten explants were in each group.
[b] Cultures which survived 3 or more weeks following removal of the explant.
[c] Cultures surviving 5 repeated subcultures.
[d] Defined as producing at least one tumor per 4 inoculations of 10^6 cells i.m. into immunosuppressed isogenic hosts.

Modified from Steele, V. E., Marchok, A. C., and Nettesheim, P.[47]

of densely packed atypical cells appeared approximately 2 months earlier than in the cultures exposed to MNNG only (Table 7). In addition, cultures derived from explants, exposed to both initiator and promoter, grew at a considerably faster rate than cultures derived from initiator exposed or from promoter exposed explants; they required only 34 days to be carried from the first to fifth passage while the other cultures required twice that long. Finally,

Table 7
EFFECT OF PROMOTION ON TIME REQUIRED BY TRACHEAL CULTURES TO REACH VARIOUS STAGES IN THE ESTABLISHMENT OF CELL LINES

		Average no. of days ± SE to		
MNNG (ng/mℓ)	TPA (μg/mℓ)	Appearance of atypical foci[a]	First passage[b]	Fifth passage
0	0	—	—	—
0.1	1.0	132 ± 11	167 ± 26	201 ± 33
0	1.0	190 ± 21	312 ± 15	287 ± 22
0.1	0	209 ± 10	242 ± 14	315 ± 12

[a] Atypical foci contained cells with increased nuclear-to-cytoplasmic ratios which were also more rounded and refractile, and had a higher frequency of mitotic figures than cells in control cultures.

[b] The cultures were first passaged when the atypical foci had reached a size of 2 cm in diameter.

Modified from Steele, V. E., Marchok, A. C., and Nettesheim, P.[50]

significantly more transformed cell lines developed from the explants receiving sequential MNNG-TPA treatment and neoplastic transformation became detectable much earlier than in the cultures derived from MNNG exposed explants (150 vs. 365 days) (Table 8). No neoplastic cell lines developed in the cultures derived from TPA treated explants. It seems quite clear that the sequential MNNG-TPA exposures had all the effects characteristic of promotion.

Besides the promotion activity of TPA for rat tracheal epithelium in vitro, the studies established another important finding, namely, that TPA, even though it does *not* cause neoplastic transformation, causes escape of the cultures from senescence and immortalization.[51] This suggests that TPA has some effects which are similar to those of carcinogens while it lacks their capacity to neoplastically transform. Studies to elucidate this immortalization effect of TPA and of carcinogens are currently underway. To date, it has been found that multiple exposures to TPA are much more effective than single exposures in causing this escape from senescence.[52] Of the proposed weak or nonpromoters, phorbol and 4-*O*-methyl-TPA induced immortalization at only low frequencies, while mezerine and acetic acid did not induce it at all (Table 9).

The studies involving organ cultures to study neoplastic transformation have been an important first step in developing epithelial transformation systems. However, the limitations inherent in this approach are related to the lack of quantitation. Therefore, to study the cellular events during neoplastic transformation of epithelial cells quantitatively, a primary tracheal epithelial cell culture system was developed which allows clonal analysis of the events occurring during transformation.[53] Using such cultures, neoplastic transformation was demonstrated with MNNG as the carcinogen.[54,55] The same system is currently being used to investigate the effects of TPA on normal and initiated epithelial cells.[56] Briefly, the method involves plating of freshly isolated tracheal cells on collagen substratum. Control cells exposed to solvent only reach confluency between 1 and 2 weeks, senesce, and exfoliate from the dish. Cells given one or more exposures to MNNG escape the senescence process to progressively grow and acquire immortality. Multiple exposures are more effective than single exposures in inducing cell lines, some of which are tumorigenic in nude mice. Twice

Table 8
THE TUMORIGENICITY OF TRACHEAL EPITHELIAL CELL LINES AT VARIOUS TIMES FOLLOWING INITIATION AND PROMOTION

Days after MNNG exposure	No. of tumorigenic[a] cell lines/No. of cell lines inoculated		
	TPA	MNNG	MNNG + TPA
0—150	0/0	0/0	1/1
151—200	0/0	0/0	3/3
201—250	0/0	0/0	3/4
251—310	0/6	0/2	6/7
311—365	0/14	3/10	8/11

[a] All tumorigenic cell lines produced invasive carcinomas.

Modified from Steele, V. E., Marchok, A. C., and Nettesheim, P.[50]

Table 9
ESTABLISHMENT OF CELL LINES FOLLOWING MULTIPLE EXPOSURE OF TRACHEAL EXPLANTS TO TUMOR PROMOTERS AND NONPROMOTERS

Agent	Concentration[a]	No. cell lines per no. explants exposed	%
Solvent			
DMSO	0.2%	1/15	7
Nonpromoters or weak promoters			
Acetic acid	0.012%	0/8	0
Mezerine	1 μg/mℓ	0/8	0
4-*O*-methyl TPA	1 μg/mℓ	1/9	11
Phorbol	1 μg/mℓ	2/12	17
Strong Promoter			
TPA	1 μg/mℓ	6/8	75
TPA	0.1 μg/mℓ	5/5	100

[a] Four exposures of 1-hr duration were given on days 9, 15, 21, and 27 of culture.

Modified from Steele, V. E., Topping, D. C., and Pai, S. B.[53]

weekly dosing with TPA from day 6 to 30 without prior MNNG exposure leads to the establishment of cell lines.[68] Experiments now in progress show that sequential MNNG and TPA exposures lead to a two- to sevenfold enhancement of colony forming efficiency. We are currently assessing the sensitivity of MNNG exposed cultures to be released by TPA from anchorage dependent growth. The data so far indicate that initiated tracheal epithelial cells have an enhanced responsiveness to TPA.

V. CONCLUSIONS

From the evidence gained through retrospective epidemiological analysis in humans, it is recognized that the etiology of lung cancer is multifactorial in nature. It is now realized that exogenous and possibly endogenous modifiers of carcinogenesis may be important factors in determining cancer incidence in humans. To understand the role of tumor promoters in the induction of respiratory tract neoplasms in humans and to identify specific modifying factors, animal and tissue culture model systems have been developed as described in this chapter. It has been known for a number of years that contaminants of breathing air, such as tobacco smoke, contain promoting agents and substances cocarcinogenic for mouse skin.[2,4,5] What has not been known, however, until recently, is whether the phenomenon of tumor promotion occurs in respiratory tract epithelium, and which substances can act as promoters on this tissue. Only recently, two-stage carcinogenesis studies in vitro and in vivo, have established that the principles of initiation and promotion apply to this tissue also, and that the classical promoter TPA and possibly asbestos have promoting effects on airway mucosa. We do not yet know how promoting substances shorten tumor latency or increase tumor frequency. A common feature of known promoters is their ability to induce cell proliferation and to interfere with normal cell differentiation.[48,57] A number of mechanisms can be envisaged to explain the promoter-induced loss of differentiation and growth controls: (1) following exposure to promoters, cells may act autonomously, because they are making their own growth stimulating substances (autocrine promotion); such substances may also inhibit the differentiation process; (2) promoters may cause cells to become insensitive to growth/differentiation regulating substances (e.g., chalones, retinoids), or (3) local growth restricting forces (e.g., cell-cell interactions) may be disrupted by the promoting agent allowing proliferation of the transformed phenotype in the initiated cells. Similarly, the removal and disruption of initiated tissue from the host animal and placing the cells in vivo or into culture induces rapid cellular proliferation and results in enhanced expression of neoplastic potential.[61-63] Certain pathological conditions may also render ineffective the growth restrictive host controls on initiated cells. Bacteria or viral infections causing tissue damage and cell proliferation have been shown to enhance tumor response.[64,65] Similarly, vitamin A deficiency[66,67] can also lead to enhanced tumor yields. Such conditions also allow or favor the expression of neoplastic potential in initiated cells which might otherwise remain dormant for the life of the animal.

Much remains to be done to understand the role of tumor promotion in respiratory tract carcinogenesis. The tracheal transplant, organ culture, and cell culture systems described here provide a means to study tumor promotion and identify those substances which have a potential to promote respiratory cancer.

REFERENCES

1. **Bock, F. G.,** The nature of tumor-promoting agents in tobacco products, *Cancer Res.*, 28, 2363, 1968.
2. **Van Duuren, B. L., Sivak, A., Langseth, L., Goldschmidt, B. M., and Segal, A.,** Initiators and promoters in tobacco carcinogenesis, *Natl. Cancer Inst. Monogr.*, 28, 173, 1967.
3. **Van Duuren, B. L.,** Tumor promoting agents in two-stage carcinogenesis, *Prog. Exp. Tumor Res.*, 11, 31, 1969.
4. **Van Duuren, B. L., Sivak, A., Katz, C., and Melchionne, S.,** Cigarette smoke carcinogenesis: importance of tumor promoters, *J. Natl. Cancer Inst.*, 47, 235, 1971.
5. **Wynder, E. L. and Hoffman, D.,** *Tobacco and Tobacco Smoke,* Academic Press, New York, 1967.
6. **Berenblum, I.,** A re-evaluation of the concept of cocarcinogenesis, *Prog. Exp. Tumor Res.*, 11, 21, 1969.

7. **Nettesheim, P. and Griesemer, R. A.,** Experimental models for studies of respiratory tract carcinogenesis, in *Pathogenesis and Therapy of Lung Cancer,* Harris, C. C., Ed., Marcel Dekker, New York, 1978, chap. 4.
8. **Nettesheim, P. and Schreiber, H.,** *Advances in Experimental Lung Cancer Research,* Springer-Verlag, Berlin, 1975.
9. **Nettesheim, P., Klein-Szanto, A. J. P., Marchok, A. C., Steele, V. E., Terzaghi, M., and Topping, D. C.,** Studies of neoplastic development in respiratory tract epithelium, *Arch. Pathol. Lab. Med.,* 105, 1, 1981.
10. **Selikoff, I. J., Churg, J., and Hammond, E. C.,** Asbestos exposure and neoplasia, *JAMA,* 188, 22, 1964.
11. **Wagner, J. C.,** Asbestos cancers — guest editorial, *J. Natl. Cancer Inst.,* 64, V, 1971.
12. **Selikoff, I. J., Hammond, E. C., and Churg, J.,** Asbestos exposure and smoking, *JAMA,* 204, 104, 1968.
13. **Hammond, E. C., Selikoff, I. J., and Seidman, H.,** Asbestos exposure, cigarette smoking, and death rates, *Ann. N.Y. Acad. Sci.,* 330, 473, 1979.
14. **Berry, G., Newhouse, M. L., and Turok, M.,** Combined effect of asbestos exposure and smoking on mortality from lung cancer in factory workers, *Lancet,* 2, 476, 1972.
15. **Lundin, F. E., Lloyd, J. W., Smith, E. M., Archer, V. E., and Holaday, D. A.,** Mortality of uranium miners in relation to radiation exposure, hard-rock mining, and cigarette smoking — 1950 through September, 1967, *Health Phys.,* 16, 571, 1969.
16. **Band, P., Feldstein, M., Saccomanno, G., Watson, L., and King, G.,** Potentiation of cigarette smoking and radiation, *Cancer,* 45, 1273, 1980.
17. **Saccomanno, G., Saunders, R. P., Archer, V. E., Auerbach, O., Kuschner, M., and Beckler, P. A.,** Cancer of the lung: the cytology of sputum prior to the development of carcinoma, *Acta Cytol.,* 9, 413, 1965.
18. **Saccomanno, G., Archer, V. E., Auerbach, O., Saunders, R. P., and Brennan, L. M.,** Development of carcinoma of the lung as reflected in exfoliated cells, *Cancer,* 33, 256, 1974.
19. **Godbold, J. H. and Tompkins, E. A.,** A long-term mortality study of workers occupationally exposed to metallic nickel at the Oak Ridge Tennessee USA Gaseous Diffusion Plant, *Occup. Med.,* 21, 799, 1979.
20. **Langer, A. M., Rohl, A. N., Selikoff, I. J., Harlow, G. E., and Prinz, M.,** Asbestos as a cofactor in carcinogenesis among nickel-processing workers, *Science,* 209, 420, 1980.
21. **Miller, L., Smith, W. E., and Berliner, S. W.,** Tests for effect of asbestos on benzo(a)pyrene carcinogenesis in the respiratory tract, *Ann. N.Y. Acad. Sci.,* 132, 489, 1965.
22. **Pylev, L. N. and Shabad, L. M.,** Some results of experimental studies in asbestos carcinogenesis, in *Biological Effects of Asbestos,* Bogovski, P., Timbrell, V., Gilson, J. C., and Wagner, J. C., Eds., International Agency for Research on Cancer, Lyon, 1973, 99.
23. **Mossman, B. T. and Craighead, J. E.,** Use of hamster tracheal organ cultures for assessing the cocarcinogenic effects of inorganic particulates on the respiratory epithelium, *Prog. Exp. Tumor Res.,* 24, 37, 1979.
24. **Harrington, J. S. and Smith, M.,** Studies of hydrocarbons on mineral dusts, *Arch. Environ. Health,* 8, 453, 1964.
25. **Shabad, L. M., Pylev, L. N., and Kolesnichenko, T. S.,** Importance of the deposition of carcinogens for cancer induction in lung tissue, *J. Natl. Cancer Inst.,* 33, 135, 1964.
26. **Lakowicz, J. R. and Hylden, J. L.,** Asbestos-mediated membrane uptake of benzo(a)pyrene observed by fluorescence spectroscopy, *Nature (London),* 275, 446, 1978.
27. **Thomson, R., Webster, I., and Kilroe-Smith, T. A.,** The metabolism of benzo(a)pyrene in rat liver microsomes: the effect of asbestos-associated metal ions and pH, *Environ. Res.,* 7, 149, 1974.
28. **Mossman, B. T., Landesman, J. M., and Craighead, J. E.,** Asbestos stimulates ornithine decarboxylase (ODC) activity in hamster tracheal epithelial cells, *J. Cell Biol.,* 87, 307, 1980.
29. **Topping, D. C. and Nettesheim, P.,** Two stage carcinogenesis studies with asbestos in Fischer 344 rats, *J. Natl. Cancer Inst.,* 65, 627, 1980.
30. **Topping, D. C., Nettesheim, P., and Martin, D. H.,** Toxic and tumorigenic effects of asbestos on tracheal mucosa, *Environ. Pathol. Toxicol.,* 3, 261, 1980.
31. **Mossman, B. T., Kessler, J. B., Ley, B. W., and Craighead, J. E.,** Interaction of crocidolite asbestos with hamster respiratory mucosa in organ culture, *Lab. Invest.,* 36, 131, 1977.
32. **Kennedy, A. R. and Little, J. B.,** Radiation carcinogenesis in the respiratory tract, in *Pathogenesis and Therapy of Lung Cancer,* Harris, C. C., Ed., Marcel Dekker, New York, 1978, chap. 5.
33. **Little, J. B., Grossman, B. N., and O'Toole, W. E.,** Factors influencing the induction of lung cancer in hamsters by intratracheal administration of ^{210}Po, in *Radionuclide Carcinogenesis,* Saunders, C. L., Busch, R. H., Ballou, J. E., and Mahlum, D. D., Eds., U.S. Atomic Energy Commission, Oak Ridge, Tenn., 1973, 119.

34. **McGrandy, R. B., Kennedy, A. R., Terzaghi, M., and Little, J. B.,** Experimental respiratory carcinogenesis: interaction between alpha radiation and benzo(a)pyrene in the hamster, in *Experimental Lung Cancer. Carcinogenesis and Bioassays,* Karbe, E. and Park, J. F., Eds., Springer-Verlag, Berlin, 1974, 485.
35. **Topping, D. C. and Nettesheim, P.,** Promotion-like enhancement of tracheal carcinogenesis in rats by 12-O-tetradecanoyl-phorbol-13-acetate, *Cancer Res.,* 40, 4352, 1980.
36. **Topping, D. C., Griesemer, R. A., and Nettesheim, P.,** Quantitative assessment of generalized epithelial changes in tracheal mucosa following exposure to 7,12-dimethylbenz(a)anthracene, *Cancer Res.,* 39, 4023, 1979.
37. **Klein-Szanto, A. J. P. and Nettesheim, P.,** unpublished data, 1981.
38. **Armuth, V. and Berenblum, I.,** Systemic promoting action of phorbol in liver and lung carcinogenesis in AKR mice, *Cancer Res.,* 32, 2259, 1972.
39. **Armuth, V. and Berenblum, I.,** Tritiated thymidine as a broad spectrum initiator in transplacental two-stage carcinogenesis with phorbol as promoter, *Int. J. Cancer,* 24, 355, 1979.
40. **Theiss, J. C., Arnold, L. J., and Shimkin, M. B.,** The effect of commercial saccharin preparations on urethan-induced lung tumorigenesis in strain A mice, *Cancer Res.,* 40, 4322, 1980.
41. **Witschi, H. P., Williamson, D., and Lock, S.,** Enhancement of urethan tumorigenesis in mouse lung by butylated hydroxytoluene, *J. Natl. Cancer Inst.,* 58, 310, 1977.
42. **Marchok, A. C., Cone, V., and Nettesheim, P.,** Induction of squamous metaplasia in tracheal organ cultures, *Lab. Invest.,* 33, 451, 1975.
43. **Crocker, T. T., Nielsen, B. I., and Lasnitzki, I.,** Carcinogenic hydrocarbons: effect on suckling rat trachea in organ culture, *Arch. Environ. Health,* 10, 240, 1965.
44. **Lane, B. P. and Miller, S. L.,** Preparation of large numbers of uniform tracheal organ cultures for long-term studies. I. Effects of serum on establishment in culture, *In Vitro,* 12, 147, 1976.
45. **Mossman, B. T. and Craighead, J. E.,** Long term maintenance of differentiated respiratory epithelium in organ cultures. I. Medium composition, *Proc. Soc. Exp. Biol. Med.,* 149, 227, 1975.
46. **Steele, V. E., Marchok, A. C., and Nettesheim, P.,** Transformation of tracheal epithelium exposed *in vitro* to N-methyl-N′-nitro-N-nitrosoguanidine (MNNG), *Int. J. Cancer,* 20, 234, 1977.
47. **Steele, V. E., Marchok, A. C., and Nettesheim, P.,** Oncogenic transformation in epithelial cell lines derived from tracheal explants exposed *in vitro* to N-methyl-N′-nitro-N-nitrosoguanidine, *Cancer Res.,* 39, 3805, 1979.
48. **Steele, V. E., Marchok, A. C., and Nettesheim, P.,** An organ culture-cell culture system for studying multistage carcinogenesis in respiratory epithelium, in *Mechanisms of Tumor Promotion and Co-Carcinogenesis,* Slaga, T. J., Boutwell, R. K., and Sivak, A., Eds., Raven Press, New York, 1978, 289.
49. **Heckman, C. A., Marchok, A. C., and Nettesheim, P.,** Respiratory tract epithelium in primary cultures: concurrent growth and differentiation during establishment, *J. Cell. Sci.,* 32, 269, 1978.
50. **Steele, V. E., Marchok, A. C., and Nettesheim, P.,** Enhancement of carcinogenesis in cultured respiratory tract epithelium by 12-O-tetradecanoylphorbol-13-acetate, *Int. J. Cancer,* 26, 343, 1980.
51. **Steele, V. E., Marchok, A. C., and Nettesheim, P.,** Establishment of epithelial cell lines following exposure of cultured tracheal epithelium to 12-O-tetradecanoylphorbol-13-acetate, *Cancer Res.,* 38, 3563, 1978.
52. **Steele, V. E. and Beeman, D. K.,** Relationships of increased growth capacity and tumor promotion in cultured rat tracheal cells, *In Vitro,* 17, 202, 1981.
53. **Steele, V. E., Topping, D. C., and Pai, S. B.,** Tumor promotion studies in rat tracheal epithelium, *Environ. Health Perspect.,* in press.
54. **Wu, R., Groelke, J. W., Chang, L. H., Porter, M. E., Smith, D., and Nettesheim, P.,** Effects of hormones on the multiplication and differentiation of tracheal epithelial cells in culture, in *Growth of Cells in Hormonally Defined Media,* Cold Spring Harbor Conf. on Cell Proliferation, Sirbasku, D., Sato, G. H., and Pardee, A., Eds., Vol. 9, Cold Spring Harbor Laboratory, Cold Spring Harbor, New York, 1982, 641.
55. **Pai, S. B., Steele, V. E., and Nettesheim, P.,** Quantitation of early cellular events during neoplastic transformation of tracheal epithelial cell cultures, submitted, 1982.
56. **Steele, V. E., Beeman, D. K., and Nettesheim, P.,** Altered sensitivity of initiated tracheal epithelial cells to the effects of TPA, *Proc. Am. Assoc. Cancer Res.,* 23, 98, 1982.
57. **Diamond, L., O'Brien, T., and Rovera, G.,** Tumor promoters inhibit terminal differentiation in culture, in *Mechanisms of Tumor Promotion and Co-Carcinogenesis,* Slaga, T. J., Boutwell, R. K., and Sivak, A., Eds., Raven Press, New York, 1978, 335.
58. **Murray, A. W. and Fitzgerald, D. J.,** Tumor promoters inhibit metabolic cooperation in cocultures of epidermal and 3T3 cells, *Biochem. Biophys. Res. Commun.,* 91, 395, 1979.
59. **Yotti, L. P., Chang, C. C., and Trosko, J. E.,** Elimination of metabolic cooperation in Chinese hamster cells by a tumor promoter, *Science,* 206, 1089, 1979.
60. **Newbold, R. F. and Amos, J.,** Inhibition of metabolic cooperation between mammalian cells in culture by tumour promoters, *Carcinogenesis,* 2, 243, 1981.

61. **Medina, D.,** Enhancement of the tumorigenicity of preneoplastic mammary nodule lines by enzymatic dissociation, *J. Natl. Cancer Inst.*, 60, 1121, 1978.
62. **Terzaghi, M. and Nettesheim, P.,** Dynamics of neoplastic development in carcinogen-exposed tracheal mucosa, *Cancer Res.*, 39, 4003, 1979.
63. **Nettesheim, P., Terzaghi, M., and Klein-Szanto, A. J. P.,** Development and progression of neoplastic disease. Morphologic and cell culture studies with airway epithelium, in *Mechanisms of Chemical Carcinogenesis,* Harris, C. C., Ed., A. R. Liss, New York, 1982, 473.
64. **Schreiber, H. P., Nettesheim, P., Lijinsky, R., Richter, C. B., and Wolburg, H. E.,** Induction of lung cancer in germ free, specific-pathogen-free, and infected rats by N-nitrosoheptamethyleneimine: enhancement by respiratory infection, *J. Natl. Cancer Inst.*, 49, 1107, 1972.
65. **Nettesheim, P., Topping, D. C., and Jamasbi, R.,** Host and environmental factors enhancing carcinogenesis in the respiratory tract, *Annu. Rev. Pharmacol. Toxicol.*, 21, 133, 1981.
66. **Nettesheim, P., Snyder, C., and Kim, J. C. S.,** Vitamin A and the susceptibility of respiratory tract tissues to carcinogenic insults, *Environ. Health Perspect.*, 29, 89, 1979.
67. **Nettesheim, P. and Williams, M. L.,** The influence of vitamin A on the susceptibility of the rat lung to 3-methylcholanthrene, *Int. J. Cancer*, 17, 351, 1976.
68. **Steele, V. E., Beeman, D. K., and Nettesheim, P.,** Altered sensitivity of initiated tracheal epithelial cells to the effects of 12-O-tetradecanoylphorbol-13-acetate, manuscript submitted.

Chapter 5

TUMOR PROMOTION IN COLON CARCINOGENESIS

Bandaru S. Reddy

TABLE OF CONTENTS

I. INTRODUCTION

Rapid progress has been made in basic concepts concerning carcinogenesis.[1,2] There are agents which are genotoxic, which by definition interact with the gene to yield an abnormal genetic material. In the classic Berenblum-Shubik terminology, such agents would be considered initiating agents.[1,3] It is thought that cancer causation requires the action of such an agent that alters the genetic material in specific ways. The second broad class of agents acts by epigenetic mechanisms and tends to increase the development of lesions initiated by genotoxic carcinogens. Thus, this list includes cocarcinogens which operate at the same time as genotoxic carcinogens and can alter the metabolism of a genotoxic agent with an increased ratio of activation/detoxification metabolites. Such agents can also act as more classic tumor promoters that exhibit their effect after the action of a genotoxic carcinogen.

During the past 2 decades, epidemiological studies have investigated the influence of environmental factors on the occurrence of cancer of the large bowel. These studies suggest that diets particularly high in total fat and low in certain fibers, vegetables, and micronutrients are generally associated with an increased incidence of large bowel cancer in man.[4-10] Dietary fat may be a risk factor in the absence of factors that are protective, such as use of high fibrous foods and fiber.[7,10,11]

The importance of dietary factors in the development of experimentally induced cancer was realized in connection with the early studies involving carcinogenic azo dye, 4-dimethylaminoazobenzene.[12] Recent studies have demonstrated that diet can affect chemical carcinogenesis at every critical step in the process, namely formation of activated carcinogens, interaction of the activated metabolite with cellular targets, enhanced sensitivity to carcinogens, and expression of initiated tumor cell.[13]

Another way in which diet can affect chemical carcinogenesis is by interfering with the interaction of ultimate carcinogens with cellular macromolecules as proposed by Miller and Miller.[12] In addition, diet can affect carcinogenesis by altering the tissue sensitivity to carcinogens. This hypothesis was studied in experiments aimed at examining the role of diet-induced liver cirrhosis in liver cancer development.[15] Finally, the fact that diet can alter the process of tumor development has been extensively studied in experiments designed to examine the role of dietary fat in mammary and colon tumorigenesis in animal models.[8,16] In these situations, the high-fat diet appears to enhance carcinogenesis through its elevation of agents that act as promoters of tumor development. In many instances, liver and extrahepatic tissue enzymes, which are broadly known as mixed function oxidases (MFO) responsible for the metabolism of a variety of substances such as carcinogens and cocarcinogens and diet-induced endogenous compounds which act as promoters, may be the mediating factors in the relationship between diet and carcinogenesis.[8]

This brief review evaluates current research, both epidemiological and experimental, on the relation between dietary factors and large bowel cancer, including the use of animal models to determine if implicated factors can be modified experimentally. The review also evaluates various initiators and promoters involved in colon carcinogenesis. Finally, it presents an evaluation of the mechanism whereby dietary factors translate to high risk for the development of this important cancer.

II. EPIDEMIOLOGY OF COLON CANCER

A. Inter- and Intracountry Differences

Cancer of the large bowel has been the subject of several epidemiological reviews.[6,17] The major differences in intracountry and intercountry distribution, as well as differences in religious groups having this cancer, have been detailed in recent publications.[10,18,19] In the past, rectal cancer was often considered together with colon cancer as colorectal or large bowel cancer. Current evidence indicates that a distinction needs to be made between colon cancer and rectal cancer.[20] The male/female ratio is about 1:4 for rectal cancer, but is near unity for colon cancer. The difference in incidence of colon cancer between a high-risk country like the U.S. and a low-risk country like Japan is about 4:1, but for the rectal cancer, this difference is merely in the order of 1.1:1, thus suggesting that the etiologies for colon and rectal cancer may be different.

In general, with few exceptions, the more economically developed a society, the greater the incidence of colon cancer, although not necessarily cancer of the rectum. The highest incidence rates are found in North America, New Zealand, and Western Europe, with the exception of Finland where the incidence is one of the lowest in the developed countries. Intermediate rates are found in eastern Europe and the Balkans, and the lowest incidences are found in Africa, Asia, and Latin America (the exception being Uruguay and Argentina, where mortality rates are similar to those found in North America). Marked differences in the age-adjusted incidence rates exist among the four countries in Scandinavia.[21] The rate is highest in Denmark and lowest in Finland. There is also an urban-rural gradient in these countries in that urban populations generally have higher risks than rural populations.[21]

Further evidence for the importance of environmental dietary factors in colon cancer is provided by studies of migrants to the U.S. and Australia from Japan and Poland, respectively.[22,23] Colon cancer incidence is higher in the first and second generation Japanese immigrants to the U.S. and in Polish immigrants to Australia than in native Japanese in Japan and in the native Poles from Poland, respectively. Of equal interest is the fact that in Israel, colon cancer incidence in Jews from Yemen and North Africa is half that of Jews from Europe and North America.[24] Further support for environmental dietary influence in the development of colon cancer is derived from the time-trend in Japan; colon cancer seems to be increasing in Japan itself, a finding consistent with the increasing westernization of the Japanese diet.[25]

Further support for lifestyle in colon cancer risk is derived from studies of special religious groups within a small geographical area. The incidence of colon cancer in Mormons (members of The Church of Jesus Christ of Latter-Day Saints) is lower than other U.S. white population with the exception of Seventh-Day Adventists (SDA).[19] Traditionally, Mormons eat more whole grain breads, fruits, and vegetables.[10] Studies by Phillips et al.[18] indicate that the SDA, who consume less meat and adhere to a lacto-ovo-vegetarian diet, are reported to have about 60% of the colon cancer death rates for total California. Jussawalla and Jain[26] found that the Parsis in Bombay exhibited a higher risk for colon cancer than the other religious groups such as Hindus and Moslems. Since the Parsis lean more toward a Western diet, the dietary habits between these two Indian populations could account for differences in colon cancer rates.

B. Etiological Factors

Cross-national correlations between colon cancer frequency and diet have been used to select from possible hypotheses for testing in case-control and cohort studies. Wynder[27] and Wynder and Reddy[28] proposed that colon cancer incidence is mainly associated with total dietary fat. They further suggested that dietary fat influences the metabolic activity of the gut microflora and thus may be involved in the pathogenesis of cancer of the colon. A world-wide correlation between colon cancer incidence and total fat consumption has been established.[16] Enig et al.[29] examined the fat-cancer relationship in the U.S. and found an equally strong, significant, positive correlation of colon cancer with total fat and vegetable fat; but no correlation was found between animal fat and colon cancer mortality and incidence. Several investigators have shown that the dietary variables chiefly associated with large bowel cancer rates were meat, other animal protein, and total fat.[4,30] These results support a role for total dietary fat in the incidence of colon cancer.

Burkitt[31] recognized the rarity of large bowel cancer in most African populations and suggested that countries consuming a diet rich in fiber have a low incidence of large-bowel cancer, whereas those eating refined carbohydrates with little fiber have a higher incidence of the disease. A recent study comparing populations in Kuopio, Finland (low-risk), Copenhagen, Denmark (high-risk), and New York (high-risk) indicated that one of the factors contributing to the low-risk of colon cancer in Kuopio appears to be high dietary fiber intake.[32,33]

Studies attempting to explain the frequency of large bowel cancer have used both correlation and case-control studies. Wynder et al.[34] conducted a large-scale retrospective study on large-bowel cancer patients in Japan, which suggested a correlation between the westernization of the Japanese diet and colon cancer. Haenszel et al.[22] demonstrated an association between colon cancer and dietary beef in Hawaiian Japanese cases and Hawaiian Japanese controls. A case-control study of cancer of the colon in Canada indicated an elevated risk for those with an increased intake of calories, total fat, and saturated fat.[35] A recent study by Williams et al.[36] using few cases of colon cancer indicated an inverse relationship between colon cancer and serum cholesterol in man.

In case-control studies in Israel and in San Francisco area American blacks, it was found that among a large variety of dietary constituents investigated, those that were lowest in the diets of patients with colon cancer as compared with controls were those containing fiber.[37,38] Bjelke[39] found less frequent use of vegetables among colorectal cancer patients; another case-control study on a series of cases and controls from Roswell Park Memorial Institute at Buffalo, N.Y., showed a lower risk of colon cancer for individuals ingesting vegetables such as cabbage, broccoli, and Brussels sprouts.[48]

The studies cited lead us to accept diet as a major etiological factor in large bowel cancer. Diets high in total fat and low in fiber are associated with an increased incidence of large-bowel cancer in man.

C. Concept of Dietary Factors and Colon Cancer

Aries et al.[41] have suggested that (1) the amount of dietary fat determines the levels of intestinal bile acids and cholesterol metabolites as well as the composition of the gut microflora and (2) the gut microflora metabolize these acid and neutral sterols to carcinogens active in the colon. Investigators have examined the potential carcinogenic activity of certain bile acids because they may be converted to potentially carcinogenic compounds and several bile acids induced sarcomas at the site of injection in experimental animals.[42] It may be noted that such reactions are unlikely to yield carcinogenic compounds from bile salts, but are much more likely to yield products which act as colon tumor promoters or cocarcinogens rather than complete carcinogens. Furthermore, the evidence of oncogenic effect — that several bile acids induce sarcomas at the injection site — does not answer and, in fact, is not relevant to the question whether select bile acids can induce carcinomas in the colon. There is no evidence that bile acids or cholesterol per se can initiate a carcinoma in either man or animals.

The possible mechanism of protective effect of dietary fiber against colon cancer has been the subject of a recent workshop.[43] Dietary fiber has been defined as that part of ingested plant material that is resistant to digestion by the secretions of the gastrointestinal tract. It comprises a heterogeneous group of carbohydrates, including cellulose, hemicellulose and pectin, and a noncarbohydrate substance, lignin.

The protective effect of dietary fiber may be due to adsorption, dilution, or metabolism of cocarcinogens, promoters and yet-to-be-identified carcinogens by the components of the fiber.[11,44,45] Different types of nonnutritive fibers possess specific binding properties. Dietary fiber could also affect the enterohepatic circulation of bile salts.[46] Fiber not only influences bile acid metabolism, thereby reducing the formation of tumor promoters in the colon, but also exerts a solvent-like effect in that it dilutes potential carcinogens and cocarcinogens by its bulking effect and is able to bind bile acids and certain carcinogenic compounds.[11,47,48]

Thus, it has been suggested that (1) the extent of the carcinogenic stress from the exogenous source is probably rather weak, (2) high fat diet alters concentration of bile acids and the activity of gut microflora which may in turn produce tumor-promoting substances from bile acids in the lumen of the colon, (3) certain dietary fibers not only enhance binding of tumorigenic compounds in the gut, but also dilute them so that their effect on the colonic mucosa is minimal, and (4) dietary fat, fiber, and certain vegetables modify the intestinal mucosal as well as hepatic enzyme inhibitors or inducers that alter the capacity of the animal to metabolize the tumorigenic compounds[8,49-51] (Table 1).

D. Dietary Fat and Fiber and Bile Acid Excretion

Studies in man were carried out in our laboratory and elsewhere on the excretion of bile acids in high- and low-risk population for colon cancer development, and to determine whether changes in the diet in terms of fat and fiber can alter the concentration of colonic bile acids. This subject has been reviewed recently.[52,53] Briefly, the population with a high risk for colon cancer have an increased amount of colonic secondary bile acids, namely deoxycholic acid and lithocholic acid, and metabolic activity of gut microflora. In addition, people on a high fat diet appear to have a higher level of fecal secondary bile acids and gut microbial activity compared to those on a low-fat diet. In a recent study, comparison of fecal bile acids was carried out between SDAs who are lacto-ovo-vegetarians, and age- and sex-matched nonSDAs consuming a high-fat, mixed-western diet. The fat intake was 28% lower and fiber intake was 2.5-fold higher in SDAs, but the total protein and calorie consumption was similar between the two groups. The fecal excretion of deoxycholic acid and lithocholic acid was lower in SDAs as compared with nonSDAs.

The effect of dietary fiber on fecal bile acids has been studied in many laboratories. Reddy et al.[33] studied the fecal bile acid excretion in healthy controls of Kuopio (Finland), a low-risk population for colon cancer development. The dietary histories indicate that the total fat and protein consumption in Kuopio is quite similar to the New York population, but the consumption of fiber, mainly cereal type, is threefold higher in Kuopio compare to the New York population. The daily output of feces is three times higher in Kuopio than that of healthy individuals in the U.S. The concentration of fecal secondary bile acids — deoxycholic acid and lithocholic acid — is decreased in Kuopio due to high fecal bulk, but the daily output remained the same in the two groups because the dietary intake of fat is the same in Kuopio and New York. Cummings et al.[54] and Kay and Truswell[55] reported that an increase in wheat bran intake increased the fecal weight and diluted the fecal bile acids. This suggests that increased fecal bulk dilutes suspected carcinogens and promoters that may be in direct contact with large bowel mucosa.

E. Two-Stage Carcinogenesis in Human Colon Cancer

Currently, much of our knowledge of the stages of carcinogenesis is based on experiments concerning the genesis of epidermoid carcinoma in the mouse skin.[3] The major significance of this type of observation is that carcinogenesis occurs as a multistep process in which the first step is possibly mutational and the other(s) can be promoted by a variety of compounds which are not necessarily carcinogenic. Two-stage carcinogenesis in which initiation and promotion are separate events mediated by different agents is distinct from experimental protocols in which a single, high dose of a carcinogen is sufficient to elicit tumor formation without subsequent promoter treatment. With two-stage system of mouse skin carcinogenesis, the first tumors to be observed are papillomas. After continued promoter treatment, malignant

Table 1
MODIFYING FACTORS IN COLON CANCER

Dietary fat[a]	Dietary fibers[a,b]	Micronutrients
Increases bile acid secretion into gut	Certain fibers increase fecal bulk and dilute carcinogens and promoters	(Include vitamins, minerals, anti-oxidants, etc.)
Increases metabolic activity of gut bacteria	Modify metabolic activity of gut bacteria	Modify carcinogenesis at activation and detoxification level
Increases secondary bile acids in colon	Modify the metabolism of carcinogens and/or promoters	Act also at promotional phase of carcinogenesis
Alters immune system		
Stimulation of mixed function oxidase system		

[a] Dietary factors, particularly high total dietary fat and a relative lack of certain dietary fibers and vegetables have a role.
[b] High dietary fiber or fibrous foods may be a protective factor even in the high dietary fat intake.

tumors appear on the skin. Several other model systems that also demonstrate the two distinct stages of carcinogenesis, initiation and promotion, have been reviewed recently.[56] Although for some of the models it is not clear whether the initiator and promoter are acting in the true sense, this model system is not limited to skin, but can be extended to many other species and tissues.[3] The fact that large number and diversity of experimental models proceed through promotion strongly suggests that diet-induced human cancer involves similar stages in the development.

Multistage models derive considerable support from epidemiology, and specific aspects of multistage models for cancer induction can sometimes be tested by epidemiological and metabolic epidemiological observations of populations subject to different doses of carcinogenic (initiating) insult or varying dose rates of promoting insult. For example, epidemiological and metabolic epidemiological investigations have indicated the importance of diet in human colon cancer, and the changes in incidence of colon cancer reflect migration from low-risk regions to regions of high-risk within the same generation.[8] This suggests that (1) the initiating insult for colon cancer is similar in populations in low- and high-risk areas and (2) when the population from low-risk countries migrates to high-risk regions, they follow the dietary practices of adopted countries which often lead to increased levels of promoters in the colon.[8]

There has been considerable controversy over the years as to whether colon adenomas can transform into carcinomas in humans.[57] Generally, there has been no major disagreement regarding the cancer risk of villous adenomas or villous papillomas. However, the cancer risk for simple tubular adenomatous polyps has been unclear. Although most investigators agree that all adenomas are qualitatively potential carcinomas, the quantitative magnitude of the risk for malignant transformation of colon adenomas into adenocarcinomas is a basis for some disagreement. Morson[58] has reported the risk to be 40% for villous adenomas, as compared to a risk of 5% for tubular adenomas and 22% for tubulovillous (mixed-type) adenomas. The potential for malignant transformation has been reported to be greater when the adenoma has more villous features.[59] Morson[58] has also reported a definite correlation of increasing epithelial atypia with increasing malignant potential.

From an epidemiological point of view, the association between adenomatous polyps and colon cancer has been reinforced by the following characteristics: (1) the incidence of adenomatous polyps closely parallels the prevalence of colon cancer in all populations so far studied; (2) in the populations studied, the risk of colon cancer increases with size and multiplicity of polyps, thus suggesting a dose-effect; (3) prospective studies in the U.S. and

Sweden have shown persons with adenomatous polyps to be at higher risk to colon cancer; (4) whites, blacks, and orientals have a lower prevalence of adenomatous polyps while living in areas of low colon cancer frequency, but display high polyp prevalence if they migrate to areas of high colon cancer risk; and (5) there is an inverse socioeconomic gradient found for both conditions (colon cancer and adenomatous polyps) in Cali, Colombia, a city in a developing country that has large social class differences in diet.[6]

The above epidemiological and clinical observations point to the possibility that there are two stages in human colon cancer which probably result from a complex interaction of yet-to-be-identified carcinogens, cocarcinogens, and tumor promoters. The extent of carcinogenic stress is rather weak, and whether or not a given individual is at high risk for colon cancer may depend more on the rather important promoting stimulus from the nutritional factors.

F. Fecal Mutagens (Presumptive Carcinogens)

Until recently, the nature of the carcinogens responsible for colon cancer not only were obscure, but there were no real leads. Recently, Nagao et al.,[60] Commoner et al.,[61] and Weisburger et al.[62] demonstrated the presence of mutagens in fried fish and meat, fried hamburgers, and broiled foods. Because of potential importance of fecal mutagens in the genesis of large bowel cancer and of the possible role of dietary factors in the induction of colon cancer, the fecal mutagenic activity of various population groups with distinct dietary habits and varied colon cancer incidences was determined by several investigators. Ehrich et al.[63] have demonstrated that the stools of South African urban whites who are at high risk for colon cancer development were higher in mutagenic activity with *Salmonella typhimurium* strains TA98 and TA100 without microsomal activation compared to South African urban and rural blacks who are at low-risk. Bruce et al.[64] were the first to show that the feces of some normal humans contained compounds that caused direct mutagenesis in the Ames assay. They have also demonstrated that increased dietary fiber, α-tocopherol, or vitamin C reduced fecal mutagens. Recently, Wilkins et al.[65] demonstrated that the mutagenicity in the ether extracts of feces of certain donors can be increased by anaerobic incubation for about 96 hr and claimed that the major mutagenicity appears to be due to a single type of compound which may be produced by anaerobic bacteria. The structure is believed to be a macrocyclic polyunsaturated compound with hydroxyl groups on the ring, at least one nitrogen function, possibly a phosphate group, one or more carbonyl group, and possibly an epoxide group. Kuhnlein et al.[66] compared fecal mutagens (water extracts) from a group of vegetarians with those from persons on typical North American diets containing meat. On TA100 and TA98, ovo-lacto-vegetarians and strict vegetarians had lower levels of fecal mutagens than nonvegetarians. Correlation studies between the pH of the fecal homogenate and mutagenicity indicate the presence of several fecal mutagens.

Recently, we have studied fecal mutagens of three populations with distinct risk for the development of colon cancer, a high-risk population in New York (nonSDA) consuming a mixed-western diet, a low-risk vegetarian SDAs, and a low-risk population in Kuopio, Finland.[67] Fecal samples of nonSDAs were highly mutagenic in TA98 without microsomal activation, followed by TA100 without activation and TA100 with activation. None of the samples of SDAs tested showed mutagenic activity in any of the tester systems, whereas Kuopio samples exhibited activity only in TA98 with microsomal activation. In general, the fecal extracts of nonSDAs consuming a high-fat mixed-western diet showed a higher mutagenic activity than did volunteers from Kuopio consuming a high-fat/high-fiber diet (Table 2).

It has been reported that certain compounds are noncarcinogenic or mutagenic alone, but enhance the tumorigenic or mutagenic properties of carcinogens and are termed as comutagens.[68-70] We have studied two groups of volunteers, namely SDAs and nonSDAs who

Table 2
MUTAGENIC ACTIVITY OF FECAL SAMPLES COLLECTED FROM HEALTHY MALE SUBJECTS FROM KUOPIO (FINLAND) AND NEW YORK METROPOLITAN AREA[a]

	% Samples with mutagenic ratio greater than 3[b]					
	TA98		TA100		TA98 & TA100	% Samples showing mutagenic activity in at least one test system
Population group	+S9	−S9	+S9	−S9		
New York nonSeventh-Day Adventists (18)	0	22	6	11	11	22
Kuopio (15)	13	0	0	0	0	13
New York Seventh-Day Adventists (11)	0	0	0	0	0	0

[a] Values represent samples which showed a mutagenic ratio of three or more in *Salmonella*/mammalian microsomal assay system.
[b] Mutagenic ratio is the number of his+ revertant colonies on the test plate divided by the number of his+ spontaneous revertant colonies on control plates.
[c] Samples showing activity both in TA98 and TA100 tester systems.

did not show any fecal mutagenic activity in our earlier study.[71] Samples collected from nonSDAs exhibited a significantly higher comutagenic activity in both TA100 and TA98 with S9 activation than did SDAs (Table 3). This is the first demonstration that the fecal samples contain comutagenic activity and that this activity differs in high- and low-risk population for the development of colon cancer.

Based on these studies, it appears that there is more than one specific mutagen present in the feces, and the lesions in somatic cells may be the product of the mutagenic activities of many substances rather than the result of one predominating compound.

III. EXPERIMENTAL STUDIES IN ANIMAL MODELS

A. Initiators of Colon Carcinogenesis

Studies on the mechanisms of colon carcinogenesis have been assisted by the discovery of several animal models that show the type of lesions observed in man.[72] These models are (1) induction of colon cancer in rats through aromatic amines such as 3,2′-dimethyl-4-aminobiphenyl (DMAB) or 3-methyl-4-naphthalamine; (2) derivatives and analogues of cycasin such as methylazoxymethanol (MAM), azoxymethane (AOM), and 1,2-dimethylhydrazine (DMH) in rats and mice of selected strains; and (3) intrarectal administration of direct-acting carcinogens of the type of alkylnitroureas, such as methylnitrosourea (MNU) or *N*-methyl-*N*′-nitro-*N*-nitrosoguanidine (MNNG) that lead to cancer of the descending colon in every species tested so far. The spectrum of lesions obtained is similar to the various types of neoplastic diseases observed in the colon and rectum of humans. The animal models are now being used effectively to study the multiple environmental factors involved in the pathogenesis of large bowel cancer.

B. Two-Stage Carcinogenesis in Colon Cancer Model

On the basis of a quantitative analysis of colon tumor multiplicity in DMH-treated rats, it has been suggested that this carcinogen is capable of producing intestinal tumors via a two-stage mechanism.[73] Each DMH injection induces a first stable and transmissible change in a number of colon epithelial cells. In rats receiving small doses or one single injection of the carcinogen, the number of such pretransformed cells will be limited and so, too, the

Table 3
COMUTAGENIC ACTIVITY OF FECAL EXTRACTS FROM NONSDAS AND SDAS IN *SALMONELLA*/MAMMALIAN MICROSOMAL ASSAY SYSTEM

	Number of his+ revertants/(plate 230—250 mg dry feces)[b]			
	TA98		TA100	
Population group[a]	Without S-9 MNNG-induced	With S9 2-AAF-induced	Without S-9 MNNG-induced	With S9 AAF-induced
NonSDAs (18)	8 ± 4[c]	1832 ± 250[d]	218 ± 98	1157 ± 140
SDAs (16)	7 ± 3	846 ± 106	104 ± 37	627 ± 104

[a] NonSDAs were consuming a high-fat, high-meat diet and SDAs were consuming a vegetarian diet. These two groups were age-matched volunteers from New York metropolitan area and did not exhibit any fecal mutagenic activity in our previous screening.
[b] Comutagenic activity is the number of his+ revertant colonies obtained with the combination of MNNG or 2-AAF and fecal extract minus the number of his+ revertant colonies induced by MNNG or 2-AAF alone.
[c] Mean ± SEM.
[d] Significantly different from SDAs $p<0.01$.

risk of further transformation. Frequent injections of DMH would result in the accumulation of pretransformed cells with a rapidly increasing risk of tumor development. Finally, treated animals would be expected to develop new tumors even at long intervals after the last injection.[73] Using CF_1 mice and DMH, it has also been shown that (1) with increased doses of DMH, there was an increased tumor yield and decreased latency period, (2) with repeated doses, there was a rapidly cumulative tumor yield, and (3) new tumors continued to accumulate in the colon even at long intervals after DMH treatment.[74] Recent study by Maskens[75] also indicates that DMH carcinogenesis in the rat colon is a two-step process. The first change is caused by DMH, the effect of which is additive when similar doses are repeated. This change is transmissible within the renewing mucosa for prolonged periods, and the affected cells have no phenotypic expression in terms of proliferative advantage. The second stage does not require carcinogen exposure, although continued presence of the carcinogen can probably contribute to it.

The above approach to two-stage carcinogenesis in the colon differs from the classical initiation-promotion experiments[3] in which the first step is probably mutational and the other one can be promoted by a variety of agents which are not necessarily carcinogens per se. However, several ways in which promotion could be involved in experimental colon carcinogenesis can be visualized.[75] Factors such as activators of carcinogen metabolism as well as hyperplasia and benign tumor formation will increase the risk of cancer. It has been shown that colon tumorigenesis can be enhanced by such promoters of colon epithelial proliferation as bile acids.

C. Dietary Fat and Colon Carcinogenesis

The stage of carcinogenesis at which the effect of dietary fat is exerted appears to be during the promotional phase of carcinogenesis rather than during initiation phase.[8] Enhancement of carcinogenesis by high-fat diet can be blocked by some, but not all, antioxidants and may be related to the ability of antioxidants to induce mixed function oxidases (MFO) or other enzymes. In addition, absorption, distribution, metabolic activation and inactivation, as well as excretion of carcinogens may be influenced by the actions of dietary fat. However, definitive pharmacokinetic and metabolic data are not available to give a complete view of the influence of dietary fat on the metabolism of any one carcinogen.

Nigro et al.[76] induced intestinal tumors in male Sprague-Dawley rats by subcutaneous administration of AOM and compared animals fed Purina® chow with 35% beef fat to those fed Purina® chow containing 5% fat. Animals fed the high fat developed more intestinal tumors and more metastases into abdominal cavity, lungs, and liver than the rats fed the low-fat diet. In another study, W/Fu rats fed a 30% lard diet had an increased number of DMH-induced large-bowel tumors compared to the animals fed the standard diet.[77] Rogers et al.[78] found that a diet, marginally deficient in lipotropes but high in fat, enhanced DMH-induced colon carcinogenesis in Sprague-Dawley rats. These results suggest that total dietary fat may have a function in the pathogenesis of colon cancer.

Reddy et al.[79] designed experiments to study the effect of a particular type and amount of dietary fat for two generations before animals were exposed to treatment with a carcinogen. Animals fed 20% lard or 20% corn oil were more susceptible to colon tumor induction by DMH than those fed 5% lard or 5% corn oil. The type of fat appears to be immaterial at the 20% level, although at the 5% fat level, there is a suggestion that unsaturated fat (corn oil) predisposes to more DMH-induced colon tumors than saturated fat (lard). Broitman et al.[80] showed that rats fed a 20% safflower oil diet had more DMH-induced large bowel tumors than the animals fed either the 5% or 20% coconut oil diets. These studies provide no evidence that dietary polyunsaturated fat per se is more effective than saturated fat in augmenting tumorigenesis by DMH. However, these data indicate that at low dietary fat levels, diets rich in polyunsaturated fats are more effective tumor promoters than diets rich in saturated fats.

Investigations were also carried out to test the effect of high dietary fat on colon tumor induction by a variety of carcinogens, DMH, MAM acetate, DMAB or MNU, which not only differ in metabolic activation, but also represent a broad spectrum of exogenous carcinogens.[81,82] Male F344 weanling rats were fed semipurified diets containing 20 or 5% beef fat. At 7 weeks of age, animals were given DMH (s.c., 150 mg/kg body weight, one dose), MAM acetate (i.p., 35 mg/kg body weight, one dose), DMAB (s.c., 50 mg/kg body weight, weekly for 20 weeks), or MNU (intrarectal, 2.5 mg per rat weekly for 2 weeks), and autopsied 30 to 35 weeks later. Irrespective of the colon carcinogen, animals fed a diet containing 20% beef fat had a greater incidence of colon tumors than did rats fed a diet containing 5% beef fat (Figure 1).

D. Dietary Fat as a Promoting Agent

The suggestion that promotion may be involved in intestinal cancer has been supported by the observation that the carcinogenic response to a variety of intestinal carcinogens is enhanced by the dietary fat which in itself is not carcinogenic. Recent studies indicate that the enhanced tumorigenesis in the animals fed the high-fat diet is due to promotional effects.[83] Ingestion of high-fat diet increased the intestinal tumor incidence when fed after AOM (carcinogen) administration, but not during or before AOM treatment. Therefore, the high-fat diet in this model exhibited most of the properties of promoters developed from mouse-skin cancer.

The carcinogenic process in the human may have similar characteristics since there is a good correlation between the findings in a variety of animal studies and those done in humans.[56] The fact that ubiquitous environmental carcinogens are present at very low concentrations suggests that promoting factors may have a preponderant influence on the eventual outcome of the neoplastic process in humans. Due to the wide variety of initiating agents and the possible difficulties in removing them from the environment, the promotional phase of carcinogenesis may be a more promising area for development of preventive measures.

E. Dietary Fiber and Colon Carcinogenesis

The relation between dietary fiber consumption and colon cancer has been studied in

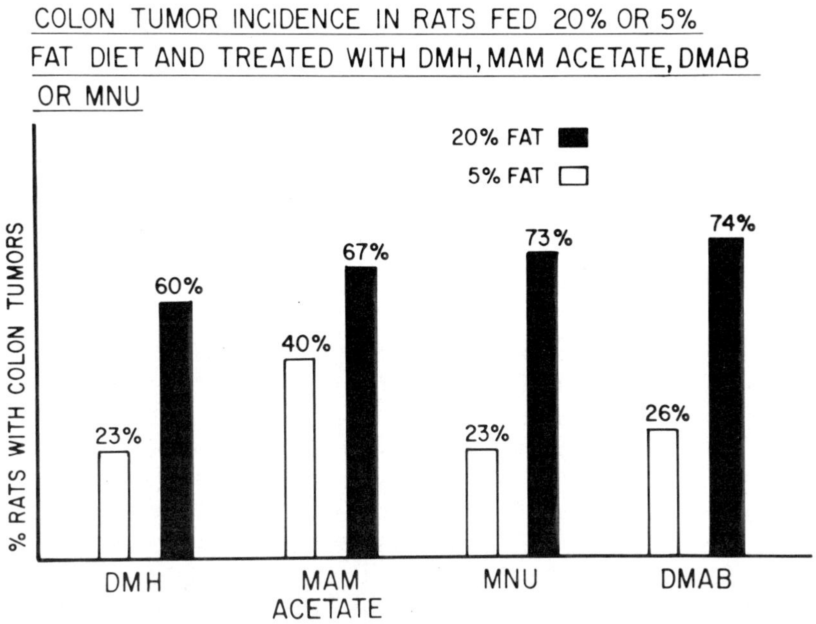

FIGURE 1. Colon tumor incidence in F344 rats fed diets containing 20% or 5% fat diet and treated with a variety of carcinogens. DMH, 1,2-dimethylhydrazine; MAM acetate, methylazoxymethanol acetate; MNU, methylnitrosourea; DMAB, 3,2′-dimethyl-4-aminobiphenyl.

experiments with animals. Wilson et al.[84] found that Sprague-Dawley rats fed a diet containing 20% corn oil or beef fat and 20% wheat bran had fewer colon tumors induced by DMH than rats fed a control diet containing 20% fat and no bran. There was no difference in the incidence of colon cancer between the rats fed corn oil and those fed beef fat. Recently, Freeman et al.[85] compared the incidence of colon tumors induced by DMH in Sprague-Dawley rats fed either a fiber-free diet or a diet containing 4.5% purified cellulose. Among the animals ingesting cellulose, fewer had colonic neoplasms, and the total number of colon tumors in this group was lower. This protective effect appeared to be associated with a shift in tumor distribution from the proximal colon to a more distal site.

In another study, Cruse et al.[86] found that a diet containing 20% wheat bran had no effect on colon carcinogenesis induced by DMH in rats. However, the doses of the chemical in this experiment were so high that any protective effect of bran might have been unobservable. In a study of the effect of diet on chemical carcinogenesis, it is important to avoid exposing the animal to an excessive level of carcinogen for a long period, as this may obscure more subtle changes induced by certain dietary modifications. In fact, the data presented by Cruse and associates suggest that a high-fiber diet reduces the frequency of death due to DMH in rats.

The effect of a diet containing 15% alfalfa, pectin, or wheat bran on colon carcinogenesis by MNU or AOM was studied in F344 rats by Watanabe et al.[87] The animals fed the alfalfa diet and treated with MNU had a higher incidence of colon tumors than those fed a control diet containing only 5% cellulose or containing pectin or wheat bran; there was no difference in the frequency of colon carcinogenesis between the rats fed a diet containing pectin and those fed a diet containing wheat bran. The frequency of colon carcinogenesis induced by AOM in rats fed a diet containing pectin or wheat bran was lower than that in rats fed a control diet or the alfalfa diet.

The effect of alfalfa, wheat bran, and cellulose on the incidence of intestinal tumors induced by AOM was further studied in Sprague-Dawley rats fed diets containing 10% fiber and 30% beef fat, 20% fiber and 6% beef fat, or 30% fiber and 6% beef fat.[44] The presence of 10% fiber in the high-fat diet did not reduce the frequency of intestinal tumors. Apparently, the effect of AOM plus the high dietary intake of fat was too great to be affected by the dietary fiber. The presence of 20% bran or cellulose or 30% of any fiber in a diet containing 6% fat significantly reduced the frequency of intestinal tumors. All the groups except those with a diet containing 20% alfalfa had a lower frequency of tumors in the proximal half of the large bowel than the groups not ingesting fiber. The concentration, but not the total daily excretion of fecal steroids, was significantly lower in the groups with a lower tumor frequency.

The effect of dietary wheat bran (15%) and dehydrated citrus fiber (15%) on AOM or DMAB-induced intestinal tumors was studied in male F344 rats.[88] Animals fed the wheat bran and citrus fiber diets and treated with AOM had a lower incidence of colon and small intestinal tumors than did those fed the control diet and treated with AOM (Table 4). On the other hand, the animals fed the wheat bran and treated with DMAB developed fewer colon and small intestinal tumors than did the rats fed the control diet; animals fed the diet containing citrus fiber and treated with DMAB had a lower incidence of small intestinal tumors. This study thus indicates that diets containing wheat bran reduce the risk of chemically induced colon cancer and that the protection against colon cancer depends on the type of fiber.

Bauer et al.[89] have demonstrated that the protective effect of dietary fiber against colon carcinogenesis probably occurs at the promotional stage rather than in the initiating period. Rats were fed a fiber-free diet or diets containing 20% wheat bran, 20% carrot fiber, or 6.5% citrus pectin from 3 days before the first injection of DMH until 14 days after the last injection. They were then transferred to a standard rat pellet diet for 10 to 12 weeks. There was no difference in the incidence of colorectal tumors between the groups fed a fiber-free diet and those fed a diet containing wheat bran or carrot fiber. However, it is possible that the high tumor yield resulting from large doses of the carcinogen in this study masked any protective effect of dietary fiber. In addition, these results and those of others reported above have suggested that the continual feeding of a high-fiber diet protects against colon carcinogenesis, while a switch from a high-fiber to a low-fiber diet after administration of the carcinogen has no observable effect. These observations imply that dietary fiber protects against tumorigenesis during the promotional phase.

IV. BILE METABOLITES AND TUMOR PROMOTION

Within the past 10 years, it has become apparent that the two-stage phenomenon in the development of neoplasms is not restricted to the skin but the other organs such as liver, bladder, and colon, to cite a few, exhibit more or less similar mechanisms.[90,91] The role of nutritional influences through the bile acids and cholesterol metabolites as promoting stimuli has been noted for the colon and will be discussed with experimental evidence. Taking a lead from human epidemiological and metabolic epidemiological information, a test system was devised in rats to demonstrate the effect of various bile metabolites in colon carcinogenesis.

A. Bile Acids and Colon Tumor Promotion

The role of bile acids in colon carcinogenesis has received some support from studies in animal models. Chomchai et al.[92] demonstrated that the carcinogenic effect of AOM in rats was increased by surgically diverting bile to the middle of the small intestine, a procedure that also raised the fecal excretion of bile salts. Nigro et al.[93] observed that feeding of a nonabsorbable resin, cholestyramine, which increases bile salt excretion, enhanced AOM-induced colon tumors in rats. Watanabe et al.[94] demonstrated that the undegraded carrageenan

Table 4
COLON TUMOR INCIDENCE IN F344 MALE RATS FED DIETS CONTAINING WHEAT BRAN OR CITRUS FIBER AND TREATED WITH AZOXYMETHANE

	Animals with colon tumors						Colon tumors per tumor bearing rat		
	Total[a]		Adenoma		Adenocarcinoma				
Diet	No.	%	No.	%	No.	%	Total	Adenoma	Adenocarcinoma
Control (96)[b]	86	90	83	86	60	63	3.45 ± 0.16[c]	2.37 ± 0.16	1.08 ± 0.18
Wheat bran (51)	36	71[d]	24	47[d]	20	39[d]	1.55 ± 0.12[e]	0.94 ± 0.13[e]	0.61 ± 0.11[e]
Citrus pulp (51)	32	63[d]	21	41[d]	20	39[d]	1.78 ± 0.18[e]	0.90 ± 0.14[e]	0.88 ± 0.16

[a] Total represents animals with adenomas and/or adenocarcinomas.
[b] Effective number of animals in each group is shown in parentheses.
[c] Mean ± SEM.
[d] Significantly different from the group fed the control diet by X^2 test ($p<0.05$ or better).
[e] Significantly different from the group fed the control diet by student's *t*-test ($p<0.05$ or better).

in the diet, which increased bile salt excretion, had an enhancing effect in colorectal carcinogenesis in rats evoked by AOM or MNU. Although this effect was mediated through an increased fecal bile salt excretion, one could not exclude the possibility of some direct effect of cholestyramine or carrageenan itself in stimulating cell duplication.

The evidence of the importance of bile acids as colon tumor promoters came from our studies (Table 5).[95,97] The development of adenomas increased significantly among those conventional rats initiated with limited amounts of intrarectal MNNG to give a definite low yield of colon cancer and administered with intrarectal lithocholic acid or taurodeoxycholic acid as promoters, compared with the group that was given only the carcinogen. Lithocholic acid applied topically to the colon increased MNNG-induced colon adenocarcinomas in rats. The bile acids themselves did not produce any tumors. A recent study also indicates that the primary bile acids, cholic acid and chenodeoxycholic acid, given intrarectally to conventional rats are subjected to bacterial 7α-dehydroxylation to deoxycholic acid and lithocholic acid, respectively.[98] Cohen et al.[99] reported that cholic acid in the diet increased MNNG-induced colon carcinogenesis in rats. Total fecal bile acids, particularly deoxycholic acid output, were elevated in animals fed cholic acid as compared with controls. This increase in fecal deoxycholic acid was due to bacterial 7α-dehydroxylation of cholic acid in the colonic contents. These studies demonstrate that these secondary bile acids have a promoting effect in colon carcinogenesis.

Various in vitro tests have been used to test the role of bile acids in carcinogenesis. Silverman and Andrews[100] examined 30 bile acids for bacterial mutagenicity and found that all were negative with eight strains of *S. typhimurium*, both with and without metabolic activation. However, when bile acids were tested with 2-aminoanthracene or benzo(a)pyrene and a phenobarbitol S-9 activation system, an enhancement of mutagenicity was found with lithocholic acid, suggesting comutagenic activity. Using the hamster embryo transformation system, lithocholic acid also was active by itself.[101]

The mechanism of action of bile acids in colon carcinogenesis has not been elucidated. Bile acids have been shown to affect cell kinetics in the intestinal epithelium, although the structural specificity of this effect has not been examined extensively.[102] In the intestine, the data do not permit the critical distinction to be made between a direct effect of bile acids on cell division and an indirect or physiological stimulus secondary to increased cell loss from sloughing or damage.[102] The cell renewal system is dynamic and may be influenced by changes in a number of factors, including the gut microflora[103] and bile acids in the intestine.[104] It has been shown that, with proper modification of the microenvironment of the intestinal tract, it is possible to alter the cellular kinetics of the mucosa. Recently, Cohen et al.[99] reported an enhanced colonic cell proliferation in rats fed cholic acid, as well as in animals treated with intrarectal MNU. This increased cell proliferation involved in DNA synthesis by cholic acid feeding would favor the expression of damage at a far higher level than with the carcinogen MNU alone, bringing about not only a greater overall incidence of MNU-induced colon tumors, but also an enhanced number of tumors in rats fed cholic acid. Lipkin[105] demonstrated that, during neoplastic transformation of colonic cells, a similar sequence of changes leading to uncontrolled proliferative activity develops in colon cancer in humans and in rodents given a colon carcinogen.

Although the molecular mechanisms of tumor-promoting action of bile acids are incompletely understood, recent studies of Takano et al.[106] suggest that the induction of colonic epithelial ornithine decarboxylase and *S*-adenosyl-L-methionine decarboxylase activities by the bile acids may play a role in these mechanisms. The studies reported indicate that the colonic epithelial responses of the polyamine biosynthetic enzymes, to applications of bile acids, are among the earliest changes to occur in this tissue in response to promoting agents.

Irrespective of the mechanism by which bile acids enhance cell proliferation and (or) decrease the generation time of proliferating cells and affect DNA repair, the phenomenon

Table 5
COLON TUMOR INCIDENCE IN GERMFREE AND CONVENTIONAL RATS TREATED WITH INTRARECTAL MNNG AND/OR BILE ACIDS

	Germfree[a]		Conventional[a]	
	Rats with tumors (%)	Tumors/rat	Rats with tumors (%)	Tumors/rat
CA (10—12)[b]	0	0	0	0
CDC (10—12)	0	0	0	0
LC (10—12)	0	0	0	0
MNNG (22—30)	27	0.27	37	0.55
MNNG + CA (24—30)	50	0.63	67[c]	0.87
MNNG + CDC (24—30)	54	1.08	70[c]	1.23
MNNG + LC (24)	71[c]	1.04	83[c]	1.83

[a] CA, CDC, or LC group received intrarectally 20 mg of sodium salt of respective bile acid three times weekly for 48 weeks; MNNG group received intrarectally 2 mg of MNNG twice a week for 2 weeks followed by vehicle for 46 weeks; MNNG + CA, MNNG + LC or MNNG + CDC group received intrarectally MNNG for 2 weeks and bile acid thereafter for 46 weeks.

[b] CA, cholic acid; CDC, chenodeoxycholic acid; LC, lithocholic acid. Number of rats are shown in parentheses.

[c] Significantly different from rats given MNNG alone by X^2 test, $p < 0.05$.

may have important implications for colon carcinogenesis. Obviously, further studies are warranted on the mechanism of tumor-promoting activity of various bile acids.

B. Cholesterol and Colon Tumor Promotion

Cruse et al.[107] proposed that prolonged exposure of dietary cholesterol is cocarcinogenic for human colon cancer, in that it facilitates the development, growth, and spread of the disease because dietary fats promote the action of several experimental carcinogens. Broitman et al.[80] studied the effect of polyunsaturated fat and cholesterol on colon tumorigenesis and demonstrated that the interaction between dietary polyunsaturated fat and dietary cholesterol and/or tissue cholesterol may promote tumorigenesis when compared with dietary saturated fat and cholesterol in the animal model.

Bischoff[108] has reviewed the carcinogenic effects of steroids and reported that cholesterol epoxide administered in an aqueous vehicle was carcinogenic in both rats and mice, but not carcinogenic to the colon. Cholesterol 3β,5α,6β-triol, a principal metabolite of cholesterol epoxide, has been found in increased levels in feces of patients of colon cancer and ulcerative colitis.[109,110]

The mutagenic, as well as colon tumor-promoting activity of cholesterol and its metabolites, has been tested by Smith et al.[111] and Reddy and Watanabe.[112] Naturally air-aged commercial samples of cholesterol contain components that are mutagenic towards *S. typhimurium* TA1537, TA1538, and TA98; however, cholesterol epoxide is nonmutagenic towards these strains.[111] Our recent studies also indicate that cholesterol, cholesterol epoxide, and triol do not exhibit any colon tumor-promoting activity in both germfree and conventional rat models (Table 6).[112] These observations suggest that cholesterol or its metabolites produced by the colonic bacteria are not detectably either a carcinogen or a promoter to the colonic mucosa.

Table 6
COLON TUMOR INCIDENCE IN GERMFREE AND CONVENTIONAL RATS TREATED INTRARECTALLY WITH MNNG AND (OR) CHOLESTEROL METABOLITES

Treatment[a,b]	Germfree rats with colon tumors (%)	Conventional rats with colon tumors (%)
Cholesterol (15)	0	0
Epoxide (21)	0	0
Triol (15)	0	0
MNNG (26)	46	71
MNNG + cholesterol (24)	46[c]	71[c]
MNNG + epoxide (24)	58[c]	58[c]
MNNG + triol (24)	46[c]	58[c]

[a] Epoxide is cholesterol-α-epoxide; triol is cholestane-3,5,6-triol.

[b] Cholesterol, epoxide, or triol group received 20 mg of respective compound three times weekly for 48 weeks; MNNG group received intrarectally 2.5 mg of MNNG twice a week for 2 weeks, followed by vehicle for 46 weeks; MNNG + cholesterol, MNNG + epoxide, or MNNG + triol group received intrarectally MNNG for 2 weeks and cholesterol metabolites thereafter for 46 weeks.

[c] Not significantly different from the group given MNNG alone by chi-square test; $p>0.05$.

V. PRENEOPLASTIC CHANGES IN COLON CARCINOGENESIS

In recent years, studies describing the proliferation and differentiation of colonic cells have focused on the changes that take place during neoplastic transformation. Earlier reviews have already dealt with preneoplastic changes in the process of colon carcinogenesis and other aspects of the natural history of neoplastic development.[20,113,114] However, a brief recapitulation of preneoplastic or precancerous changes in colon tissue will be presented here.

The evolution of ordinary large bowel carcinoma from its precursor tissue is best understood by looking into a few features of normal colon. In normal colon of man, after pulse labeling with tritiated thymidine, proliferative cells occupy about three quarters of the colonic crypt column. About 15 to 20% of the cells in the proliferative zone are in DNA synthesis, and the mean duration of the proliferative cell cycle is about 2 days. As cells migrate to the upper portions of crypts, they rapidly leave the proliferative cycle within hours, as cell differentiation takes place. The rapidly proliferating cells lining the colonic mucosa of man are largely replaced in 4 to 8 days. However, a small fraction of cells remains for a longer period.

In the normal rodents, rapidly renewing colonic epithelial cells also proliferate in the lower portion of the colonic crypts, but more rapidly and with a shorter cell cycle than in man.[115] The mucosa of the rectosigmoid colon is renewed more slowly than mucosa of other regions of the intestinal tract. Epithelial cells in the rectosigmoid region appear to have a longer time in which to maintain in contact with carcinogens and/or promoters before being extruded than proliferating cells in other regions. In man, a large fraction of all colonic carcinomas has been seen in the rectosigmoid region.

In man, abnormal cell proliferation in colonic epithelial cells eventually leads to a failure of the cells to repress DNA synthesis. Some epithelial cells continue to synthesize and fail to repress formation of new DNA during their migration to the surface of mucosa. During the evolution of benign and malignant neoplasms of the colon, metabolic abnormalities, such as changes in enzyme activity, develop, and increased biochemical and morphological expressions of abnormal proliferation and differentiation are observed. Thus, persistent DNA synthesis during migration of colonic epithelial cells by itself is not typical only of the development of neoplasia. However, some migrating cells that fail to repress DNA synthesis also develop additional properties that enable them to be retained in the colonic mucosa in increasing numbers. Cells with these proliferative and characteristic morphological changes progress into pathologically defined neoplasms.

A. Human Model

1. Hereditary Precancerous Lesions

In individuals with dominant-inherited disease, familial polyposis who are at high risk for colon cancer development, patches of flat mucosa can be detected having epithelial cells that fail to repress DNA synthesis during migration to the surface of the mucosa.[116,117] This finding has been observed in normal appearing colonic epithelial cells of subjects with familial polyposis before as well as after the cells develop adenomatous changes and begin to accumulate as polyps. Current observations also have indicated a significantly higher frequency of abnormal proliferative activity of this type in high-risk colon cancer-prone families in which individuals do not develop polyposis, and where the pattern of cancer inheritance resembles the autosomal dominant pattern of familial polyposis.[117] In familial polyposis, as colonic epithelial cells which do not repress proliferative activity undergo abnormal maturation and accumulate in the mucosa, they develop morphological changes characteristic of adenomas; these further develop into the tubular or villous structures. Most epithelial cells in these adenomas are extruded, whereas only a minor fraction are retained to proliferate and induce growth. Carcinomas develop with increasing frequency as these adenomatous excrescenses enlarge. This concept allows for a contribution of endogenous and/or exogenous carcinogenic or promoter elements to interact with the cells having a hereditary predisposition to neoplasia. It also allows for the introduction of preventive measures to block the steps leading to malignant transformation of cells.

2. Nonhereditary Precancerous Lesions

In terms of cancer incidence, adenomatous polyps are implicated in colon carcinogenesis. As discussed elsewhere in this review, it is suspected of being a precursor in the great majority of cases of colon cancer, although this subject constitutes an old medical controversy familiar to many investigators. Recent advances in our knowledge of the pathology and epidemiology of polyps have clarified considerably some of the obscure points of the controversy.[6] Adenomatous polyps are crowded accumulations of tubular glands with little or no stroma between them. Their surface is composed of the same type of glands found in the deeper portions of the polyp. Some of the adenomatous polyps have areas of villous or papillary architecture, the villi being lined by the same type of epithelial cells lining the tubular glands. Pure villous adenomas are recognized as having marked propensity for malignant transformation. In adenomas, the control mechanisms governing DNA synthesis are largely lost, so that thymidine uptake and cell division occur at all levels in adenomatous tissue.[114] The significance of the geographical associations in the occurrence of adenomatous polyps and colon cancer is enhanced by the multiplicity of polyps in populations at higher risk to large bowel cancer, a feature consistent with the observations that larger and more numerous polyps have a greater tendency for malignant transformation.[118]

B. Animal Models

The effect of a chemical carcinogen on the proliferation of colonic cells has now been observed in several studies using DMH. In the mouse after DMH administration, tumor nodules appear predominantly in the distal colon that is similar to the distribution found in man. Multifocal tumors ranging from adenomatous polyps to metaplasias and carcinomas grow from the mucosa, protruding into the lumen of the rectosigmoid region. In DMH-induced adenomas in the mouse, cell proliferation also proceeded more rapidly than in flat adjacent mucosa similar to the observation on inherited adenomatosis of man noted above.[122] The repeated delivery of DMH resulted in the expression of DNA synthesis cells to the upper third of the glands, but with the middle third of the crypt the most active proliferative zone. Twenty weeks later, mice with abnormal proliferative pattern had adenomas and carcinomas present primarily in the distal portion of the colon. In DMH-induced tumors, the growth rate was more rapid in small tumor nodules than in larger ones.

In mice and rats, treatment with DMH results in progressive changes, from early focal atypias and hyperplasias, located mainly on the mucosal folds, to adenomatous polyps and carcinomas. The development of these changes appears to be accompanied by impairment of cell differentiation and also by abnormal tritiated thymidine autoradiographic findings. Thurnherr et al.[121] noted a broadening of the proliferative zone in some areas of mucosa, together with a shift of tritiated thymidine-labeled epithelial cells to proliferate in expanding adenomas and carcinomas. In mice, as cells continued to synthesize DNA throughout most of their life span, both the position up from the base of the crypts and total number of thymidine-labeled cells increased. This widening of the proliferative colonic crypt compartment, and persistent tritiated thymidine incorporation into the DNA of cells migrating towards the crypt surfaces and in expanding adenomas, are similar to changes seen in man. DMH-induced tumors developed with thymidine-labeled cells near the surfaces of the lesions, which continued to expand into the lumen of the colon. In these animal models, some species differences have been recorded on the effect of DMH on the development of tumors.

VI. CONCLUSION

During the last decade, some progress has been made in the understanding of the role played by the dietary constituents in general, and specifically the role of lipids and fibers in colon cancer. The population with high incidences of cancer of the large bowel are characterized by consumption of a high level of dietary fat. Furthermore, dietary fat may be a risk factor for the colon cancer in the absence of factors that are protective, such as use of high fibrous foods and fiber. Thus, alteration of dietary habits leading to a lower intake of fat and higher intake of certain fibers would be indicated to decrease the risk of this important cancer. Beginning this dietary pattern early in life may prove most beneficial.

The demonstration of two stages in experimentally induced cancer in animal models suggests that there are two stages in environmentally induced cancer in humans. Most human cancers in reality result from a complex interaction of carcinogens, cocarcinogens, and tumor promoters. However, the understanding of post-initiating events appears to offer some promise that intervention in the cancer process in man prior to the occurrence of overt tumors may be an achievable and realistic goal.[91] Most of the nutritional or dietary factors act at the promotional phase of carcinogenesis. Because promotion is a reversible process, in contrast to the rapid, irreversible process of initiation by carcinogens, manipulation of promotion would seem to be the best method of cancer prevention.

Although there is much need for further research to understand the modification of the carcinogenic process, the successes thus achieved have expanded into some understanding of the numerous steps involved in the activation and detoxification of various chemical carcinogens and promoters by a variety of means. Application of a number of such basic tools, elimination of harmful agents from the environment, reduction of biochemical activation processes and a concomitant increase in detoxification reactions, as well as trapping of active intermediates by harmless nucleophilic reagents, point to a promising future for preventive efforts. Thus, there is hope that this important cancer can be controlled by modifying not only environment with respect to genotoxic carcinogens, but also that of epigenetic carcinogens and, thus, human cancer risk feasibly can be reduced.

ACKNOWLEDGMENTS

This research was supported in part from grants CA-16382, CA-12376, CA-32617, and CA-17613, contract CP-33208, CP-85659, and CP-05721 from the National Cancer Institute. The author acknowledges the expert assistance of Ms. Arlene Banow in preparation of the manuscript.

REFERENCES

1. **Griffin, A. C. and Shaw, C. R., Eds.,** *Carcinogenesis: Identification and Mechanism of Action,* Raven Press, New York, 1979.
2. **Emmelot, P. and Kriek, E., Eds.,** *Environmental Carcinogenesis: Occurrence, Risk, Evaluation and Mechanism,* Elsevier, Amsterdam, 1979.
3. **Slaga, T. J., Sivak, A., and Boutwell, R. K.,** Eds., *Carcinogenesis,* Vol. 2, Raven Press, New York, 1978.
4. **Armstrong, D. and Doll, R.,** Environmental factors and cancer incidence and mortality in different countries, with special reference to dietary practices, *Int. J. Cancer,* 15, 617, 1975.
5. **Burkitt, D. P.,** Colonic-rectal cancer; fiber and other dietary factors, *Am. J. Clin. Nutr.,* 31, S58, 1978.
6. **Correa, P. and Haenszel, W.,** The epidemiology of large bowel cancer, *Adv. Cancer Res.,* 26, 1, 1978.
7. **Graham, S. and Mettlin, C.,** Diet and colon cancer, *Am. J. Epidemiol.,* 109, 1, 1979.
8. **Reddy, B. S., Cohen, L., McCoy, G. D., Hill, P., Weisburger, J. H., and Wynder, E. L.,** Nutrition and its relationship to cancer, in *Advances in Cancer Research,* Vol. 32, Klein, G. and Weinhouse, S., Eds., Academic Press, New York, 1980, 237.
9. **Wynder, E. L., Kajitani, T., Ishekawa, S., Dodo, H., and Takano, A.,** Environmental factors of cancer of the colon and rectum. II. Japanese epidemiological data, *Cancer,* 23, 1219, 1969.
10. **West, D. K.,** in *Banbury Report #4: Cancer Incidence in Defined Populations,* Cairns, J., Lyon, J. L., and Skolnick, M., Eds., Cold Spring Harbor Laboratory, Cold Spring Harbor, N.Y., 1980, 31.
11. **Reddy, B. S., Hedges, A. R., Laakso, K., and Wynder, E. L.,** Metabolic epidemiology of large bowel cancer. Fecal bulk and constituents of high-risk North American and low-risk Finnish population, *Cancer,* 42, 2832, 1978.
12. **Miller, E. C. and Miller, J. A.,** The presence and significance of bound aminoazo dyes in the livers of rats fed ρ-dimethylaminoazobenzene, *Cancer Res.,* 7, 468, 1947.
13. **Wattenberg, L. W.,** Inhibitors of chemical carcinogenesis, *Adv. Cancer Res.,* 26, 197, 1975.
14. **Miller, E. C.,** Some current perspectives on chemical carcinogenesis in humans and experimental animals: presidential address, *Cancer Res.,* 38, 1479, 1978.
15. **Warwick, G. P.,** Effect of the cell cycle on carcinogenesis, *Fed. Proc.,* 30, 1760, 1971.
16. **Carroll, K. K. and Khor, H. T.,** Dietary fat in relation to tumorigenesis, *Prog. Biochem. Pharmacol.,* 10, 308, 1975.
17. **Doll, R.,** General epidemiologic considerations in etiology of colorectal cancer, in *Colorectal Cancer: Prevention, Epidemiology and Screening,* Winawer, S., Schottenfeld, D., and Sherlock, P., Eds., Raven Press, New York, 1980, 3.
18. **Phillips, R. L., Garfinkel, L., Kuzma, J. W., Beeson, W. L., Lotz, T., and Brin, B.,** Mortality among California Seventh-Day Adventists for selected cancer sites, *J. Natl. Cancer Inst.,* 65, 1097, 1980.
19. **MacMahon, B., Copley, G., Fraumeni, J. F., Jr., Greenwald, P., and Haenszel, W., Eds.,** Populations at low risks of cancer, N.C.I. monograph, *J. Natl. Cancer Inst.,* 65, 1055, 1980.
20. **Weisburger, J. H., Reddy, B. S., and Joftes, D., Eds.,** Colorectal Cancer, UICC Technical Report Series, Vol. 19, Union Internationale Contre le Cancer, Geneva, 1975, 1.
21. **Teppo, L. and Saxen, E.,** Epidemiology of colon cancer in Scandinavia, *Isr. J. Med. Sci.,* 15, 322, 1979.
22. **Haenszel, W., Berg, J. W., Segi, M., Kurihara, M., and Locke, F. B.,** Large bowel cancer in Hawaiian Japanese, *J. Natl. Cancer Inst.,* 51, 1765, 1973.
23. **Staszewski, J., McCall, M. G., and Stenhouse, N. S.,** Cancer mortality in 1962—66 among Polish migrants to Australia, *Br. J. Cancer,* 25, 599, 1971.
24. **Doll, R., Muir, C., and Waterhouse, J., Eds.,** *Cancer Incidence in Five Continents,* Vol. II, International Union Against Cancer, Berlin, 1970, 463.
25. **Hirayama, T.,** Epidemiology of breast cancer with special reference to the role of diet, *Prev. Med.,* 7, 173, 1978.

26. **Jussawalla, D. J. and Jain, D. K.,** *Cancer Incidence in Greater Bombay,* 1970—1972, Indian Cancer Society, Bombay Cancer Registry, India, 1976.
27. **Wynder, E. L.,** Dietary habits and cancer epidemiology, *Cancer,* 43, 1955, 1979.
28. **Wynder, E. L. and Reddy, B. S.,** Studies of large bowel cancer: human leads to experimental application, *J. Natl. Cancer Inst.,* 50, 1099, 1973.
29. **Enig, M. G., Mann, R. J., and Keeney, M.,** Dietary fat and cancer trends — a critique, *Fed. Proc.,* 37, 2215, 1978.
30. **Howell, M. A.,** Diet as an etiological factor in the development of cancers of the colon and rectum, *J. Chron. Dis.,* 28, 67, 1975.
31. **Burkitt, D. P.,** Some neglected leads to cancer causation, *J. Natl. Cancer Inst.,* 47, 913, 1971.
32. International Agency for Research on Cancer Intestinal Microecology Group, Dietary fibre transit time, faecal bacteria, steroids and colon cancer in two Scandinavian populations, *Lancet,* 2, 207, 1977.
33. **Reddy, B. S., Hedges, A. R., Laakso, K., and Wynder, E. L.,** Metabolic epidemiology of large bowel cancer. Fecal bulk and constituents of high-risk North American and low-risk Finnish population, *Cancer,* 42, 2832, 1978.
34. **Wynder, E. L., Kajitani, T., Ishikawa, S., Dodo, H., and Takano, A.,** Environmental factors of cancer of the colon and rectum, *Cancer,* 23, 1210, 1969.
35. **Jain, M., Cook, G. M., Davis, F. G., Grace, M. G., Howe, G. R., and Miller, A. B.,** A case-control study of diet and colorectal cancer, *Intl. J. Cancer,* 26, 757, 1980.
36. **Williams, R. R., Sorlie, P. D., Feinleib, M., McNamara, P. M., Kannel, W. B., and Dawber, T. R.,** Cancer incidence by levels of cholesterol, *JAMA,* 245, 247, 1981.
37. **Modan, B., Barrel, V., Lubin, F., Modan, M., Greenberg, R. A., and Graham, S.,** Low fibre intake as an etiologic factor in cancer of the colon, *J. Natl. Cancer Inst.,* 55, 15, 1975.
38. **Dales, L. G., Friedman, G. D., Wry, H. K., Grossman, S., and Williams, S. R.,** Case-control study of relationships of diet and other traits to colorectal cancer in American blacks, *Am. J. Epidemiol.,* 109, 132, 1979.
39. **Bjelke, E.,** Epidemiological studies of cancer of the stomach, colon and rectum, *Scand. J. Gastroenterol.,* 9 (Suppl. 31), 1, 1974.
40. **Graham, S., Dayal, H., Swanson, M., Mittelman, A., and Wilkinson, G.,** Diet in the epidemiology of cancer of the colon and rectum, *J. Natl. Cancer Inst.,* 61, 709, 1978.
41. **Aries, V., Crowther, J. S., Drasar, B. S., Hill, M. J., and Williams, R. E. O.,** Bacteria and etiology of cancer of the large bowel, *Gut,* 10, 334, 1969.
42. **Reddy, B. S., Weisburger, J. H., and Wynder, E. L.,** Colon cancer: bile salts as tumor promoters, in *Carcinogenesis,* Vol. 2, Slaga, T. J., Boutwell, R. K., and Sivak, A., Eds., Raven Press, New York, 1978, 453.
43. **Talbot, J. M.,** *The Role of Dietary Fiber in Diverticular Disease and Colon Cancer,* Life Sciences Research Office, Federation of American Societies for Experimental Biology, Bethesda, Md.
44. **Nigro, N. D., Bull, A. W., Klopfer, B. A., Pak, M. S., and Campbell, R. L.,** Effect of dietary fiber on azoxymethane-induced intestinal carcinogenesis in rats, *J. Natl. Cancer Inst.,* 62, 1097, 1979.
45. **Spiller, G. A.,** Interaction of dietary fiber with the dietary components: a possible factor in certain cancer etiology, *Am. J. Clin. Nutr.,* 31 (Suppl.), S231, 1979.
46. **Kern, F., Birkner, H. J., and Ostrower, V. S.,** Binding of the bile acids by dietary fiber, *Am. J. Clin. Nutr.,* 31, S175, 1979.
47. **Cummings, J. H., Hill, M. J., Jivraj, T., Houston, H., Branch, W. J., and Jenkins, D. J. A.,** The effect of meat protein and dietary fiber on colonic function and metabolism. I. Changes in bowel habit, bile acid excretion and calcium absorption, *Am. J. Clin. Nutr.,* 32, 2086, 1979.
48. **Rubino, M. A., Pethica, B. A., Zuman, P., in** *Dietary Fibres: Chemistry and Nutrition,* Inglett, G. and Falkehag, I., Eds., Academic Press, New York, 1979, 251.
49. **Hill, M. J., Drasar, B. S., Aries, V. C., Crowther, J. S., Hawksworth, G. B., and Williams, R. E. O., Bacteria and aetiology of cancer of large bowel,** *Lancet,* 1, 95, 1971.
50. **Goldin, B. R. and Gorbach, S. L.,** The relationship between diet and rat fecal bacterial enzymes implicated in colon cancer, *J. Natl. Cancer Inst.,* 57, 371, 1976.
51. **Campbell, T. C.,** Influence of nutrition on metabolism of carcinogenesis, *Adv. Nutr. Res.,* 2, 29, 1979.
52. **Reddy, B. S.,** Dietary fat and its relationship to large bowel cancer, *Cancer Res.,* 41, 000, 1981.
53. **Reddy, B. S.,** Diet and excretion of bile acids, *Cancer Res.,* 41, 000, 1981.
54. **Cummings, J. H., Wiggins, H. S., Jenkins, D. J. A., Houston, H., Jivraj, T., Drasar, B. S., and Hill, M. J.,** Influence of diets high and low in animal fat on bowel habit, gastrointestinal transit time, fecal microflora, bile acid and fat excretion, *J. Clin. Invest.,* 61, 953, 1978.
55. **Kay, R. M. and Truswell, A. S.,** Effect of wheat fibre on plasma lipids and faecal steroid excretion in man, *Br. J. Nutr.,* 37, 227, 1977.

56. **Diamond, L., O'Brien, T. G., and Baird, W. M.,** Tumor promoters and the mechanism of tumor promotion, *Adv. Cancer Res.*, 32, 1, 1980.
57. **Rawson, R. W.,** Colonic polyps: antecedent- or associated-lesions of large bowel cancer, *Semin. Oncol.*, 3, 361, 1976.
58. **Morson, B. C.,** Precancerous conditions of the large bowel, *Proc. R. Soc. Med.*, 64, 7, 1971.
59. **Appel, M. F., Spjut, H. J., and Estrada, R. G.,** The significance of villous component in colonic polyps, *Am. J. Surg.*, 134, 770, 1977.
60. **Nagao, M., Honda, M., Seino, Y., Yahagi, T., and Sugimura, T.,** Mutagenicity of smoke condensates and the charred surfaces of fish and meat, *Cancer Lett.*, 2, 221, 1977.
61. **Commoner, B., Vithayathil, A. J., Dolara, P., Nair, S., Madyastha, P., and Cuca, G. C.,** Formation of mutagens in beef and beef extract during cooking, *Science*, 201, 913, 1978.
62. **Weisburger, J. W., Reddy, B. S., Spingarn, N. E., and Wynder, E. L.,** Current views on the mechanisms involved in the etiology of colorectal cancer, in *Colorectal Cancer: Prevention, Epidemiology and Screening*, Winawer, S., Schottenfeld, D., and Sherlock, P., Eds., Raven Press, New York, 1980, 19.
63. **Ehrich, M., Ashell, J. E., Van Tassell, R. L., Wilkins, T. D., Walker, A. R. P., and Richardson, N. J.,** Mutagens in the feces of 3 South African populations at different levels of risk for colon cancer, *Mutat. Res.*, 64, 231, 1979.
64. **Bruce, W. R., Varghese, A. J., Furrer, R., and Land, P. C.,** A mutagen in the feces of normal humans, in *Origins of Human Cancer*, Vol. 4, Cold Spring Harbor Conf. Cell Proliferation, Hiatt, H. H., Watson, J. P., and Winston, J. A., Eds., Cold Spring Harbor Laboratory, Cold Spring Harbor, N.Y., 1977, 1641.
65. **Wilkins, T. D.,** Microbiological considerations in interpretation of data obtained with experimental animals, in *Banbury Report #7*, Bruce, W. R., Correa, P., Lipkin, M., Tannenbaum, S. R., and Wilkins, T. D., Eds., Cold Spring Harbor Laboratory, New York, 1981, 3.
66. **Kuhnlein, U., Bergstrom, D., and Kuhnlein, H.,** Mutations in feces from vegetarians and non-vegetarians, *Mutat. Res.*, 85, 1, 1981.
67. **Reddy, B. S., Sharma, C., Darby, L., Laakso, K., and Wynder, E. L.,** Metabolic epidemiology of large bowel cancer: fecal mutagens in high- and low-risk population for colon cancer, a preliminary report, *Mutat. Res.*, 72, 511, 1980.
68. **Rao, T. K., Young, J. A., Weeks, C. E., Slaga, T. J., and Epler, J. L.,** Effect of the co-carcinogen benzo(a)pyrene on microsome-mediated chemical mutagenesis on *Salmonella typhimurium*, *Environ. Mutagenesis*, 1, 105, 1979.
69. **Nagao, M., Yahagi, T., Kawachi, T., Kosuge, K., Tsuji, K., Wakabayashi, S., Mizusaki, S., and Matsumoto, T.,** Co-mutagenic action of norharman and harman, *Proc. Jpn. Acad.*, 53, 95, 1977.
70. **Matsumoto, T., Yoshida, D., and Mizusaki, S.,** Enhancing effect of harman on mutagenicity in *Salmonella*, *Mutatet. Res.*, 56, 85, 1972.
71. **Reddy, B. S., Sharma, C., and Wynder, E. L.,** Fecal factors which modify the formation of fecal co-mutagens in high- and low-risk populations for colon cancer, *Cancer Lett.*, 10, 123, 1980.
72. **Bralow, S. P. and Weisburger, J. H.,** Experimental carcinogenesis, *Clin. Gastroenterol.*, 5, 527, 1976.
73. **Maskens, A. P.,** Mathematical models of carcinogenesis and tumor growth, in *Gastrointestinal Tract Cancer*, Lipkin, M. and Good, R., Eds., Plenum Press, New York, 1978, 361.
74. **Deschner, E. E., Long, F. C., and Maskens, A. P.,** Relationship between the dose, time and tumor yield in mouse dimethylhydrazine-induced colon tumorigenesis, *Cancer Lett.*, 8, 23, 1979.
75. **Maskens, A. P.,** Confirmation of the two-step nature of chemical carcinogenesis in the rat colon adenocarcinoma model, *Cancer Res.*, 41, 1240, 1981.
76. **Nigro, N. D., Singh, D. V., Campbell, R. L., and Pak, M. S.,** Effect of dietary beef fat on intestinal tumor formation by azoxymethane in rats, *J. Natl. Cancer Inst.*, 54, 429, 1975.
77. **Bansal, B. R., Rhoads, J. E., Jr., and Bansal, S. C.,** Effects of diet on colon carcinogenesis and the immune system in rats treated with 1,2-dimethylhydrazine, *Cancer Res.*, 38, 3293, 1978.
78. **Rogers, A. E. and Newberne, P. M.,** Dietary effects on chemical carcinogenesis in animal models for colon and liver tumors, *Cancer Res.*, 35, 3427, 1975.
79. **Reddy, B. S., Narisawa, T., Vukusich, D., Weisburger, J. H., and Wynder, E. L.,** Effect of quality and quantity of dietary fat and dimethylhydrazine in colon carcinogenesis in rats, *Proc. Soc. Exp. Biol. Med.*, 151, 237, 1976.
80. **Broitman, S. A., Vitale, J. J., Vavrousek-Jakuba, E., and Gottlieb, L. S.,** Polyunsaturated fat, cholesterol and large bowel tumorigenesis, *Cancer*, 40, 2455, 1977.
81. **Reddy, B. S., Mangat, S., Weisburger, J. H., and Wynder, E. L.,** Effect of high-risk diets for colon carcinogenesis or intestinal mucosal and bacterial β-glucuronidase activity in F344 rats, *Cancer Res.*, 37, 3533, 1977.
82. **Reddy, B. S. and Ohmori, T.,** Effect of intestinal microflora and dietary fat on 3,2′-dimethyl-4-aminobiphenyl-induced colon carcinogenesis in F344 rats, *Cancer Res.*, 41, 1363, 1981.

83. **Bull, A. W., Soullier, B. K., Wilson, P. S., Hayden, M. T., and Nigro, N. D.,** Promotion of azoxymethane-induced intestinal cancer by high-fat diets in rats, *Cancer Res.*, 39, 4956, 1979.
84. **Wilson, R. B., Hutcheson, D. P., Wideman, L.,** Dimethylhydrazine-induced colon tumors in rats fed diets containing beef fat or corn oil with and without wheat bran, *Am. J. Clin. Nutr.*, 30, 176, 1977.
85. **Freeman, H. J., Spiller, G. A., and Kim, Y. S.,** A double-blind study on the effect of purified cellulose dietary fiber on 1,2-dimethylhydrazine-induced rat colonic neoplasia, *Cancer Res.*, 38, 2912, 1978.
86. **Cruse, J. P., Lewin, M. R., and Clark, G. G.,** Failure of bran to protect against experimental colon cancer in rats, *Lancet*, 2, 1278, 1978.
87. **Watanabe, K., Reddy, B. S., Weisburger, J. H., and Kritchevsky, D.,** Effect of dietary alfalfa, pectin and wheat bran on azoxymethane- or methylnitrosourea-induced colon carcinogenesis in F344 rats, *J. Natl. Cancer Inst.*, 63, 141, 1979.
88. **Reddy, B. S., Mori, H., and Nicolais, M.,** Effect of dietary wheat bran and dehydrated citrus fiber on azoxymethane-induced intestinal carcinogenesis in F344 rats, *J. Natl. Cancer Inst.*, 66, 553, 1981.
89. **Bauer, H. G., Asp, N., Oste, R., Dahlqvist, A., and Fredlund, P. E.,** Effect of dietary fiber on the induction of colorectal tumors and fecal β-glucuronidase activity in the rat, *Cancer Res.*, 39, 3752, 1979.
90. **Pitot, H. C. and Serica, A.,** Two states of initiation and promotion in hepatocarcinogenesis, *Biochim. Biophys. Acta*, 605, 191, 1980.
91. **Sivak, A.,** Cocarcinogenesis, *Biochim. Biophys. Acta*, 560, 67, 1979.
92. **Chomchai, C., Bhadrachari, N., and Nigro, N. D.,** The effect of bile on the induction of experimental intestinal tumors in rats, *Dis. Colon Rectum*, 17, 310, 1974.
93. **Nigro, N. D., Bhadrachari, N., and Chomchai, C.,** A rat model for studying colonic cancer: effect of cholestyramine on induced tumors, *Dis. Colon Rectum*, 16, 438, 1973.
94. **Watanabe, K., Reddy, B. S., Wong, C. Q., and Weisburger, J. H.,** Effect of undegraded carrageenan on colon carcinogenesis in F344 rats treated with azoxymethane or methylnitrosourea, *Cancer Res.*, 38, 4427, 1978.
95. **Narisawa, T., Magadia, N. E., Weisburger, J. H., and Wynder, E. L.,** Promoting effect of bile acid on colon carcinogenesis after intrarectal instillation of MNNG in rats, *J. Natl. Cancer Inst.*, 53, 1093, 1974.
96. **Reddy, B. S., Narisawa, T., Weisburger, J. H., and Wynder, E. L.,** Promoting effect of deoxycholic acid on colonic adenocarcinomas in germfree rats, *J. Natl. Cancer Inst.*, 56, 441, 1976.
97. **Reddy, B. S., Watanabe, K., Weisburger, J. H., and Wynder, E. L.,** Promoting effect of bile acids in colon carcinogenesis in germfree and conventional F344 rats, *Cancer Res.*, 37, 3238, 1977.
98. **Reddy, B. S. and Watanabe, K.,** Effect of cholesterol metabolites and promoting effect of lithocholic acid in colon carcinogenesis in germfree and conventional F344 rats, *Cancer Res.*, 39, 1521, 1979.
99. **Cohen, B. I., Raicht, R. F., Deschner, E. E., Takahashi, M., Sarwal, A. N., and Fazzini, E.,** Effect of cholic acid feeding on N-methyl-N-nitrosourea-induced colon tumors and cell kinetics in rats, *J. Natl. Cancer Inst.*, 64, 573, 1980.
100. **Silverman, S. J. and Andrews, A. W.,** Bile acids: comutagenic activity in Salmonella-mammalian microsome mutagenicity test: brief communication, *J. Natl. Cancer Inst.*, 59, 1557, 1977.
101. **Kelsey, M. I., Andrews, A. W., Pienta, R. J., and Kawalek, J. C.,** in *1980 Workshop on Bile Acids and Large Bowel Carcinogenesis*, National Large Bowel Cancer Project, Houston, January 17 to 19, 1980, 38.
102. **Bagheri, S. A., Bolt, M. G., Boyer, J. L., and Palmer, R. H.,** Stimulation of thymidine incorporation in mouse liver and biliary tract epithelium by lithocholate and deoxycholate, *Gastroenterology*, 7, 188, 1978.
103. **Matsuzawa, T. and Wilson, R.,** The intestinal mucosa of germfree mice after whole body X-irradiation with the kalorventgens, *Radiat. Res.*, 25, 15, 1965.
104. **Meslin, J. C., Sacquet, E., and Raiband, P.,** Action d'une flore microbienne qui ne deconjuque pas les sels biliaries sur la morphologie et le renouvellement callulaire de la muqueuse de l'intestin grele du rat, *Ann. Biol. Anim. Biochim. Biophys.*, 14, 709, 1974.
105. **Lipkin, M.,** Biology of large bowel cancer. Present status and research frontiers, *Cancer*, 36, 2319, 1975.
106. **Takano, S., Matsushima, M., Erturk, E., and Bryan, G. T.,** Early induction of rat colonic epithelial ornithine and S-adenyl-L-methionine decarboxylase activities by N-methyl-N′-nitro-N-nitrosoguanidine or bile salts, *Cancer Res.*, 41, 624, 1981.
107. **Cruse, J. P., Lewin, M. R., and Clark, C. G.,** Dietary cholesterol is co-carcinogenic for human colon cancer, *Lancet*, 1, 152, 1979.
108. **Bischoff, F.,** Carcinogenic effects of steroids, *Adv. Lipid Res.*, 7, 165, 1969.
109. **Reddy, B. S., Martin, C. W., and Wynder, E. L.,** Fecal bile acids and cholesterol metabolites of patients with ulcerative colitis, a high risk group for development of colon cancer, *Cancer Res.*, 37, 1697, 1977.
110. **Reddy, B. S. and Wynder, E. L.,** Metabolic epidemiology of colon cancer — fecal bile acids and neutral sterols in colon cancer patients and patients with adenomatous polyps, *Cancer*, 39, 2533, 1977.

111. **Smith, L. L., Smart, V. B., and Ansari, G. A. S.,** Mutagenic cholesterol preparations, *Mutatat. Res.*, 68, 23, 1979.
112. **Reddy, B. S. and Watanabe, K.,** Effect of cholesterol metabolites and promoting effects of lithocholic acid in colon carcinogenesis in germfree and conventional F344 rats, *Cancer Res.*, 39, 1521, 1979.
113. **Lipkin, M.,** Susceptibility of human population groups to colon cancer, *Adv. Cancer Res.*, 27, 281, 1978.
114. **Lane, N., Fenoglio, C. M., Kaye, G. I., and Pascal, R. R.,** Defining the precursor tissue of ordinary large bowel carcinoma: implications for cancer prevention, in *Gastrointestinal Tract Cancer*, Lipkin, M. L. and Good, R., Eds., Plenum Press, New York, 1978, 295.
115. **Lipkin, M.,** Proliferation and differentiation of gastrointestinal cells, *Physiol. Rev.*, 53, 891, 1973.
116. **Deschner, E. and Lipkin, M.,** Proliferative patterns in colonic mucosa of polyposis families, *Cancer*, 35, 413, 1975.
117. **Lipkin, M.,** Measurement of risk factors in identifying population with increased susceptibility to colon cancer, in *Colorectal Cancer: Prevention, Epidemiology and Screening*, Winawer, S., Schottenfeld, D., and Sherlock, P., Eds., Raven Press, New York, 1980, 143.
118. **Silverberg, E. and Holleb, A.,** Cancer statistics, *CA Cancer J. Clin.*, 25, 8, 1975.
119. **Lohrs, U., Wiebecke, B., and Edgar, M.,** Morphologische und autoradiographische untersuchung der darmschleim — haut- veranderringen nach einmaliger injektion von DMH, *Z. Gesamte Exp. Med.*, 151, 297, 1969.
120. **Springer, P., Springer, J., and Oehlert, W.,** Early stages of DMH-induced carcinoma of the small and large intestine of the rat, *Z. Krebsforsch.*, 74, 236, 1970.
121. **Thurnherr, N., Deschner, E. E., Stonehill, E. H., and Lipkin, M.,** Induction of adenocarcinomas of the colon in mice by weekly injection of 1,2-dimethylhydrazine, *Cancer Res.*, 33, 940, 1973.
122. **Deschner, E. E. and Lang, F. C.,** Colonic neoplasms in mice produced with six injections of 1,2-dimethylhydrazine, *Oncology*, 36, 255, 1977.

Chapter 6

TUMOR PROMOTION IN BLADDER CARCINOGENESIS

Samuel M. Cohen, Gen'i Murasaki, Leon B. Ellwein, and Robert E. Greenfield

TABLE OF CONTENTS

I. INTRODUCTION

Bladder cancer represents a small proportion of the total incidence of human cancer, but it has been intensively studied because of the known relationship of specific chemicals to the etiology of the disease. It has been a useful model for the study of chemical carcinogenesis in animals and for relating degree of exposure to carcinogens to the incidence of disease in humans. The induction of human bladder cancer may occur as the result of prolonged or repeated exposure to large doses of a single carcinogen, or more commonly, it appears to be induced by exposure to low doses of multiple agents in an additive or synergistic manner. The interaction of these various agents and factors in the etiology and mechanism of bladder cancer will be discussed in this chapter.

II. URINARY BLADDER CARCINOGENESIS

A. Historical

The relationship of chemicals to urinary bladder carcinogenesis was initially observed in humans. Rehn, in 1895, identified an increased incidence of cancer of the urinary bladder in workers in the aniline dye industry in Germany.[1,2] In 1937, Hueper and colleagues[3] were able to demonstrate that 2-naphthylamine, one of the chemicals to which these workers were exposed, induced bladder tumors when administered to dogs. Dogs as an experimental animal have proven to be of use in the study of other aromatic amines, in the identification of carcinogens of the urinary bladder, and in the study of carcinogen metabolism.[4] However, generalized use of dogs as an experimental tool is extremely limited because of the long induction period required and because of the high cost involved in maintaining sufficiently large numbers of dogs to perform experiments with statistically significant results. The use of smaller experimental animals, such as rats or mice, would be more useful for detailed studies concerning metabolism of carcinogens and especially in studying the mechanisms of the disease, but the administration of most aromatic amines or amides results in liver tumors rather than urinary bladder tumors in rodents.[1,2] 2-Acetylaminofluorene (AAF), an aromatic amide, was reported in 1941 to induce tumors of several tissues including the urinary bladder in rodents.[1,2] Initially it was demonstrated in rats, and subsequently it has been demonstrated in other rodent species including mice and hamsters. Thus, an experimental model for small animal species in which tumors can be induced within a relatively short period of time became available for studies of bladder carcinogenesis. However, AAF induced tumors of other tissues in addition to tumors of the urinary bladder, especially the liver, mammary gland, and ear duct.

In the 1960s, three bladder specific carcinogens were eventually discovered in rats which have provided the animal models necessary for the detailed evaluation of bladder carcinogenesis. Dibutylnitrosamine was shown to induce tumors of the urinary bladder, but also tumors of other tissues including the esophagus and liver.[5] However, *N*-butyl-*N*-(4-hydroxybutyl)nitrosamine (BBN), a metabolite of dibutylnitrosamine, administered in the drinking water, was specific for the urinary bladder.[5] *N*-[4-(5-Nitro-2-furyl)-2-thiazolyl]formamide (FANFT), a 5-nitrofuran, also induced bladder tumors in a number of species when administered in the diet.[6] It was initially demonstrated as a bladder carcinogen in female Sprague-Dawley rats,[6] but has subsequently been shown to be a bladder carcinogen in other strains of rats as well as in mice, hamsters, and dogs.[7] The guinea pig, however, appears to be resistant to FANFT and other nitrofurans.[7] Intravesical instillation of *N*-methyl-*N*-nitrosourea (MNU), a direct acting carcinogen, also was shown to be carcinogenic for the urinary bladder.[8] A dose-related response has been reported for all three of these chemicals in the induction of urinary bladder cancer.[9-11]

Other nitrosamines[12] and nitrofurans[7] have been shown to be carcinogenic toward the bladder, particularly the former class of compounds. The nitrosamines appear to require at least one of the aliphatic chains of the secondary nitroso compound to be an even numbered chain with a minimum of four carbons in the chain. It would appear that metabolism is through sequential hydroxylation and oxidation with cleavage of the acetyl groups gradually shortening the chain. The carboxypropyl metabolite of BBN is also carcinogenic for the urinary bladder,[9] but the ultimate metabolite is not yet definitely known. In mice, the urinary bladder appears to be susceptible only to the nitrofuran FANFT. In rats, FANFT and its deformylated analogue, 2-amino-4-(5-nitro-2-furyl)thiazole, are carcinogenic to the bladder.[7,13] The other nitrofurans induce tumors of other tissues, occasionally of the upper urinary tract, but not the urinary bladder. However, in hamsters[14] and in dogs,[15] the urinary bladder appears to be a common target tissue for thiazole substituted 5-nitrofurans. The ultimate metabolite of FANFT is not yet known, but a number of enzyme systems have been known to activate this chemical including the microsomal mixed function oxidase,[16] xanthine oxidase,[16] and prostaglandin endoperoxide synthetase.[17] Which of these is biologically significant in the metabolic activation of FANFT has not yet been determined.

Occasionally, other compounds have been shown to induce bladder tumors in some species, but none appear to be more potent or more organ specific than the three described above.[1,2]

B. Histogenesis of Rodent Bladder Cancer

The epithelial lining of the lower urinary tract has been referred to as the urothelium and consists of three cell layers.[1] The basal layer consists of round to oval cells with centrally placed nuclei and rests on a basement membrane. The intermediate cell layer consists of somewhat larger cells that are also round to oval. The most superficial cell layer consists of large umbrella-like cells which are polygonal and extend over multiple intermediate cells. This superficial cell is unique for the urothelium and is distinguished by the asymmetric unit membrane that lines its luminal surface.[18] In rodents, the asymmetric unit membrane remains on the luminal surface and in fusiform vesicles throughout the life span of the animals. It can be used as a marker of terminal differentiation and can be detected by transmission electron microscopy; the characteristic microridge pattern that it forms on the luminal surface can be observed more readily by scanning electron microscopy.[18] The superficial cells are joined by a junctional complex which forms a tight junction between the cells; this complex forms part of the barrier to urine.[19]

Following the oral administration of a urinary bladder carcinogen, the urothelium proliferates more rapidly than the normally quiescent urothelium, and a simple hyperplasia is formed.[9,20,21] During carcinogenesis, nodular and papillary hyperplasia gradually evolve with the eventual formation of a papilloma. The papilloma is followed by noninvasive carcinoma and eventually by invasion. Distant metastases occasionally are found if the animals are kept alive long enough. Most of the animals, however, die of massive hematuria. Ureteral obstruction is only occasionally observed with resulting hydronephrosis, except it occurs frequently in Sprague-Dawley rats. Histologically, most of the tumors induced in rodents are transitional cell carcinomas, and many of these are papillary.[9,20,21] Frequently, there is squamous differentiation within these tumors, but squamous cell carcinomas are infrequent except in mice.[9,22] Thus, there is considerable similarity between the animal model and the human disease, although differences are present and must be considered in extrapolating results from the animal model to the human situation.

Ultrastructurally, there is a progressive loss in the number and size of the tight junctions during carcinogenesis.[19] There is progressive loss of the features of differentiation, including the formation of fusiform vesicles and asymmetric unit membranes.[18] With the loss of differentiation to superficial cells, the surface of the bladder becomes lined by intermediate cells and/or basal cells. The luminal surface of these cells is characterized by having short, uniform microvilli covered with a glycocalyx fuzz.[23] With progression to more advanced hyperplastic lesions, there is the appearance of pleomorphic microvilli which are longer than the usual microvilli; they vary in size and shape and many branched forms appear.[18] Similar surface features are present on transitional cell carcinoma cells in animals as well as in humans. However, these changes are not specific for neoplasia as they also are seen in the marked nodular and papillary hyperplasia during regeneration and repair of severe damage to the bladder epithelium, such as following freeze ulceration[24] or cyclophosphamide administration.[25] In these latter instances, the lesions are totally reversible and nonneoplastic.

During carcinogenesis, there have been several histochemical changes observed, most notably alkaline phosphatase[26,27] that is rapidly lost early in carcinogenesis and is also absent in tumor cells. However, similar loss of activity is seen in the marked regenerative hyperplasia following freeze ulceration or cyclophosphamide.[26] A similar loss of beta-glucuronidase activity is seen in both neoplastic and regenerative hyperplastic proliferations. A more variable change has been observed in the activities of succinic dehydrogenase[27] and alpha-naphthyl esterase.[26] Unfortunately, no histochemical or ultrastructural feature marker has been identified that is specific for neoplasia. However, these changes can be used in specific studies in following the course of the disease and in identifying early changes in the bladder epithelium. Also, the number of cells involved with these particular changes can be quantified.

III. MULTISTAGE CARCINOGENESIS

A. Administration of Multiple Bladder Carcinogens

The administration of multiple carcinogens has been shown in other tissue systems to result in additive or synergistic effects.[28] The simultaneous administration of low doses of bladder carcinogens, at doses which individually do not induce tumors within the time of the study, were shown to have a synergistic effect in the induction of bladder cancer by Tsuda and colleagues.[29] The carcinogens, BBN, FANFT, AAF, and 3,3′-dichlorobenzidine, were administered to male Wistar rats for 4 weeks followed by 36 weeks of control diet. At the end of the experiment, there was a significant incidence of bladder cancer in the groups administered multiple chemicals, but not in the groups receiving only one of the chemicals. These same investigators[30] also demonstrated that sequential administration of the same four carcinogens at the same doses for the same periods of time produced similar results. The administration of other bladder carcinogens together, such as phenacetin and BBN,[31] or MNU and 2-naphthylamine,[32] has also been reported to result in an increased incidence of tumors. It is unclear in these studies whether the sequence of administration of the chemicals is important to whether they could be administered in a random order.

B. Initiation and Promotion in Bladder Carcinogenesis

The model of initiation and promotion originally described in the mouse skin model takes into consideration that the sequence of administration of specific agents is important in the carcinogenic sequence.[28] Thus, the administration of one chemical, the initiator, must precede the administration of the second agent, the promoter, for tumors to appear. In the classical model, if the sequence is reversed, tumors do not appear.

In the 1960s, there became available evidence that the multistage model of carcinogenesis may also be applicable to the urinary bladder. Bryan and Springberg[33] demonstrated that the insertion of a cholesterol pellet containing the 8-methyl ether of xanthurenic acid (XAE), a tryptophan metabolite, into the urinary bladder of mice resulted in a 33% incidence of bladder carcinoma compared to an 8% incidence in mice having only the cholesterol pellet without XAE inserted. However, if the XAE was administered as a single subcutaneous injection with the cholesterol pellet present in the urinary bladder (the pellet not containing XAE), a similar incidence of bladder cancer, 30%, was induced. A subcutaneous injection of XAE by itself did not induce tumors, but the insertion of a pure pellet of XAE into the urinary bladder did result in induction of one bladder carcinoma in 63 mice (1.6%). In this study, the XAE, which eluted rapidly from the cholesterol pellet, possibly acted as an initiating agent, whereas the vehicle, continuing intact in the bladder for prolonged periods of time, acted as the promoting agent, perhaps by mechanical irritation. Similarly, Clayson and colleagues[34] demonstrated that the administration of a small dose of 2-aminodiphenylene oxide by stomach tube followed by the implantation of a paraffin wax pellet into the lumen of the mouse urinary bladder resulted in significantly more bladder carcinomas than administration of either the chemical alone or the implanted pellet alone.

The role of the pellet in these experiments has remained incompletely defined,[35] but at least it provides a prolonged mitotic stimulus to the bladder mucosa. Also, the process of inserting the pellet into the bladder provides a burst of mitotic activity since the bladder must be incised and sutured closed. This results in a marked regenerative hyperplasia with tissue kinetics similar to that following ulceration by freezing or by cyclophosphamide injection.[24] As shown below, this type of activity appears to provide a stimulus for the induction of bladder cancer if the mitotic activity is maintained at above normal levels.

A more classical model of initiation-promotion for the urinary bladder was established by Hicks et al.[36] in 1973 using the intravesical instillation of a single dose of MNU as the initiator followed by either sodium saccharin or sodium cyclamate in the diet as the promoter. Administration of only the MNU did not result in tumors. The rats fed only sodium saccharin or sodium cyclamate without prior initiation with MNU developed a low incidence of bladder tumors, 2 and 1%, respectively. MNU followed by cyclophosphamide, however, did not result in an increased incidence of tumors. Additional evidence that two-stage carcinogenesis occurred in the urinary bladder was provided using the FANFT and BBN animal models in rats. Cohen et al.[37] reported that the administration of 6 weeks of FANFT at a level of 0.2% followed immediately by either sodium saccharin or D,L-tryptophan in the diet resulted in an increased incidence of bladder tumors compared to the group fed FANFT for 6 weeks followed by control diet. The latter group had an incidence of 20%. However, by using 4 weeks of FANFT administration as the initiator, tumors were still induced when followed by either sodium saccharin or L-tryptophan as the promoter, but no tumors were induced when the brief feeding of FANFT was followed by control diet.[38] The incidence of bladder tumors in the groups receiving either sodium saccharin or L-tryptophan after FANFT was considerably lower than in the experiment using 6 weeks of FANFT as the initiator. If FANFT was administered for only 2 weeks followed by sodium saccharin, there was no significant incidence of tumors compared to FANFT followed by control diet.[39] This dose response for an initiating agent is similar to that seen in experiments in other tissues.[28]

If the sodium saccharin or tryptophan was not administered until 6 weeks after the FANFT was discontinued in the diet, during which time the rats received control diet, the incidence of tumors was also increased compared to the administration of FANFT only.[37] During the 6-week period between the administration of FANFT and the administration of the second compound, the FANFT is cleared from the body[16] and the urothelial hyperplasia regresses to normal.[40] This provides some evidence that initiation in the bladder is irreversible as in the mouse skin model.[28]

BBN has also been shown to act as initiator in the rat bladder cancer model and sodium saccharin[41] and phenacetin[31] have been shown to be promoters. More recently, Ito and colleagues[42] demonstrated that sodium ascorbate also had promoting activity in this model although sodium cyclamate was inactive. However, the dose of sodium cyclamate was low compared to the experiments using MNU as the initiator.[36]

In all of these experiments, the incidence of tumors with sodium saccharin, sodium cyclamate, tryptophan, or sodium ascorbate when administered alone was either zero or less than 3%, as would be expected of a promoting agent. Thus, the model of initiation and promotion in the urinary bladder has many similarities to the model in mouse skin, but the experiment of reversing the order of administration of the two chemicals has yet to be performed.

C. Sodium Saccharin

Saccharin (1,2-benzisothiazol-3(2H)-one, 1,1-dioxide) is a weak acidic compound which is weakly soluble in water.[43] The sodium salt, sodium saccharin, is considerably more soluble and is the form consumed by humans as a nonnutritive sweetening agent. The widespread use of the chemical by humans and the high doses generally used in experimental studies have engendered considerable controversy with regard to extrapolation of the results of the animal studies to the potential risks in humans. We will discuss here only the results in animal studies and their possible interpretations with regard to mechanisms of carcinogenesis.

Sodium saccharin administered orally, in the drinking water or in the diet, has been reported to be weakly carcinogenic in one generation studies in rats[43] and to induce greater incidences of bladder tumors in two generation studies.[44] The greatest activity of tumor induction by sodium saccharin, however, has been in experiments utilizing a two-stage model with sodium saccharin being the second chemical administered. Increased incidences have resulted if MNU,[11,36] FANFT,[37,38] or BBN[31,41] were used as initiators. In most instances, the length of time required for the induction of tumors in rats, whether sodium saccharin was used as the only agent or as a promoter, has been quite long, usually 18 months to 2 years. Also, the carcinogenesis studies have involved high doses of the chemical in the diet, usually 5 or 7.5%, or in the drinking water.

In animal experiments, sodium saccharin has displayed many of the properties that one would expect for a promoting agent. It is not metabolized in rats, and it is excreted in high concentration in the urine.[43] By itself, it is considered at most a weak carcinogen.[43,44] Also, it does not appear to have mutagenic activity in in vitro assays,[43] but it does appear to increase the rate of recombination in certain yeast species.[45] Also, similar to promoters in other tissue models, sodium saccharin inhibits cell to cell communication.[46] In addition, sodium saccharin induces a high incidence of mild hyperplasia in the target organ,[47-49] the urothelium, even without prior initiation. The induction of hyperplasia by sodium saccharin is related to dose, but long-term studies evaluating the dose response of sodium saccharin as a promoter have not yet been reported.

The mechanism by which sodium saccharin acts remains unclear. Some investigators postulated that it causes bladder tumors by the induction of calculi.[43] However, long-term, longitudinal, prospective studies evaluating urine have been performed in rats fed sodium saccharin, and no increased crystalluria or calculus formation was observed.[50] Other changes in the urine which might indirectly result in the induction of bladder cancer following sodium saccharin administration have not yet been identified. The changes in the urine that have been observed are those to be anticipated following the administration of high doses of the sodium salt of a weak acid. The total sodium excretion increases markedly and the pH increases slightly. Since the animals administered sodium saccharin in the diet have a markedly increased intake of water, the amount of water excreted in the urine is also increased and this results in a slightly decreased osmolality and only slight increases in the concentration of sodium. No changes were observed in potassium excretion. For unknown reasons, there was a persistent decrease in the concentration of glucose in the urine and a corresponding hypoglycemia. Hypoglucosuria and hypoglycemia were also observed in rats fed L-tryptophan in the diet, although the other changes in the urine following sodium saccharin feeding were not found after L-tryptophan.

Direct interactions of sodium saccharin with cell components have not yet been identified.[51-54] Sodium saccharin does not appear to bind to DNA and it is not metabolically activated to a reactive electrophile. However, a recent study using taste receptors on the tongue demonstrate that sodium saccharin can bind to the plasma membrane of such cells. It is not known at the present time whether it binds to receptors on the bladder cell membrane.

D. Tryptophan

The relationship of tryptophan and its metabolites to the etiology of human bladder cancer has remained an enigma[1,2] since the original observation by Dunning et al.[55] in 1950 that D,L-tryptophan administered simultaneously with AAF increased the bladder carcinogenicity of AAF. Tryptophan by itself did not induce bladder tumors. Additional stimulus for trying to relate urinary bladder carcinogenesis to tryptophan and its metabolites came from studies in the 1950s showing that metabolites of tryptophan along the niacin pathway were aromatic amines similar to those already known as bladder carcinogens in humans.[1,2] These metabolites included anthranilic acid and kynurenine. In addition, the ortho-aminophenol analogues of these two compounds, also metabolites of tryptophan, were present in the urine of humans. It was shown by Price and colleagues[2] at the University of Wisconsin that the excretion of certain tryptophan metabolites, including kynurenine, 3-hydroxykynurenine, acetylkynurenine, and kynurenic acid, in the urine was increased in approximately 50% of the patients with bladder cancer seen at that institution. Extensive studies were performed at Wisconsin and at other laboratories concerning the metabolism of tryptophan along the niacin pathway and the relationship of these metabolites in bladder cancer patients and other diseases. During these studies, it was demonstrated that vitamin B_6, pyridoxine, was involved along the tryptophan metabolic pathway, and that the abnormal tryptophan metabolite levels seen in some patients could be corrected by the oral administration of pyridoxine.[2]

The insertion into the bladder of mice of cholesterol or paraffin wax pellets containing various chemicals, including various tryptophan metabolites, gave rise to increased incidences of bladder tumors compared to mice having the pellet alone.[1,2,33,56,57] However, as mentioned above, interpretation of these studies remains difficult since a large proportion of animals with only the pellet eventually developed bladder tumors, particularly if observed over long periods of time rather than the usual 50 to 60 weeks of many of the earlier reported studies.[35] It was observed in other studies that tryptophan administered orally to animals induced hyperplasia of the urinary bladder, but in none of these studies was the administration of even large doses of tryptophan shown to induce cancer by itself.[1,2,57,58] Several other studies were performed which were unable to demonstrate any kind of a relationship. In addition, alternative explanations of the original observation by Dunning et al.[55] were subsequently suggested. For example, it was noted in the study by Dunning et al.[55] that tryptophan administration decreased the incidence of liver tumors in response to AAF, enabling the animals to live longer. Possibly the increased longevity was responsible for the eventual increased incidence of bladder tumors which tend to appear later than the liver tumors. Also, another metabolite of tryptophan, indole, which is not derived from the niacin pathway but rather arises from the serotonin pathway, can act as a sulfate trap for AAF.[1,2,59-61] It was demonstrated that the sulfate ester of the *N*-hydroxylated metabolite of AAF was the most likely ultimate metabolite leading to AAF liver carcinogenesis.[59,62] Any substance which would deplete the sulfate pool would be able to inhibit the liver carcinogenicity of AAF, resulting in more of the compound excreted in the urine where it could be metabolized by other pathways, generating an ultimate reactive electrophile in the bladder.[60] However, this mechanism could not definitely be demonstrated experimentally.

The induction of hyperplasia by orally administered tryptophan and the tenuous relationship of tryptophan and its metabolites to bladder carcinogenesis in animals and in humans suggested to us the possibility that tryptophan could act as a promoting substance for bladder carcinogenesis. Thus, D,L-tryptophan was administered to rats after FANFT initiation and an increased incidence of bladder tumors was demonstrated.[37] This type of experiment is quite distinct from the original Dunning et al.[55] experiment in which tryptophan and AAF were simultaneously administered. With the advent of the ready availability of pure L-tryptophan rather than the D,L-racemic mixture of tryptophan, the experiment was repeated.[38] Although there was an increased incidence of bladder lesions with L-tryptophan after 4 weeks of FANFT initiation, increase was not at a statistically significant level. However, promoting activity was observed with L-tryptophan after FANFT initiation in mice[63] and with D,L-tryptophan in dogs after initiation with aromatic amines.[64]

Again, these data suggest a relationship for tryptophan with bladder cancer, but are not definitive. Similarly, subsequent studies in humans have shown a relationship with tryptophan metabolites and bladder cancer which would be consistent with a promoting effect. Thus, patients with low-grade, low-stage bladder cancer who had abnormal levels of tryptophan metabolites in the urine at the time of their initial diagnosis were shown to have a significantly higher rate of recurrence that patients who had normal levels.[65] Also, Byar and Blanchard[66] reported that patients with low-grade, low-stage bladder carcinoma treated with pyridoxine after transuretheral resection of the bladder lesion had a significantly lower rate of recurrence than patients treated with placebo. Unfortunately, in the latter study, there was no attempt to identify the tryptophan metabolite status of the patients, or whether those that benefited from the pyridoxine were those with abnormal tryptophan metabolite levels. Nevertheless, these experimental and clinical studies are provocative and require more systematic evaluation.

Tryptophan and its metabolites have many of the properties that one would anticipate for a tumor promoter. The administration of tryptophan in the diet results in increased levels of metabolites in the urine and also induces a mild hyperplasia of the bladder.[1,2,58] By itself, however, it does not induce bladder tumors.[1,2,56,57] Tryptophan and its metabolites have not been shown to be mutagenic in in vitro assays and covalent binding to DNA has not been demonstrated.[67]

IV. URINE

The urogenous theory of bladder carcinogenesis predicts that carcinogens arrive at the bladder mucosa via the urine rather than via the bloodstream. Ample evidence for this has been reported beginning in 1953 with the observation in dogs that urinary diversion of the ureters during the time of administration of the bladder carcinogen prevented the appearance of bladder tumors.[68] In addition to this direct evidence for the urogenous theory, support for the theory is indirectly suggested by the increased concentration of carcinogens or metabolites in the urine compared to the blood.[1,2]

More recently, evidence has been presented which suggests that a substance or substances in urine are directly involved in the carcinogenic process. Chapman et al.[69] demonstrated that in a bladder divided in half by a suture, a wax pellet inserted into either half induced bladder tumors only if urine was present. Thus, in the half of bladder without urine, no tumors arose. Again, there is the problem of determining the role of the pellet. More direct evidence for the role of urine in carcinogenesis and a determination of the stage during which it is important was described by Rowland et al.[70] In their experiment, FANFT was administered in the diet for 14 weeks. This had previously been shown to be a "carcinogenic" dose of FANFT. Thus, if the animals were allowed to live for sufficient periods of time, bladder tumors should have developed. In a group of rats in which urine continued to go through the urinary bladder, tumors did develop. However, after the 14 weeks of FANFT, if the ureters were diverted by performing bilateral ureterosigmoidostomies, no tumors developed in the urinary bladder after 30 weeks, or significantly fewer tumors developed after longer periods of time compared to rats with urine still flowing through the bladder.

Oyasu et al.[71] provided additional evidence that a factor or factors in urine are important in the later phases of carcinogenesis. Utilizing the heterotopic bladder model developed by them, they were able to show that bladders exposed initially to BBN and then exposed to saline developed significantly fewer bladder tumors than bladders which were exposed to BBN and then exposed to urine of equal osmolality and pH as the saline. Using an in vitro assay[72] for the stimulation of ornithine decarboxylase and cell proliferation, they were able to demonstrate that the enhancing activity in the urine for bladder carcinogenesis resided in two molecular weight fractions: one being macromolecular and of molecular weight greater than 10,000 daltons, and one less than 1000 daltons. They have presented some evidence that the macromolecular component is a peptide.[73] The smaller molecular species has not yet been identified, but a number of candidates are possible. In their in vitro assay system, they have identified that anthranilic acid, a tryptophan metabolite, enhances activity.[72] Other possibilities include other tryptophan metabolites, various polyamines, or a variety of other substances, such as urea or creatinine that are normally present in the urine. It must be emphasized that the urine used as the enhancing agent in these experiments was normal rat urine, not urine from animals administered carcinogens. Similar enhancing activity has also been identified in normal human urine.[87]

The question arises that, if components of normal urine have enhancing activity in carcinogenesis, why are there are not more tumors spontaneously? Although the answer to such a question is not yet definitively known, likely explanations involve the changes in the urothelium that are observed following the administration of carcinogens. The most likely of these possibilities is that the administration of a carcinogen produces what would be considered a "leaky" epithelium.[19] As described above, the normal urinary bladder epithelium provides a barrier to urine, which, although not perfect, is adequate for avoiding the toxic effects of the very concentrated levels of certain substances in the urine. One of the first changes to occur during carcinogenesis is a breakdown in this barrier.[19] This includes a decrease in the formation of the asymmetric unit membrane and a decrease in the tight junctions between the superficial cells. The tight junctions become less numerous and individually become attenuated as the administration of the carcinogen continues. This would allow for increased exposure to substances in the urine, particularly macromolecular species.

V. REGENERATIVE HYPERPLASIA AND BLADDER CARCINOGENESIS

Regenerative hyperplasia of the urinary bladder epithelium can be induced by several chemical and physical methods. Chemically it can be induced by either the intravesical instillation of chemically reactive compounds such as MNU,[8,11] or by the instillation of corrosive compounds such as acetic acid or formalin.[24] Also, it can be induced chemically by the systemic administration of compounds that excrete an active metabolite in the urine, such as the intraperitoneal injection of cyclophosphamide.[25] Physical means include the stripping of the bladder epithelium,[74] incising the bladder with the placement of a suture,[24] and the method developed by Shirai et al.[75] that involves the application to the serosal surface of a frozen metal rod. By whatever method, the process of regeneration and repair and the tissue kinetics are similar. Differences in the time involved for the mucosa to return to normal depend on the extent of the ulceration and the strain and species of test animals used. Following the initial insult to the bladder, there is necrosis of the epithelium which lasts from several minutes to a few days depending on the inciting agent. This is followed by a period of rapid cell proliferation of the epithelium and the generation of marked hyperplasia, including nodular and papillary formation similar in appearance to that seen during the course of chemically induced bladder carcinogenesis. The ulcer is eventually repaired and the hyperplasia regresses so that eventually the bladder epithelium appears morphologically normal, and remains so for the lifetime of the animal (up to 2 years of observation).

The urinary bladder epithelium is normally a mitotically quiescent tissue, the turnover rate estimated at 50 to 200 days.[1,76] If it is assumed that the initiation event requires a cell to be in the process of replication,[77-79] little initiation would be anticipated to occur in the urinary bladder under normal circumstances with a short period of administration of an initiator. This may explain why initiation in the bladder appears to require a relatively long period of time compared to the mitotically active mouse skin. Thus, in the BBN model, a week of administration in the drinking water is required,[31,41] and 4 to 6 weeks of feeding are required for initiation in the FANFT model.[37,38] With MNU, only a single intravesical instillation is required, but this may be related to the marked regenerative hyperplasia following the extensive ulceration induced by this chemical.[11] To determine whether the period of initiation in the FANFT model could be shortened by administering it to a rat with a rapidly proliferating bladder, we performed the experiment[39] depicted in Figure 1. Ulceration and regenerative hyperplasia was induced either by the freeze ulceration method of Shirai et al.[75] or by the i.p. injection of cyclophosphamide. In the test group, the FANFT was administered for 2 weeks at a level of 0.2% of the diet, and promotion was to be produced by the subsequent administration of sodium saccharin as 5% of the diet. The other groups represent appropriate controls. The results are summarized in Table 1.

As expected, the animals administered FANFT immediately after ulceration and then promoted with sodium saccharin developed bladder tumors. It did not make any difference whether the ulceration was by the freeze ulceration technique or whether it was by cyclophosphamide injection. However, quite surprisingly, animals administered saccharin either immediately after ulceration or after a 2-week delay, during which time the animals received only control diet, developed bladder tumors at approximately the same incidence that the groups of rats fed FANFT for those 2 weeks. Groups administered either the ulceration, sodium saccharin, or FANFT alone, did not develop bladder cancer. Although not conclusive, these data would suggest that mutation, at least as defined by the Ames assay, is not a necessary part of the carcinogenic process in the urinary bladder epithelium. Neither the addition of FANFT for 2 weeks compared to control diet for 2 weeks nor cyclophosphamide compared to freeze ulceration increased the incidence of bladder tumors, despite the fact that FANFT[80] and cyclophosphamide[81] administration produce urine with strong mutagenic activity. This mutagenic activity is present in the urine of FANFT-fed animals in the form of a compound which requires metabolic activation, presumably by the bladder epithelium itself. In the present experiment, the metabolic machinery needed to activate FANFT may not be present during the repair of the ulcer. However, cyclophosphamide produces a mutagenic urine with a compound, presumably acrolein,[82] which does not require metabolic activation.

Induction of bladder tumors with sodium saccharin administered to animals with a rapidly proliferating bladder mucosa also suggests an explanation for previous studies with sodium saccharin involving the pellet implantation technique[83] and two-generation administration.[44] In each of these experiments, sodium saccharin is administered to an animal with a rapidly proliferating bladder epithelium induced either by freeze ulceration or cyclophosphamide in the present experiments, by surgical incision and implantation of a pellet in the pellet implantation experiments, or through the embryonic and fetal development of the bladder in utero in the two-generation experiment. The pellet implantation experiments would also suggest that sodium saccharin need not be present for long periods of time as long as a continued stimulus for cell proliferation, the pellet, is present. In the pellet implantation experiments, sodium saccharin is leached from the pellet within a short period of time, within several days, and is not present thereafter. Other experiments utilizing the MNU-sodium saccharin model also suggest that sodium saccharin administration is not necessary for prolonged periods of time.[84] In that model it would appear that several weeks of administration of sodium saccharin, possibly less than 20, are sufficient for inducing an irreversible change in the urinary bladder which then can presumably be completed by the enhancing substance(s) present in urine.

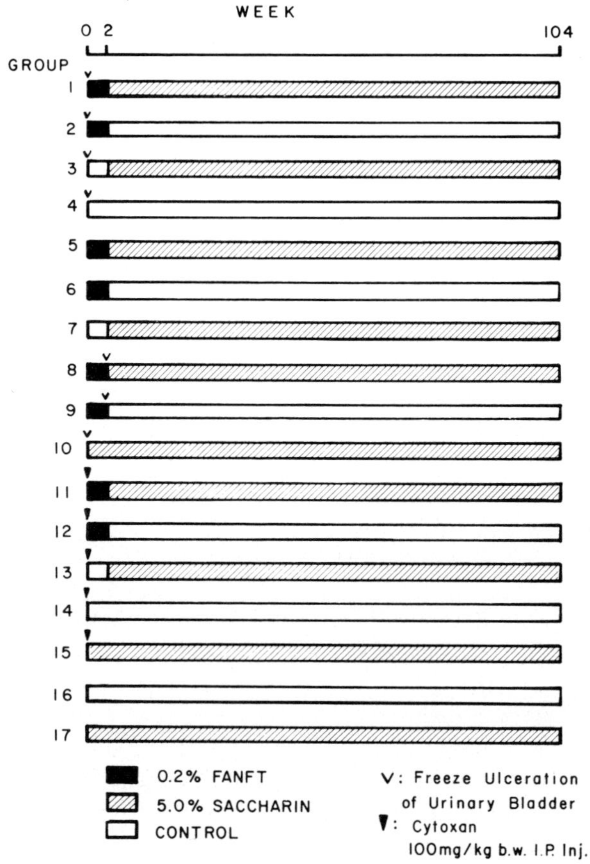

FIGURE 1. Experimental design to determine the effect of regenerative hyperplasia on urinary bladder carcinogenesis. (From Cohen, S. M., Murasaki, G., Fukushima, S., and Greenfield, R. E., *Cancer Res.*, 42, 66, 1982. With permission.)

Table 1
EFFECT OF REGENERATIVE HYPERPLASIA ON BLADDER CARCINOGENESIS

Group	Effective no. of rats	Bladder Tumors[a]		
		Papilloma	Carcinoma	Total
Ul→FANFT→S[b]	23	0	4(17)	4(17)
Ul→FANFT	22	0	0	0
Ul→Cont→S	20	1(5)	5(25)	6(30)
Ul	23	0	0	0
FANFT→S	21	0	1(5)	1(5)
FANFT	19	0	0	0
S	17	0	0	0
FANFT→Ul→S	22	1(5)	8(36)	9(41)
FANFT→Ul	21	0	2(10)	2(10)
Ul→S	21	2(10)	2(10)	4(20)
CP→FANFT→S	22	3(14)	4(18)	7(32)
CP→FANFT	9	0	0	0
CP→Cont→S	17	2(12)	3(18)	5(30)

Table 1 (continued)
EFFECT OF REGENERATIVE HYPERPLASIA ON BLADDER CARCINOGENESIS

Group	Effective no. of rats	Bladder Tumors[a]		
		Papilloma	Carcinoma	Total
CP	7	1(14)	0	1(14)
CP→S	17	3(18)	3(18)	6(36)
Cont	32	0	0	0
S	20	0	0	0

[a] Numbers in parentheses represent the percentage of the rats in a group with the given lesion.

[b] Ul, ulcer by freezing; S, sodium saccharin as 5% of diet; FANFT, *N*-[4-(5-nitro-2-furyl)-2-thiazolyl]formamide as 0.2% of diet for 2 weeks; CP, single i.p. injection of cyclophosphamide, 100 mg/kg.

From Cohen, S. M., Murasaki, G., Fukishima, S., and Greenfield, R. E., *Cancer Res.*, 42, 65, 1982. With permission.

VI. COMPUTER-BASED PROBABILISTIC MODEL OF URINARY BLADDER CARCINOGENESIS

The results of the above experiments and others were consistent with a two-stage process of carcinogenesis in the urinary bladder, but they offered little in the way of explaining the importance of, and the interrelationships between, the many factors which are present during the process. We have developed a probabilistic, computer-based model of the carcinogenic process utilizing data generated from several animal experiments which takes these variables into account. The model is based on a two-stage process. The cellular process of going from the normal to the initiated state is referred to as initiation, and the process of going from the initiated to the transformed state (malignant state) is referred to as transformation. It should be recognized that this two-stage theory does not exclude the possibility that the process of going from a normal cell to a transformed cell may involve more than two changes in cell structure and function; the model represents the process as involving two irreversible events, each of which may involve multiple cellular changes.

The computer-based model is a probabilistic representation of the dynamics of the normal, initiated, and transformed cell populations. It has been described in detail elsewhere,[85] but the essentials of the model will be described here along with some of the predictions obtained from the model.

The various transitions between populations of different kinds of cells are illustrated in Figure 2. Under normal circumstances, the stem cells can divide into either two stem cells or into a stem cell and a committed cell, or the stem cell can die. We make the assumption that the change from a stem cell to a committed cell is irreversible, and that once a cell is committed toward the process of differentiation it will eventually complete the process and die. Thus, any cell that progresses along this pathway will eventually be lost from the stem cell population pool. We further make the assumption that the critical events in carcinogenesis occur only within the population of stem cells. Although the model is based on urinary bladder carcinogenesis, it can be applied to other tissues, recognizing that in those tissues it may be that the target cells for carcinogenesis are not specifically stem cells. Whatever the tissue, a critical variable within the model is the population of cells that are susceptible to carcinogenic stimuli and, thus, capable of forming a neoplastic cell population.

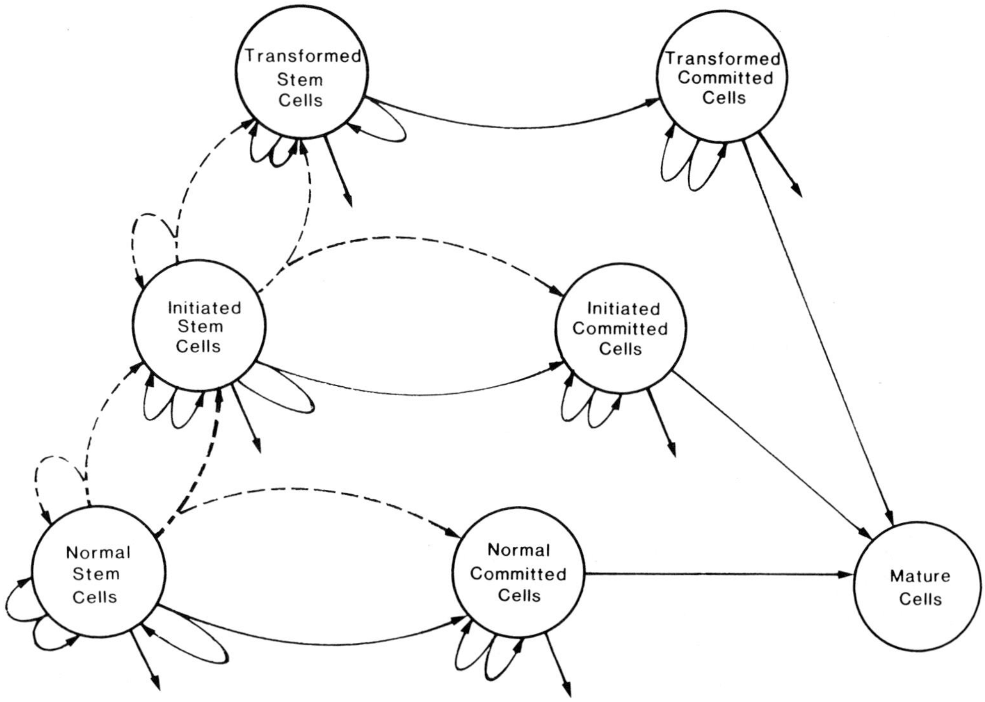

FIGURE 2. Possible cellular transitions. Arrows pointing down and to the right represent loss due to cell death. (From Cohen, S. M., Greenfield, R. E., and Ellwein, L. B., *Cancer Res.*, in press.)

We have made the assumptions that each transition event, initiation and transformation, is irreversible, that each event can only occur during a cell division (not when a cell is at rest), and that each event occurs with a certain probability. In the absence of a carcinogenic stimulus, it is obvious that this probability must be exceedingly low, and that it probably varies with different tissues and species. With these assumptions, several specific variables become essential in determining the likelihood of developing a malignancy. The likelihood of initiation occurring within a given cell population will be dependent on the number of normal stem cells present, the number of cell divisions that occur in that cell population within the time period of interest, and the probability of initiation occurring in a given cell during division. The likelihood of transformation (at least one initiated cell becoming transformed) is dependent on the number of initiated stem cells present as a function of time, the number of mitoses occurring in that cell population, and the probability of transformation occurring during the division of an initiated stem cell. Thus, any stimulus that affects any of these variables would affect the likelihood of an organism eventually developing a malignancy. The expression derived to describe the probability that a malignant cell will be present by some time m is

$$1 - \{[r_1p_{1,2}/(r_1p_{1,2} - r_2p_{2,3})]^m - [r_2p_{2,3}/(r_1p_{1,2} - r_2p_{2,3})]\,[1 - r_1p_{1,2}]^m\}^{S_1(0)}$$

where the probability of a normal stem cell becoming initiated during division is represented by $p_{1,2}$, the probability of an initiated stem cell becoming a transformed stem cell is represented by $p_{2,3}$, the mitotic rates for normal and initiated stem cells are represented by r_1 and r_2, respectively, and $S_1(0)$ represents the number of stem cells present at $m = 0$. It should be recognized that this expression is applicable only so long as the mitotic rates and transition probabilities are constant, or stationary. The computer-based model approximates nonstationary conditions by considering a series of stationary segments.

In applying this model, we used data from FANFT-induced urinary bladder carcinogenesis experiments in the rat.[18,37-40] By utilizing estimates of mitotic rates and reproducing experimentally obtained incidence data at different intervals following various times of administration of the carcinogen, we were able to estimate the transition probabilities $p_{1,2}$ and $p_{2,3}$. We estimated that the number of stem cells normally present in the urinary bladder was 100,000, since there are approximately only one million epithelial cells in the normal rat bladder, and the stem cells are only a proportion of the basal cells present in the bladder. Mitotic rates were estimated from autoradiographic data,[47,76] and the number of nonmalignant stem cells at various times after administration of the carcinogen were estimated based on histopathological evaluation of the rat bladders during the course of the FANFT experiments.[18,37-40]

During the time of administration of FANFT, there is an increase in cell number, and there is a marked increase in the mitotic rate of the bladder epithelium. Based on the results of the computer model, the probability of initiation ($p_{1,2}$) is also markedly altered during the time of administration of FANFT from the normal level of 5×10^{-6} to 1×10^{-2}. Somewhat unexpectedly, however, the second probability, the probability of transformation ($p_{2,3}$), did not change from the normal level of 5×10^{-6} during the period of administration of FANFT. In fact, for the model-based results to be comparable to the observed experimental incidences, $p_{2,3}$ could *not* be altered from normal levels.

Another set of experiments based on the feeding of FANFT followed by sodium saccharin administration[18,37-40] were considered. It was found that sodium saccharin administration did not affect $p_{1,2}$, and also did not affect $p_{2,3}$. The entire effect of sodium saccharin administration was to increase the number of cells present in the bladder (hyperplasia) and to increase the mitotic rate of the bladder epithelium. Again, it was not necessary or possible to change $p_{2,3}$ and still have the results of the computer model match the results actually observed in the experiments.

It is obvious from the modeling of the hypothesized carcinogenic process that cell mitotic rates and the number of cells present as a function of time are critical variables in predicting eventual tumor formation. Given a sufficiently long time period, the model predicts that, even in the absence of a stimulus to increase mitotic rates and stem cell number, all animals would develop bladder cancer. As is expected, however, that period of time is well beyond the normal life span of the animal: it would take 400 years before one half of an unexposed rat population develops bladder tumors!

The model provides an explanation for various observations that have been made in experimental carcinogenesis. Although the critical properties of initiation and promotion as described in the mouse skin model can be readily explained,[28] the present model is more general than the classical initiation-promotion concept of carcinogenesis. In fact, it becomes exceedingly difficult, if not impossible, to actually define promotion with the framework of our model. Experimental results other than those from the classical initiation-promotion experiments can also be explained on the basis of our model. For example, tumors are generally observed earlier in an increased number following the extended administration of a complete carcinogen, such as FANFT, compared to the incidence over time following a two-phase protocol, such as FANFT followed by sodium saccharin.[28] Since FANFT has an effect on the probability of initiation, whereas sodium saccharin does not, the number of initiated cells generated during FANFT administration will constantly increase, increasing the number of initiated cells which immediately have the potential for transformation. In contrast, initiation in the two-phase protocol is limited to the time of exposure to FANFT; the number of initiated cells increases only slowly during exposure to sodium saccharin.

The present model emphasizes the critical role of specific parameters in the carcinogenic process: the population of normal and initiated stem cells; the mitotic rates of normal, initiated, and transformed stem cells; the probabilities of cell initiation, $p_{1,2}$, and of transformation, $p_{2,3}$. Obviously, several different mechanisms may be involved in increasing any of these parameters in various experimental systems. Thus, any procedure which would result in an increase in the number of stem cells and/or the mitotic rate would be expected to increase the likelihood of developing tumors in response to that procedure. An increase in the population of normal stem cells could result either from an increased production of cells or from a decrease in cell loss. Obviously, increased production will take place only if the mitotic rate is increased. Loss of cells from the stem cell population, however, can occur by two mechanisms, either by death of the cell or by differentiation. If the process of differentiation is partially or completely inhibited, it would result in an increase in the number of normal stem cells.

It is obvious from the above description of the model and from the experiments described previously that endogenous as well as exogenous factors will have a marked influence on the process of carcinogenesis. For the urinary bladder, urine is always present and has been shown to be important in the etiology of bladder tumors following FANFT or BBN administration.[70,71] The substance(s) in urine which causes the bladder epithelium to proliferate more rapidly than normal would be expected to enhance the carcinogenic process on the basis of our model. The presence of endogenous factors, such as urine in the bladder[70,71] or bile acids in the liver,[86] has received little attention with regard to their role in carcinogenesis. Their importance in maintaining or increasing cell proliferation may be critical in the dynamics of the carcinogenic process.

We believe that synthesis of data from various animal studies through computer-based modeling is a valuable approach toward furthering the understanding of the complex relationship between multiple exposures to exogenous or endogenous agents in the development of tumors. The availability of a model applicable to both animals and man will assist in the extrapolation of animal data to human problems. It will permit a better assessment of the carcinogenic risk of a particular agent to man when only partial information is available. In the future it is hoped that such increased understanding of the multiple factors and stages in human carcinogenesis, whether exogenous or endogenous, or whether chemical, viral, or physical, will permit the development of methods to interrupt these processes and, thus, to prevent tumor formation.

ACKNOWLEDGMENTS

We gratefully acknowledge the assistant of Jeanette Leemkuil in the preparation of this manuscript. Research from our laboratories reported here were supported in part by USPHS Grants CA32513 and CA28874 from the National Cancer Institute through the National Bladder Cancer Project and RR05660 from the Division of Research Resources of the National Institutes of Health.

REFERENCES

1. **Clayson, D. B. and Cooper, E. H.,** Cancer of the urinary tract, *Adv. Cancer Res.*, 13, 271, 1970.
2. **Price, J. M.,** Etiology of bladder cancer, in *Benign and Malignant Tumors of the Urinary Bladder*, Maltry, E., Ed., Medical Examination Publishing, Flushing, N.Y., 1971, 189.
3. **Hueper, W. C., Wiley, F. H., and Wolfe, H. D.,** Experimental production of bladder tumors in dogs by administration of beta-naphthylamine, *J. Ind. Hyg. Toxicol.*, 20, 46, 1938.

4. **Radomski, J. L.,** The primary aromatic amines: their biological properties and structure-activity relationships, *Annu. Rev. Pharmacol. Toxicol.*, 19, 129, 1979.
5. **Druckrey, H., Preussmann, R., Ivankovic, S., and Schmahl, D.,** Organotrope carcinogene Wirkungen bei 65 Verschiedenen N-Nitroso-Verbindungen an BD-Ratten, *Z. Krebsforsch.*, 69, 103, 1967.
6. **Erturk, E., Price, J. M., Morris, J. E., Cohen, S., Leith, R. S., Von Esch, A. M., and Crovetti, A. J.,** The production of carcinoma of the urinary bladder in rats by feeding N-[4-(5-nitro-2-furyl)-2-thiazolyl]formamide, *Cancer Res.*, 27, 1998, 1967.
7. **Cohen, S. M.,** Toxicity and carcinogenicity of nitrofurans, in *Carcinogenesis*, Vol. 4, Bryan, G. T., Ed., Raven Press, New York, 1978, 171.
8. **Hicks, R. M. and Wakefield, J. St. J.,** Rapid induction of bladder cancer in rats with N-methyl-N-nitrosourea. I. Histology, *Chem. Biol. Interact.*, 5, 139, 1972.
9. **Ito, N., Arai, M., Sugihara, S., Hirao, K., Makiura, S., Matayoshi, K., and Denda, A.,** Experimental urinary bladder tumors induced by N-butyl N-(4-hydroxybutyl)nitrosamine, in *Gann Monograph on Cancer Research*, Vol. 17, Odashima, S., Takayama, S., and Sato, H., Eds., University of Tokyo Press, 1975, 367.
10. **Arai, M., Cohen, S. M., Jacobs, J. B., and Friedell, G. H.,** Effect of dose on urinary bladder carcinogenesis induced by rats by N-[4-(5-nitro-2-furyl)-2-thiazolyl]formamide, *J. Natl. Cancer Inst.*, 62, 1013, 1979.
11. **Hicks, R. M. and Chowaniec, J.,** The importance of synergy between weak carcinogens in the induction of bladder cancer in experimental animals and humans, *Cancer Res.*, 37, 2943, 1977.
12. **Singer, G. M., Lijinsky, W., Buettner, L., and McClusky, G. A.,** Relationship of rat urinary metabolites of *N*-nitrosomethyl-*N*-alkylamine to bladder carcinogenesis, *Cancer Res.*, 41, 4942, 1981.
13. **Wang, C. Y. and Kamiryo, Y.,** Carcinogenicity of 2-amino-4-(5-nitro-2-furyl)-thiazole in rats and metabolism of this carcinogen by cultured dog urothelial cells, *Proc. Am. Assoc. Cancer Res.*, 19, 146, 1978.
14. **Croft, W. A. and Bryan, G. T.,** Production of urinary bladder carcinomas in male hamsters by N-[4-(5-nitro-2-furyl)-2-thiazolyl]formamide, N-[4-(5-nitro-2-furyl)-2-thiazolyl]acetamide, or formic acid 2-[4-(5-nitro-2-furyl)-2-thiazolyl]hydrazide, *J. Natl. Cancer Inst.*, 51, 941, 1973.
15. **Erturk, E., Atassi, S. A., Yoshida, O., Cohen, S. M., Price, J. M., and Bryan, G. T.,** Comparative urinary and gallbladder carcinogenicity of N-[4-(5-nitro-2-furyl)-2-thiazolyl]formamide and N-[4-(5-nitro-2-furyl)-2-thiazolyl]acetamide in the dog, *J. Natl. Cancer Inst.*, 45, 535, 1970.
16. **Swaminathan, S. and Lower, G. M., Jr.,** Biotransformations and excretion of nitrofurans, in *Carcinogenesis — A Comprehensive Survey: Nitrofurans*, Vol. 4, Bryan, G. T., Ed., Raven Press, New York, 1978, 59.
17. **Zenser, T. V., Mattammal, M. B., and Davis, B. B.,** Metabolism of N-[4-(5-nitro-2-furyl)-2-thiazolyl]formamide by prostaglandin endoperoxide synthetase, *Cancer Res.*, 40, 114, 1980.
18. **Jacobs, J. B., Arai, M., Cohen, S. M., and Friedell, G. H.,** A long-term study of reversible and progressive urinary bladder cancer lesions in rats fed N-[4-(5-nitro-2-furyl)-2-thiazolyl]formamide, *Cancer Res.*, 37, 2817, 1977.
19. **Merk, F. B., Pauli, B. U., Jacobs, J. B., Alroy, J., Friedell, G. H., and Weinstein, R. S.,** Malignant transformation of urinary bladder in humans and in N-[4-(5-nitro-2-furyl)-2-thiazolyl]formamide-exposed Fischer rats: ultrastructure of the major components of the permeability barrier, *Cancer Res.*, 37, 2843, 1977.
20. **Erturk, E., Cohen, S. M., Price, J. M., and Bryan, G. T.,** Pathogenesis, histology, and transplantability of urinary bladder carcinomas induced in albino rats by oral administration of N-[4-(5-nitro-2-furyl)-2-thiazolyl]formamide, *Cancer Res.*, 29, 2219, 1969.
21. **Tiltman, A. J. and Friedell, G. H.,** The histogenesis of experimental bladder cancer, *Invest. Urol.*, 9, 218, 1971.
22. **Erturk, E., Cohen, S. M., and Bryan, G. T.,** Urinary bladder carcinogenicity of N-[4-(5-nitro-2-furyl)-2-thiazolyl]formamide in female Swiss mice, *Cancer Res.*, 30, 1309, 1970.
23. **Hicks, R. M. and Wakefield, J. St. J.,** Membrane changes during urothelial hyperplasia and neoplasia, *Cancer Res.*, 36, 2502, 1976.
24. **Fukushima, S., Cohen, S. M., Arai, M., Jacobs, J. B., and Friedell, G. H.,** Scanning electron microscopic examination of reversible hyperplasia of the rat urinary bladder, *Am. J. Pathol.*, 102, 373, 1981.
25. **Fukushima, S., Arai, M., Cohen, S. M., Jacobs, J. B., and Friedell, G. H.,** Scanning electron microscopy of cyclophosphamide-induced hyperplasia of the rat urinary bladder, *Lab. Invest.*, 44, 89, 1981.
26. **Cohen, S. M.,** Pathology of experimental bladder cancer in rodents, in *The Pathology of Bladder Cancer*, Cohen, S. M. and Bryan, G. T., Eds., CRC Press, Boca Raton, Fla., in press.
27. **Kunze, E.,** Development of urinary bladder cancer in the rat, in *Carcinogenesis*, Vol. 67, Springer-Verlag, Berlin, 1979, 145.
28. **Scribner, J. D. and Suss, R.,** Tumor initiation and promotion, *Int. Rev. Exp. Pathol.*, 18, 137, 1978.

29. **Tsuda, H., Miyata, Y., Murasaki, G., Kinoshita, H., Fukushima, S., and Ito, N.,** Synergistic effect of urinary bladder carcinogenesis in rats treated with N-butyl-N-(4-hydroxybutyl)nitrosamine, N-[4-(5-nitro-2-furyl)-2-thiazolyl]formamide, N-2-fluorenylacetamide, and 3,3′-dichlorobenzidine, *Gann,* 68, 183, 1977.
30. **Tatematsu, M., Miyata, Y., Mizutani, M., Hananouchi, M., Hirose, M., and Ito, N.,** Summation effect of N-butyl-N-(4-hydroxybutyl)-nitrosamine, N-[4-(5-nitro-2-furyl)-2-thiazolyl]formamide, N-2-fluorenylacetamide, and 3,3′-dichlorobenzidine on urinary bladder carcinogenesis in rats, *Gann,* 68, 193, 1977.
31. **Nakanishi, K., Fukushima, S., Shibata, M., Shirai, T., Ogiso, T., and Ito, N.,** Effect of phenacetin and caffeine on the urinary bladder of rats treated with N-butyl-N-(4-hydroxybutyl)nitrosamine, *Gann,* 69, 395, 1978.
32. **Hicks, R. M.,** Multistage carcinogenesis in the urinary bladder, *Br. Med. Bull.,* 36, 39, 1980.
33. **Bryan, G. T. and Springberg, P. D.,** Role of the vehicle in the genesis of bladder carcinomas in mice by the pellet implantation technic, *Cancer Res.,* 26, 105, 1966.
34. **Clayson, D. B., Lawson, T. A., and Pringle, J. A. S.,** The carcinogenic action of 2-aminodiphenylene oxide and 4-aminodiphenyl on the bladder and liver of the C57 X IF mouse, *Br. J. Cancer,* 21, 755, 1967.
35. **Jull, J. W.,** Carcinogenesis by chemicals implanted in the bladder: an evaluation, in *Gann Monograph on Cancer Research,* Vol. 17, Odashima, S., Takayama, S., and Sato, H., Eds., University of Tokyo Press, 1975, 383.
36. **Hicks, R. M., Wakefield, J. St. J., and Chowaniec, J.,** Evaluation of a new model to detect bladder carcinogens or co-carcinogens: results obtained with saccharin, cyclamate and cyclophosphamide, *Chem. Biol. Interact.,* 11, 225, 1975.
37. **Cohen, S. M., Arai, M., Jacobs, J. B., and Friedell, G. H.,** Promoting effect of saccharin and D,L-tryptophan in urinary bladder carcinogenesis, *Cancer Res.,* 39, 1207, 1979.
38. **Fukushima, S., Friedell, G. H., Jacobs, J. B., and Cohen, S. M.,** Effect of L-tryptophan and sodium saccharin on urinary bladder carcinogenesis initiated by N-[4-(5-nitro-2-furyl)-2-thiazolyl]formamide, *Cancer Res.,* 41, 3100, 1981.
39. **Cohen, S. M., Murasaki, G., Fukushima, S., and Greenfield, R. E.,** Effect of regenerative hyperplasia on the urinary bladder: carcinogenicity of sodium saccharin and N-[4-(5-nitro-2-furyl)-2-thiazolyl]formamide, *Cancer Res.,* 42, 65, 1982.
40. **Cohen, S. M., Jacobs, J. B., Arai, M., Johansson, S., and Friedell, G. H.,** Early lesions in experimental bladder cancer: experimental design and light microscopic findings, *Cancer Res.,* 36, 2508, 1976.
41. **Nakanishi, K., Hirose, M., Ogiso, T., Hasegawa, R., Arai, M., and Ito, N.,** Effect of sodium saccharin and caffeine on the urinary bladder of rats treated with N-butyl-N-(4-hydroxybutyl)nitrosamine, *Gann,* 71, 490, 1980.
42. **Ito, N., Fukushima, S., Shirai, T., Nakanishi, K., Hasegawa, R., and Imaida, K.,** Modifying factors on urinary bladder carcinogenesis, Proc. 2nd Int. Conf. Carcinogenic Mutagenic *N*-Substituted Aryl Compounds, S29, 1982.
43. Cancer Testing Technology and Saccharin, Office of Technology Assessment, U.S. Government Printing Office, Washington, D.C., 1977.
44. **Arnold, D. L., Moodie, C. A., Grice, H. C., Charbonneau, S. M., Stavric, B., Collins, B. T., McGuire, P. F., Zawidzka, Z. Z., and Munro, I. C.,** Long-term toxicity of *ortho*-toluenesulfonamide and sodium saccharin in the rat, *Toxicol. Appl. Pharmacol.,* 52, 113, 1980.
45. **Moore, C. W. and Schmick, A.,** Recombinogenicity and mutagenicity of saccharin in Saccharomyces cerevisiae, *Mutat. Res.,* 67, 215, 1979.
46. **Umeda, M., Noda, K., and Ono, T.,** Inhibition of metabolic cooperation in Chinese hamster cells by various chemicals including tumor promoters, *Gann,* 71, 614, 1980.
47. **Fukushima, S. and Cohen, S. M.,** Saccharin-induced hyperplasia of the rat urinary bladder, *Cancer Res.,* 40, 734, 1980.
48. **Murasaki, G. and Cohen, S. M.,** Effect of dose of sodium saccharin on the induction of rat urinary bladder proliferation, *Cancer Res.,* 41, 942, 1981.
49. **Nakanishi, K., Hagiwara, A., Shibata, M., Imaida, K., Tatematsu, M., and Ito, N.,** Dose response of saccharin in induction of urinary bladder hyperplasias in Fischer 344 rats pretreated with N-butyl-N-(4-hydroxybutyl)-nitrosamine, *J. Natl. Cancer Inst.,* 65, 1005, 1980.
50. **Demers, D. M., Fukushima, S., and Cohen, S. M.,** Effect of sodium saccharin and L-tryptophan on rat urine during bladder carcinogenesis, *Cancer Res.,* 41, 108, 1981.
51. **Kennedy, G., Faucher, D. E., and Calandra, J. C.,** Metabolic fate of saccharin in the albino rat, *Food Cosmet. Toxicol.,* 10, 143, 1972.
52. **Sweatman, T. W. and Renwick, A. G.,** Saccharin metabolism and tumorigenicity, *Science,* 205, 1019, 1979.
53. **Sweatman, T. W. and Renwick, A. G.,** The tissue distribution and pharmacokinetics of saccharin in the rat, *Toxicol. Appl. Pharmacol.,* 55, 18, 1980.

54. **Lutz, W. K. and Schlatter, C.,** Saccharin does not bind to DNA of liver or bladder in the rat, *Chem. Biol. Interact.*, 19, 253, 1977.
55. **Dunning, W. F., Curtis, M. R., and Maun, M. E.,** The effect of added dietary tryptophan on the occurrence of 2-acetylaminofluorene induced liver and bladder cancer in rats, *Cancer Res.*, 10, 454, 1950.
56. **Bryan, G. T.,** Role of tryptophan metabolites in urinary bladder cancer, *Am. Ind. Hyg. Assoc. J.*, 30, 27, 1969.
57. **Bryan, G. T.,** The role of urinary tryptophan metabolites in the etiology of bladder cancer, *Am. J. Clin. Nutr.*, 24, 841, 1971.
58. **Radomski, J. L., Glass, E. M., and Deichmann, W. B.,** Transitional cell hyperplasia in the bladders of dogs fed D.L-tryptophan, *Cancer Res.*, 31, 1690, 1971.
59. **DeBaun, J. R., Miller, E. C., and Miller, J. A.,** *N*-hydroxy-2-acetylaminofluorene sulfotransferase: its probable role in carcinogenesis and in protein-(methion-*S*-yl) binding in rat liver, *Cancer Res.*, 30, 577, 1970.
60. **Weisburger, J. H., Weisburger, E. K., Madison, R. M., Wenk, M. L., and Klein, D. S.,** Effect of acetanilide and *p*-hydroxyacetanilide on the carcinogenicity of *N*-2-fluorenylacetamide and *N*-hydroxy-*N*-2-fluorenylacetamide in mice, hamsters, and female rats, *J. Natl. Cancer Inst.*, 51, 235, 1973.
61. **Oyasu, R., Sumie, H., and Burg, H. E.,** Neoplasms of urinary bladders of hamsters treated with 2-acetylaminofluorene and indole, *J. Natl. Cancer Inst.*, 45, 853, 1970.
62. **King, C. M. and Phillips, B.,** Enzyme-catalyzed reactions of the carcinogen *N*-hydroxy-2-fluorenylactamide with nucleic acid, *Science*, 159, 1351, 1968.
63. **Matsushima, M.,** The role of the promoter L-tryptophan on tumorigenesis in the urinary bladder. II. Urinary bladder carcinogenicity of FANFT (initiating factor) and L-tryptophan (promoting factor) in mice, *Jpn. J. Urol.*, 68, 731, 1977.
64. **Radomski, J. L., Radomski, T., and McDonald, W. E.,** Cocarcinogenic interaction between D,L-tryptophan and 4-aminobiphenyl or 2-naphthylamine in dogs, *J. Natl. Cancer Inst.*, 58, 1831, 1977.
65. **Yoshida, O., Brown, R. R., and Bryan, G. T.,** Relationship between tryptophan metabolism and heterotopic recurrences of human urinary bladder tumors, *Cancer*, 25, 773, 1970.
66. **Byar, D. and Blanchard, C.,** Comparisons of placebo, pyridoxine, and topical thiotepa in preventing recurrence of stage I bladder cancer, *Urology*, 10, 556, 1977.
67. **Bowden, J. P., Chung, K. T., and Andrews, A. N.,** Mutagenic activity of tryptophan metabolites produced by rat intestinal microflora, *J. Natl. Cancer Inst.*, 57, 921, 1976.
68. **Scott, W. W. and Boyd, H. L.,** Study of the carcinogenic effect of beta-naphthylamine on the normal and substituted isolated sigmoid loop bladder of dogs, *J. Urol.*, 70, 914, 1953.
69. **Chapman, W. H., Kirchkin, D., and McRoberts, J. W.,** Effect of the urine and calculus formation in the incidence of bladder tumors in rats implanted with paraffin wax pellets, *Cancer Res.*, 33, 1225, 1973.
70. **Rowland, R. G., Henneberry, M. O., Oyasu, R., and Grayhack, J. T.,** Effect of urine and continued exposure to carcinogen on progression of early neoplastic urinary bladder lesions, *Cancer Res.*, 40, 4524, 1980.
71. **Oyasu, R., Hirao, Y., and Izumi, K.,** Enhancement by urine of urinary bladder carcinogenesis, *Cancer Res.*, 41, 478, 1981.
72. **Izumi, K., Hirao, Y., Happ, G., and Oyasu, R.,** *In vitro* induction of ornithine decarboxylase in urinary bladder carcinoma cells, *Cancer Res.*, 41, 405, 1981.
73. **Babaya, K., Miyata, Y., Chmiel, J. S., and Oyasu, R.,** Effect of rat urine fractionated by molecular weight on urinary bladder carcinogenesis, *Cancer Res.*, 42, 15, 1982.
74. **Hicks, R. M. and Chowaniec, J.,** Experimental induction, histology, and ultrastructure of hyperplasia and neoplasia of the urinary bladder epithelium, in *International Review of Experimental Pathology*, Vol. 18, Richter, G. W. and Epstein, M. A., Eds., Academic Press, New York, 1978, 199.
75. **Shirai, T., Cohen, S. M., Fukushima, S., Hananouchi, M., and Ito, N.,** Reversible papillary hyperplasia of the rat urinary bladder, *Am. J. Pathol.*, 91, 33, 1978.
76. **Tiltman, A. J. and Friedell, G. H.,** Effect of feeding N-[4-(5-nitro-2-furyl)-2-thiazolyl]formamide on mitotic activity of rat urinary-bladder epithelium, *J. Natl. Cancer Inst.*, 48, 125, 1972.
77. **Kennedy, A. R., Murphy, G., and Little, J. B.,** Effect of time and duration of exposure to 12-O-tetradecanoylphorbol-13-acetate on X-ray transformation of C3H 10T1/2 cells, *Cancer Res.*, 40, 1915, 1980.
78. **Tsuda, H., Sarma, D. S. R., Rajalakshmi, S., Zubroff, J., Farber, E., Batzinger, R. P., Cha, Y., and Bueding, E.,** Induction of hepatic neoplastic lesions in mice with a single dose of hycanthone methanesulfonate after partial hepatectomy, *Cancer Res.*, 39, 4491, 1979.
79. **Warwick, G. P.,** Effect of the cell cycle on carcinogenesis, *Fed. Proc.*, 30, 1760, 1971.
80. **Klemencic, J. M. and Wang, C. Y.,** Mutagenicity of nitrofurans, in *Carcinogenesis*, Vol. 4, Bryan, G. T., Ed., Raven Press, New York, 1978, 99.

81. **Mohn, G. R. and Ellenberger, J.,** Genetic effects of cyclophosphamide, ifosfamide and trofosfamide, *Mutat. Res.*, 32, 331, 1976.
82. **Brock, N., Stekar, J., Pohl, J., Niemeyer, U., and Scheffler, G.,** Acrolein, the causative factor of urotoxic side-effects of cyclophosphamide, ifosfamide, trofosfamide and sulfosfamide, *Arzneim. Forsch. Drug Res.*, 29, 659, 1979.
83. **Bryan, G. T., Erturk, E., and Yoshida, O.,** Production of urinary bladder carcinomas in mice by sodium saccharin, *Science (Washington, D.C.),* 168, 1238, 1970.
84. **Bonneville, M. A. and Caruthers, J. M. S.,** Correlations of biochemical and morphological changes during rat urinary bladder carcinogenesis, *Proc. Natl. Bladder Cancer Proj.*, p. 30, 1980.
85. **Greenfield, R. E., Ellwein, L. B., and Cohen, S. M.,** A computer-based probabilistic model of carcinogenesis and analysis of experimental urinary bladder carcinogenesis induced by N-[4-(5-nitro-2-furyl)-2-thiazolyl]formamide and sodium saccharin, *Carcinogenesis,* in press.
86. **Tsuda, H., Imaida, K., Oshima, M., Cameron, R., and Ito, N.,** Promoting effect of bile acids and related compounds in the induction of y-glutamyl transpeptidase (y-GT) positive liver cell foci as possible endogenous factors of hepatocarcinogenesis, *Proc. Am. Assoc. Cancer Res.*, 23, 103, 1982.
87. **Oyasu, R.,** personal communication.

Chapter 7

INITIATION AND PROMOTION IN PANCREATIC CARCINOGENESIS

B. D. Roebuck, Daniel S. Longnecker, and James D. Yager, Jr.

TABLE OF CONTENTS

I. INTRODUCTION

A. Epidemiology of Pancreatic Cancer

Epidemiological studies designed to identify causes of carcinoma of the pancreas in humans have implicated several risk factors. Such reports and reviews have consistently demonstrated an association of cigarette smoking, increasing age, and male sex with pancreatic cancer. Risk factors such as specific occupational chemical exposure and the presence of diabetes have been examined in smaller populations and/or fewer studies. In contrast, other implicated environmental or dietary factors, e.g., coffee drinking,[1,2] are incompletely evaluated and the focus of controversy.[3,4] Differences of opinion among epidemiologists may reflect the study of different populations or varying methods and focus. Thus there is a hierarchy among risk factors associated with pancreatic cancer as reflected in Table 1. Several factors are listed as "strongly implicated" because three or more studies have shown a positive correlation with the presence of pancreatic cancer. Other factors are listed as "weakly implicated" because they are supported by a single epidemiological study or by studies which are contradicted by other studies. Still other risk factors have been listed in an "intermediate" category when we have judged the support to be stronger or the opposition weaker. This tabulation is presented for convenience in summarizing epidemiological data and should not be accepted as reflecting an exhaustive review. Recent review articles serve the latter role.[11,16]

Identification of risk factors by epidemiological studies does not provide objective evidence for the mechanisms of effect on carcinogenesis in regard to initiation, cocarcinogenesis, or promotion. Such analysis of mechanisms may require experimental evaluation in animal models as has been done with high fat diets (see Section II.B). Other risk factors which could be evaluated in animal models include diabetes, alcohol, coffee, cigarette smoking, sex hormones, and specific chemicals. Studies in animals may help to evaluate the importance of risk factors about which there is controversy or which pertain to such small or dispersed population groups as to make conclusive epidemiological studies difficult. Other factors such as chronic pancreatitis are less amenable to experimental evaluation because of the lack of a suitable animal model for the risk factor.

B. Animal Models for Pancreatic Carcinogenesis

Prior to the last 8 years, progress and interest in pancreatic carcinogenesis had been severely limited by the lack of experimental models. The occurrence of this disease in "untreated" rodents has been reported to be very low.[17-19] For example, in the routine postmortem examination of 1252 rats of the Chester Beatty strain, only eight pancreatic tumors were found. All tumors were in rats older than 16.5 months and only three of the eight were malignant.[18] A 20% spontaneous incidence of well-differentiated acinar cell tumors in 2-year-old *Mastomys natalensis* rats has been reported.[20] The *Mastomys* is noted for the development of neoplastic disease in many organ systems.[21] An epidemiological survey of domestic animals revealed that cattle, horses, dogs, and cats had a low incidence of pancreatic cancer.[22] The dog was similar to the human with respect to the estimated relative risk by age, incidence, and frequency of pancreatic adenocarcinoma. The susceptibility of the dog to specific pancreatic chemical carcinogens has not adequately been studied,[23] and a model has not yet been developed.

In Table 2, the better characterized animal models of neoplasia of pancreatic exocrine tissue are listed, and in Figure 1 structures for selected chemicals are shown. Included in this list are two of the most extensively characterized animal models: namely, azaserine in the rat and oxidized dipropylnitrosoamines in the hamster. Subsequently, these two models will be discussed in detail.

The first report of a chemical with promise for use in the development of an animal model for pancreatic cancer was published in 1968 by Druckrey and co-workers.[31] *N*-Methyl-*N*-

Table 1
RISK FACTORS ASSOCIATED WITH CARCINOMA OF THE PANCREAS

Strongly implicated	Intermediate	Weakly implicated
Cigarette smoking[1,5,6]	High dietary fat[5]	Specific industrial and environmental chemicals[2,8,13]
Diabetes (females)[5-8]	Coffee[1,2,12]	Chronic pancreatitis[5,8,14]
Sex (male)[9-11]		Alcoholism[1,2,5,15]
Age[6,9,11]		
Race (black)[9-11]		

Table 2
ANIMAL MODELS OF NEOPLASIA OF PANCREATIC EXOCRINE TISSUE

Chemical	Species	Effect[a]	Ref.
Acinar cell[b]			
Azaserine	Rat	Ca	24,25
7,12-Dimethylbenzanthracene (DMBA)	Rat	Ca	26,27
4-Hydroxyaminoquinoline-1-oxide (HAQO)	Rat	Ad	28
		Ca	29
N^{δ}-(*N*-methyl-*N*-nitrosocarbamoyl)-L-ornithine	Rat	Ca	30
N-methyl-*N*-nitrosourea (MNU)	Guinea pig	Ca	31,32
Ductal and Ductular Cells[b]			
N-Nitrosobis(2-oxopropyl)amine (BOP)	Hamster	Ca	33
N-Nitrosobis(2-hydroxypropyl)amine (BHP)	Hamster	Ca	34
N-Nitroso(2-hydroxypropyl)(2-oxopropyl)amine (HPOP)	Hamster	Ca	35
Dimethylnitrosomorpholine	Hamster	Ca	36
N-Nitrosodimethylamine	Rat	Ca	37

[a] The type of neoplasm is abbreviated as follows: adenoma, Ad; and adenocarcinoma, Ca.
[b] The known or presumed cell of origin of the neoplasm.

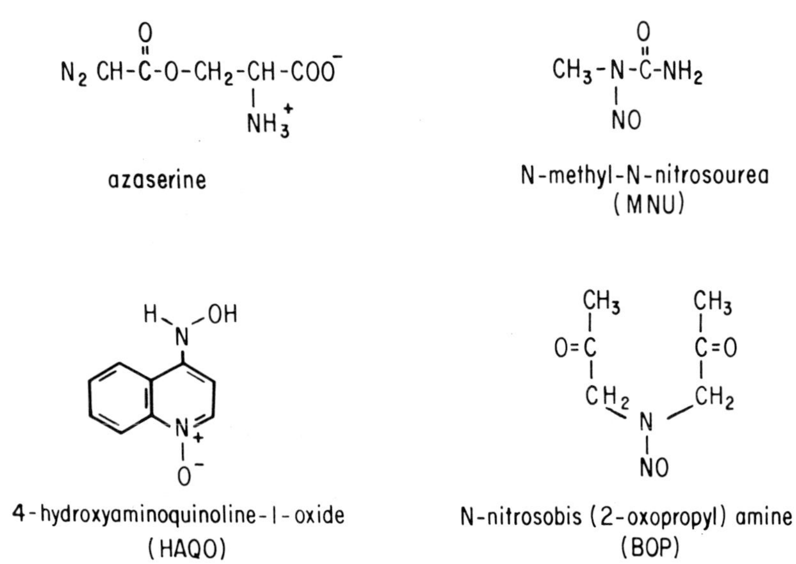

FIGURE 1. Chemical structures of selected carcinogens of the exocrine pancreas.

nitrosourea (MNU) was presented via the drinking water to guinea pigs. For pancreatic adenocarcinomas, the latent period was very long (averaging 800 days) and the incidence was low (25%). Furthermore, the incidence of cancers at other sites was greater than the incidence of pancreatic cancer. Subsequent experiments using the inbred Strain 13 guinea pig and weekly intragastric instillation of 10 mg of MNU per kilogram of body weight yielded pancreatic adenocarcinomas in 200 to 300 days.[32] However, by day 200 of the experiment, a 54% mortality in the MNU-treated animals was recorded. Among the survivors, the incidence of pancreatic adenocarcinomas was 29%. While some adenocarcinomas had duct-like characteristics, an acinar cell origin is likely since atypical acinar cells were widely observed in the pancreas of most guinea pigs.

Another early model is that in which a single injection of 4-hydroxyaminoquinoline-1-oxide (HAQO) induced hyperplastic nodules and well-differentiated adenomas of acinar cells in the rat, but not adenocarcinomas.[28] Later, Konishi et al.[29,38] produced adenocarcinomas by injecting HAQO at the peak of acinar cell DNA synthesis following a partial pancreatectomy.

Of the chemical carcinogens affecting the pancreatic acinar cells, azaserine is the best characterized. Longnecker and Curphey[24] first reported azaserine to be a carcinogen for the pancreas of the Wistar rat. Azaserine was injected i.p. at 5 mg/kg of body weight either twice (Group 1) or once weekly (Group 2) for 6 months, and the animals were autopsied between 12 and 24 months after the first azaserine injection. Pancreatic adenocarcinomas were found in 56% of Group 1 and 22% of Group 2 rats. None were found in the control group. The highest incidence of nonpancreatic tumors was in kidney, (40% in Group 1 and 24% in Group 2). Male rats had a higher incidence of both pancreatic and renal tumors than female rats. Pancreases of all azaserine-treated rats contained large numbers of hyperplastic, atypical acinar cell nodules (AACN). Individual malignant tumors measured as much as 6.5 cm in greatest diameter. Malignant tumors were found in all portions of the pancreas (head, body, and tail) with no evidence of disproportionate involvement of one region over another. Multiple hepatic metastases and invasion in regional lymph nodes were observed in several rats.

Pancreatic adenocarcinomas have been classified according to their histologic pattern.[25] Sixty-three percent of these tumors were pure acinar cell carcinomas. Of particular interest are the acinar cell carcinomas mixed with duct-like carcinomas and microadenocarcinomas. These two types constituted 21% of the azaserine-induced tumors of the rat. The proportion and types of human pancreatic adenocarcinomas which arise from acinar cells are currently a matter of controversy and speculation.

The pancreases of Wistar and Wistar/Lewis rats have similar responsiveness to azaserine in various multiple-dose protocols, but the Wistar/Lewis strain appears to develop considerably fewer renal neoplasms.[25,39] With similar multiple-dose injection protocols, the Wistar/Lewis rats fed the purified, AIN-76 diet (AIN) developed a greater incidence and number of pancreatic adenocarcinomas than rats fed commercially available laboratory chow.[25]

Considerable progress in the characterization of the rat/azaserine model of exocrine pancreatic carcinogenesis has been made by the evaluation of the presumptively preneoplastic AACN. The criteria for histopathological identification, counting methods, and sizing techniques have been described.[25,40] These focal lesions appear as early as 2 months, but are most readily identified and counted at 4 or 6 months following a single or series of azaserine injections.[40-42] A correlation between AACN number per pancreas and the incidence of pancreatic cancer has been noted. The number of AACN appears to have value in predicting carcinogenicity. For example, Roebuck and Longnecker[40] have evaluated several species and rat strains for AACN induction by azaserine. The Syrian golden hamster and the Strain 13 guinea pig were found to be refractory to the induction of AACN, the CD-1 mouse and Fischer rat were intermediate, and the Wistar and Wistar/Lewis rats were very responsive. In a subsequent carcinogenicity experiment comparing the mouse and the Wistar/Lewis rat, the mouse did not develop azaserine-induced pancreatic adenocarcinomas, whereas the rat did.[39] The average number of AACN was higher in male than in female Wistar/Lewis rats,[40] and a subsequent study showed that the male rat developed more carcinomas than the female.[39]

Though not as fully evaluated, the size of AACN has been shown to correlate with the incidence of pancreatic cancer.[25] For example, in a group of rats treated with azaserine and fed standard laboratory chow, the incidence of pancreatic adenomas and adenocarcinomas was 21% and the average cross-sectional area of an AACN was 0.20 ± 0.13 mm^2. In a comparable group of rats fed the AIN diet, the tumor incidence was 71% and the average area of AACN was 0.66 ± 0.19 mm^2. Both AACN number and size appear to have value in predicting carcinogenicity.

Of the chemical carcinogens that primarily induce ductal and/or ductular cell lesions, several oxidized dipropylnitrosamines are the best characterized (Table 2, Figure 1). In hamsters, *N*-nitrosobis(2-hydroxypropyl)amine (BHP) was first reported to yield nearly a 100% incidence of pancreatic adenocarcinomas with a latency of approximately 4 to 5 months.[34] BHP at doses as high as 500 mg/kg of body weight was administered subcutaneously to the Syrian golden hamster at weekly intervals for life. Histologically, the majority of the pancreatic adenomas and adenocarcinomas had "duct-like" characteristics. In these same hamsters, pancreatic adenocarcinomas having acinar cell characteristics were observed at an incidence of approximately 10%. Of the hamsters with pancreatic neoplasms, 72 to 100% had simultaneous tumors at other sites, especially adenocarcinomas of the nasal cavity and various hepatic and renal neoplasms.[34] *N*-nitrosobis(2-oxopropyl)amine (BOP), structurally related to BHP (Figure 1), induced a high incidence of pancreatic adenocarcinomas and a lower incidence of neoplasms of other organs.[43] With a single dose of BOP (5 to 40 mg/kg), the latency of pancreatic cancer ranged from 30 to 75 weeks and the incidence of adenocarcinomas ranged from 20 to 80%. The female hamsters were more responsive than the males. Furthermore, with a single dose of BOP, tumors in other organs were significantly reduced. In a recent review of this model, Pour et al.[35] summarized the evidence for the histogenesis of these adenocarcinomas and concluded that the earliest lesions arise from cells of the pancreatic ducts and especially of the ductules.

The hamster pancreas apparently is uniquely susceptible to the oxidized dipropylnitrosamine carcinogens. The rat,[44] mouse,[45,46] guinea pig,[47] and the tree shrew[48] are all refractory to the induction of pancreatic adenocarcinomas with these carcinogens when compared to the Syrian golden hamster. This susceptibility may be related to the relatively high incidence of spontaneous ductular neoplasms seen in this species.[49] Comparative studies of the metabolism of these carcinogens in the hamster and the rat have been completed.[50] This class of carcinogens was metabolized similarly by both rat and hamster. Thus, the resistance of the rat and perhaps the other species is not due to species specific differences in whole animal metabolism. Pancreatic neoplasms including adenocarcinomas have developed in the Wistar rat treated with BHP and fed raw soya flour.[51] It is of interest that these BHP-treated rats developed AACN and acinar cell carcinomas rather than ductal neoplasms. Raw soya flour is hypothesized to have promoted the BHP initiated pancreatic lesions. This implies that BHP is a complete carcinogen for hamster, but not for rat pancreas.

Currently, some controversy exists concerning the importance and role for these two models of pancreatic carcinogenesis. The controversy centers on the purported cell or cells or origin of human pancreatic adenocarcinoma. Human adenocarcinoma of the exocrine pancreas often has "duct-like" cellular morphology and it has been widely assumed that such cancers arise from ductal cells.[52] The hamster/BOP model clearly yields tumors with "duct-like" features and the preneoplastic lesions apparently arise from ductal and/or ductular cells. With the rat/azaserine model, approximately 20% of the adenocarcinomas (which are of acinar cell origin) have "duct-like" histological features.[25,53] Only recently has the occurrence of AACN in human pancreas been carefully described.[54] Whether human AACN progress to adenocarcinomas is unresolved. Until the histogenesis of the human adenocarcinomas is clarified, both models appear highly relevant. Furthermore, in the studies discussed below, both models have yielded similar results.

C. In Vitro Systems for Studying Pancreatic Carcinogenesis

The potential contributions of in vitro studies to the analysis of carcinogenesis in the pancreas were recognized,[55] and this has required development of methods for isolation and culture of cells of the exocrine pancreas. Methods for isolation and primary culture of pancreatic islets were developed earlier by investigators with an interest in islet function and transplantation[56] and will not be reviewed here.

1. Acinar Cells

Methods for isolation and primary culture of acinar cells have been described[57-59] and have been applied to guinea pig, rat, and hamster pancreas. Both enzymatic and mechanical approaches are utilized for isolation of cells. Oliver[59] has described culture for up to 4 weeks. No normal acinar cell lines have been reported. The limited survival of differentiated acinar cells in primary culture has permitted studies of acute biochemical effects, but not of long-term biological effects of carcinogens, inhibitors, or promoters of pancreatic neoplasia in culture. Isolated acinar cells have been exposed to carcinogens and studied by alkaline elution analysis of DNA to demonstrate damage.[42,60,61] Primary acinar cell cultures have also been used to demonstrate unscheduled DNA synthesis following carcinogen treatment[61] and for isolation of alkylated DNA and identification of *N*-7-carboxymethylation following in vitro exposure to ^{14}C-azaserine.[62]

An alternate approach, the isolation of pancreatic acini, has been described[63,64] and should be further evaluated in studies with carcinogens to see if this approach might facilitate longer survival in culture.

2. Ductal Cells

Two approaches have been described for isolation of duct cells from the pancreas of cow and human. One involves mechanical scraping of the opened duct.[65] In the second, the duct system of the intact pancreas is perfused with digestive enzymes.[66] Culture of the isolated ductal cells has been utilized in morphologic studies of the effects of several carcinogens on bovine and human cells. These methods are applicable only in large animals. The cell yields are small, in the range of 2×10^6 cells per bovine pancreas. Stoner[65] reported survival and growth of ductal cells for 30 weeks, but shorter survival has been the rule in other laboratories.[66] Biochemical studies of carcinogen effects by methods such as alkaline elution analysis are not yet practical because of the limited number of cells derived from each pancreas.

Isolation of segments of pancreatic ducts of rats and hamsters has been described.[67] The cultured ducts consist of epithelium and surrounding connective tissue. Survival in primary culture for as long as 8 weeks was described, but growth was minimal. This preparation has been used for morphologic studies of the effects of carcinogens on ductal cells. The yield of ductal cells is so low as to limit the application of this method in biochemical studies, although several enzyme activities have been assayed.

Culture of pancreatic duct explants isolated by dissection from pancreases of cows and humans has been described.[66] Bovine explants have survived as long as 4 months. It appears that successful explant cultures can be established from human pancreases with a post-mortem interval of 4 hr or less, and repair of anoxic cell injury in culture was described.[66] Explants of common duct from Syrian golden hamsters have been similarly cultured.[66] Growth of ductal epithelial cells from the explants onto the culture dish was described as a potential source of ductal cells. Characterization of carcinogen effects in bovine duct have been limited to morphologic studies which have shown growth of anaplastic ductal cells in cultures treated with *N*-methyl-*N*-nitrosoguanidine (MNNG), and lesser degrees of cellular atypia and proliferation in cultures treated with BHP, dimethylnitrosamine (DMN) and *N*-nitroso-2,6-dimethylmorpholine. Atypical cellular changes have been induced in human explants treated with MNNG or 4-nitroquinoline-1-oxide.[66]

3. Organ Culture

Organ culture of pancreatic slices or fragments has been described.[37,68,69] Survival of functionally differentiated acinar cells has been a limiting problem. Murrell et al.[69] describes 5-day survival of pancreas from 7-day-old rats using chemically defined medium containing hydrocortisone. The cultured explants were about 6 × 5 × 1 to 2 mm in size. Parsa et al.[37,68] reported survival of some ductal cells for 12 weeks in explants of human pancreas. These measured about 5 × 5 × 1 mm and were cultured in a chemically defined medium with insulin and ascorbic acid. Acinar cells underwent necrosis within 6 weeks. Intralobular ductules underwent necrosis at 7 to 9 weeks.

Parsa et al.[68] have utilized explant organ cultures of rat and human pancreas for in vitro carcinogenesis and have reported prolonged survival of atypical ducts and ductules in carcinogen-treated cultures. Growth of anaplastic cells suggested in vitro transformation which has been documented by xenotransplantation of carcinogen-treated human explants into nude mice with subcutaneous growth of carcinomas. Effective carcinogens in rat explants have been DMN, MNU, BHP, and azaserine. The first two carcinogens were also effective in human explants. Up to two thirds of DMN-treated explants have shown evidence of transformation. Parsa et al.[70] have also demonstrated the effectiveness of 12-*O*-tetradecanoylphorbol-13-acetate in promoting carcinogenesis in the rat model following a brief exposure to MNU. Based on the presence of early proliferative changes, Parsa et al.[70] suggest that many of these carcinomas arise in ductal cells.

Parsa's work offers an important approach for comparison between species of the effects of pancreatic carcinogens identified in animal studies. The fact that DMN is a carcinogen in vitro for rat pancreas, whereas it has not induced pancreatic carcinomas in vivo points out the need for caution in evaluating organ specific carcinogenicity of chemicals solely by in vitro studies.

4. General Comments

These studies of exocrine pancreas in cell and organ culture reflect a period of method development. Such studies provide approaches for separately studying carcinogenesis in ductal and acinar cells and already provide evidence that both cell types seem capable of metabolic activation of certain procarcinogens. The results reported by Parsa and co-workers are spectacular and should be useful in studies of mechanism if the method can be applied in other laboratories.

II. TWO-STAGE CARCINOGENESIS IN PANCREAS

It is widely accepted that carcinogenesis is a multistep process with each step probably representing one of an unknown total number of discontinuous rare events.[71] Experimentally, at least two and possibly more[71,72] stages can be separated, namely initiation and promotion. Initiation constitutes a persistent if not permanent event that can occur following treatment with a single subcarcinogenic dose of an appropriate agent. Most initiators are mutagens, and the process is thought to involve mutation in the target somatic cells. In contrast, promotion represents a process that is, at least for a time, reversible. It involves chronic treatment with a chemical agent that ultimately enhances tumor incidence and number.

Promoters are not mutagens, and the process probably does not involve mutation in the target cells.

Two-stage carcinogenesis was originally demonstrated in skin[73] and to date has been shown to occur in several other tissues including liver,[74,75] mammary gland,[76,77] colon,[78,79] and other organs.[75] Recently, Longnecker et al.,[25] Roebuck et al.,[53,80] and Pour et al.[35] reported the results of studies indicating that pancreatic carcinogenesis also consists of at least two separable stages.

A. Initiation Stage

1. Uptake of Pancreatic Carcinogens

The rat model for pancreatic carcinogenesis developed by Longnecker and Curphey[24] used multiple treatments with azaserine, an amino acid that is relatively selective for induction of pancreatic cancer originating in acinar cells. The exocrine pancreas is one of the most active protein synthesizing organs, and the uptake of amino acids has been shown to respond to hormones,[81,82] and feeding and fasting.[83] In fact, the sensitivity of amino acid uptake in pancreas to the availability of food can be shown in animals adapted to controlled lighting and feeding schedules. Baril and Potter[84] demonstrated systematic oscillations of amino acid transport in livers of rats adapted to an 8 + 16 feeding schedule (12 hr light, 12 hr dark with food available during the first 8 hr of the dark period). Uptake of ^{14}C-labeled α-aminoisobutyric acid (AIB) was stimulated by food intake and then declined during the subsequent fasting period. Daily oscillations in amino acid uptake can be demonstrated in the pancreas (Figure 2). In this study, Wistar rats were adapted to a 2 + 22 feeding schedule (food available for the first 2 hr of the 12 hr dark period).[85] It can be seen that AIB uptake in pancreas starts shortly before the beginning of the feeding and dark period and is somewhat out of phase with liver. Also, the pancreas maintains a higher base line level of this amino acid than liver, and concentrates it to a greater extent at the peak of the daily oscillations.

Longnecker and Curphey[24] reported that the pancreas concentrated azaserine to a greater degree than other tissues. Recently, Perantoni et al.,[86] using four cultured cell lines, demonstrated that azaserine uptake was correlated with gamma glutamyl transpeptidase activity. Pancreatic acinar cells contain high levels of this enzyme compared to, for example, adult hepatocytes in which it is absent.[75] This could result in greater accumulation of azaserine in the pancreas and thus play a role in the organotropism of this carcinogen. However, since the extent of uptake of amino acids in the pancreas is dependent on the feeding/fasting state within a single day, azaserine administration at one time would result in selective uptake, while at another time the carcinogen might be more evenly distributed. This could become important in single dose carcinogen treatment protocols, but would be less important with multiple dose protocols. Similar variation in uptake could pertain for other carcinogens.

2. Metabolism of Pancreatic Carcinogens

It is widely recognized that many chemical carcinogens require metabolic conversion to ultimate carcinogenic forms. In fact, the organ specificity of various chemical carcinogens may be largely due to the extent and nature of metabolism in that target organ. Either the pancreas has the metabolic capacity to activate chemicals or it receives activated forms of chemicals from other organs such as liver.

The ability of pancreatic tissue to metabolize various types of chemical carcinogens has been studied to a limited extent with human pancreas[87] and in greater detail in pancreas from three experimental animals: guinea pig,[88] rat,[89,90] and hamster.[50,91,92] In general, pancreatic tissue from these species has the ability to metabolize various aromatic hydrocarbons and nitrosamines, but the metabolic capacity is very low in comparison to liver. In such studies, cell fractions made from whole pancreas should be regarded as reflecting the metabolic capability of acinar cells because of their dominant number in pancreas. Bolender[93]

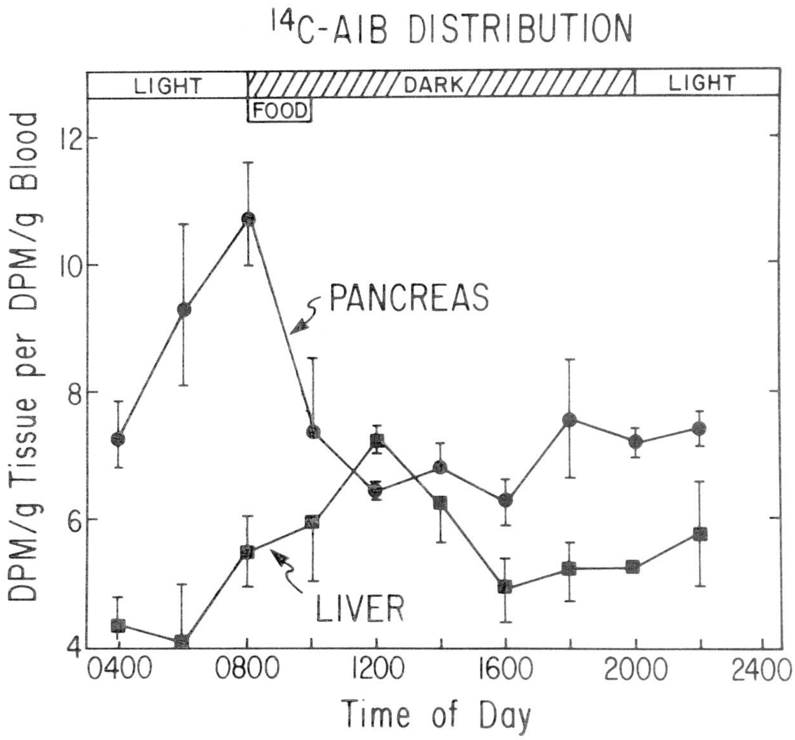

FIGURE 2. Daily oscillations in α-aminoisobutyric acid (AIB) uptake in the pancreas and liver.

found that acinar cells comprised 82% of the guinea pig pancreas, while ductal cells composed less than 4% of the total. A few specific examples will be discussed below.

Iqbal et al.[88] and Roebuck[115] found that guinea pig pancreatic tissue had low levels of benzo(a)pyrene hydroxylase (BPH) activity. Data from Roebuck are shown in Table 3. BPH activity in control pancreas is only 0.5% of that found in liver. However, pretreatment of guinea pigs with benzo(a)pyrene results in the induction of BPH activity. Iqbal et al.[88] reported similar results and also demonstrated that 3-methylcholanthrene pretreatment induced BPH. These results clearly demonstrate that guinea pig pancreatic tissue has the capacity to metabolize aromatic hydrocarbon carcinogens, and that this function is inducible, although small, compared to liver.

In rats, Dissin et al.[26] demonstrated that 7,12-dimethylbenz[a]anthracene (DMBA) induced pancreatic adenocarcinomas which were invasive, metastasized, and had duct-like characteristics. Since the carcinogen was implanted in the pancreas, this suggested that the rat pancreas had the capacity to activate DMBA to its ultimate carcinogenic form. Recently, Black et al.[89] demonstrated that the rat pancreas could metabolize DMBA to water-soluble products similar to those formed in liver. However, in the pancreas, this ability was not inducible by phenobarbital,[89] supporting the earlier observations of Lavigne and Marchand[90] that phenobarbital, while causing increased pancreatic weight, protein synthesis, and secretion of amylase, lipase, and RNase, did not enhance pancreatic drug metabolizing activity.

Gingell et al.[50] have also demonstrated that the intact rat can metabolize BOP, a chemical that is carcinogenic for hamster, but not rat pancreas. However, since the BOP metabolites formed in both species are the same, the resistance of rat to BOP appears not to be due to metabolic activity in the whole animal.

Azaserine, a carcinogen for rat pancreas, appears to be a direct acting mutagen in the

Table 3
BENZO(A)PYRENE HYDROXYLASE (BPH) ACTIVITY OF CONTROL AND BENZO(A)PYRENE PRETREATED GUINEA PIG TISSUES[a]

Benzo(a)pyrene pretreatment	Number of animals	BPH activity (pmol/mg protein per minute) Liver	Pancreas
Control	7	162 ± 26[b]	0.87 ± 0.15
2 mg/kg 1 day	5	272 ± 30	2.92 ± 1.43
20 mg/kg 1 day	3	254 ± 18	4.33 ± 1.46
20 mg/kg 4 days	3	410 ± 31	11.27 ± 2.19

[a] BPH activity was determined using the fluorometric method of Nebert and Gelboin.[94]
[b] Mean ± SEM.

Data from Roebuck, B. D., unpublished observations.

Ames assay.[24,95] However, recent studies have indicated that the ability of azaserine to damage pancreatic DNA is pyridoxal dependent.[96] Thus, the bacterial strains may be capable of generating the alkylating species. Therefore, azaserine probably requires some type of metabolic activation which is not dependent on the microsomal enzyme system.

Hamster pancreas has the capacity to metabolize various nitrosamines that are potent carcinogens for hamster pancreas and, to a lesser degree, liver.[91,92] Scarpelli et al.[92] demonstrated that this metabolic capability is located in the microsomal fraction of hamster pancreas and is enhanced by inducers of mixed function oxidase activity such as beta-naphthoflavone and 2,3,7,8-tetrachlorodibenzo-*p*-dioxin. These inducers also increase the activity of pancreatic aryl hydrocarbon hydroxylase in the hamster.

The results discussed above clearly demonstrate that human, guinea pig, rat, and hamster pancreas have the ability to metabolize pancreatic chemical carcinogens. This capability, while facilitating the detoxification of chemicals which reach the pancreas may also result in the formation of mutagenic metabolites which have the ability to initiate pancreatic carcinogenesis. Thus, it is important to demonstrate which environmental chemicals have the ability to cause pancreatic DNA damage directly or following their metabolic activation.

3. DNA Damage and Repair in Pancreatic Carcinogenesis

The most extensive studies on the role of DNA damage and repair in pancreatic carcinogenesis have been carried out in the rat/azaserine model. Using alkaline sucrose gradient centrifugation[39,97-99] and alkaline elution techniques,[42,60] we have demonstrated that azaserine causes DNA damage in pancreas, liver, and kidney of the rat. DNA damage detected by these techniques most likely represents alkaline-labile lesions caused by depurination at sites of *N*-7-guanine alkylation. In fact, Zurlo et al.[62] have recently shown that azaserine treatment of rat pancreatic acinar cells results in the formation of 7-carboxymethylguanine in DNA. The identification of other adducts in DNA from azaserine-treated acinar cells is under way. DNA damage detected by alkaline sucrose gradient centrifugation can be seen as early as 1 hr after azaserine treatment.[97] Damage in pancreas and liver persists for 4 weeks and beyond following single dose treatment with azaserine at 10 or 30 mg/kg, doses which will induce the formation of AACN.[42] However, azaserine primarily induces pancreatic tumors with only a low incidence of liver tumors. Thus, occurrence and persistence of DNA damage as detected by using alkaline sucrose or alkaline elution techniques does not explain the organotropic properties of this carcinogen. In addition, azaserine is not a pancreatic carcinogen in mice or hamsters, yet persistent pancreatic DNA damage is also detected in these non-responsive species. Thus, it is obvious that more detailed studies are required to reveal the mechanism(s) responsible for the organotropic and species specificity of azaserine. Among other things, the specific types of DNA adducts formed and their individual rates of repair may be important in this regard.

As indicated above, BOP is a pancreatic carcinogen in hamsters. Lawson et al.[100] have recently demonstrated the presence of 7-methylguanine, but not *O*-6 methylguanine, in pancreas and liver of hamsters treated with [1-C^{14}]BOP. These results demonstrate that this carcinogen is an alkylating agent in hamster. Their study also revealed that the sites of alkylation of liver and pancreas DNA differed significantly.[100] Since 7-methylguanine is not considered to be important in carcinogenesis and since *O*-6 methylguanine was not detected, other alkylated products that might have been formed, e.g., pyrimidines or phosphates, may have a role in BOP-induced carcinogenesis in the hamster.

As indicated above, BOP is metabolized to the same metabolites in hamster and rat[50] and yet, BOP does not appear to be a pancreatic carcinogen in rat. Zurlo et al.[61] recently reported that BOP induced DNA damage was detected in rat pancreas at high doses, and these doses are also capable of inducing AACN in rat pancreas.[116]

The results discussed above clearly demonstrate that the known pancreatic carcinogens cause DNA damage. While this may be important in their ability to initiate pancreatic carcinogenesis, it cannot by itself account for their organotropic properties as complete carcinogens. DNA damage is also seen in other organs, particularly liver, where these agents induce only a low incidence of cancer. In fact, Shinozuka et al.[101] and Roebuck et al.[53] have shown that feeding lipotrope-deficient diets enhances the appearance of liver neoplasms in azaserine-treated rats. Thus, at least this pancreatic carcinogen is also able to initiate hepatocarcinogenesis. However, while it is a fairly potent complete carcinogen for pancreas, it is only a weak complete carcinogen for liver. Thus, the processes of cocarcinogenesis and/or promotion also appear to be important in pancreatic carcinogenesis.

4. Single-Dose Protocols for Initiation of Pancreatic Carcinogenesis

Single-dose initiation protocols for induction of pancreatic cancer exist and are well characterized for the rat/azaserine and the hamster/BOP models. Seven-week-old, male Wistar/Lewis rats injected i.p. with 30 mg azaserine per kilogram of body weight had a 30 to 50% incidence of pancreatic adenocarcinomas at 12 months and 15 months, respectively (Table 4). Syrian golden hamsters treated subcutaneously with a single-dose of BOP in the range of 5 to 40 mg per kilogram of body weight resulted in pancreatic adenocarcinomas as early as 30 weeks; however, the majority of the adenocarcinomas were observed with a latency period close to 1 year.[33] Though less well characterized as a model, a single dose of HAQO in the rat induces AACN.[28] In the regenerating rat pancreas, a single dose of HAQO results in pancreatic adenocarcinomas.[29]

B. Postinitiation Stage

To date, factors which operate on pancreatic carcinogenesis during the postinitiation phase include dietary unsaturated fats, various retinoids, and products of raw soy beans. Most experiments have utilized a relatively short initiation phase of multiple treatments with carcinogen followed by a relatively long postinitiation phase of continuous exposure to the

Table 4
PANCREATIC NEOPLASMS INDUCED BY A SINGLE DOSE OF AZASERINE[a]

Months postinitiation	Number of rats per group	Incidence of pancreatic neoplasms	
		Adenomas	Adenocarcinomas
12	10	4	3
15	10	1	5

[a] Male Wistar/Lewis rats were injected i.p. at 7 weeks of age with 30 mg azaserine per kilogram of body weight. Throughout the study they were fed the purified AIN diet.

test agent. Often purified diets similar to those whose compositions are shown in Table 5 were fed. At the end of the experimental period, the entire pancreas was excised, fixed, processed, and stained by standard histological procedures for light microscopic examination of the incidence and number of pancreatic adenomas and adenocarcinomas. The results from several such experiments are summarized in Tables 6 and 7.

1. Promotion of Pancreatic Carcinogenesis

Our first experiments in modulation of carcinogenesis were designed to survey the effects of various diets on pancreatic carcinogenesis. In the initial experiments, separation of the stages of carcinogenesis was not made. Rats fed a diet of 20% unsaturated fat (corn oil) had a significantly higher incidence and mean number of pancreatic tumors than groups fed a comparable level of saturated fat, AIN diet (5% corn oil), or low fat diet (2% corn oil).[53] Furthermore, in the group fed unsaturated fat, there were three invasive pancreatic adenocarcinomas while none were seen in the other groups (see Table 6). The enhancement of pancreatic carcinogenesis cannot be attributed to increased caloric intake or weight gain in the rats fed unsaturated fat, as the rats fed saturated fat were similar in both respects.

To illustrate the mechanisms of the enhancement, Roebuck et al.[80] divided the experiment into two operational phases: initiation and postinitiation (Table 7). The initiation phase was composed of a short series of azaserine injections over a 6-week period followed by the postinitiation phase of several months. When either the saturated or unsaturated fat diets were fed during the initiation phase and followed by the AIN diet in the postinitiation phase, the incidence and number of pancreatic tumors was no different than for the azaserine-initiated group fed the AIN diet during both phases of carcinogenesis (Table 7). Thus, with the carcinogen azaserine, diet had no effect on the initiation of pancreatic cancer. In Table 7, one can compare the results of several experiments designed to evaluate the effect of diet on the postinitiation phase. In three separate cases, promotion has been demonstrated. In groups fed unsaturated fat (corn oil) as 20% of the diet, more pancreatic tumors were observed when compared to groups fed AIN or 20% saturated fat diets during the postinitiation phase. Thus, corn oil promoted in two slightly different initiation protocols and for postinitiation phases of differing length. The rat/azaserine model is sufficiently characterized to modulate the azaserine treatment or the length of the postinitiation phase to optimize the outcome. An additional experiment has shown that safflower oil, also an unsaturated fat, is perhaps more effective than corn oil as a promoting agent (Table 7).

The results of these dietary studies are most readily compared to the DMBA-induced breast carcinogenesis model in the rat where unsaturated fats, but not saturated fats, enhanced carcinogenesis.[103] No direct relationship between the incidence of breast tumors and the degree of lipid unsaturation was found.[104,105] Hopkins and Carroll[106] have shown that promotion of breast cancer by dietary fats probably requires at least a minimum quantity of

Table 5
COMPOSITION OF TEST DIETS

Ingredient	AIN	Low fat	Lipotrope deficient	Unsaturated fat	Saturated fat	Safflower oil
Casein	20.0	20.0	3.0	20.0	20.0	20.0
Methionine	0.3	0.3	0.0	0.3	0.3	0.3
Cornstarch	15.0	15.6	11.0	11.7	11.7	11.7
Sucrose	50.0	52.4	36.8	38.3	38.3	38.3
Cellulose	5.0	5.0	5.0	5.0	5.0	5.0
Corn oil	5.0	2.0	20.0	20.0	2.0	0.0
Coconut oil (hydrogenated)	0.0	0.0	0.0	0.0	18.0	0.0
Safflower oil	0.0	0.0	0.0	0.0	0.0	20.0
Vitamin mix[a]	1.0	1.0	1.0	1.0	1.0	1.0
Mineral mix[a]	3.5	3.5	3.5	3.5	3.5	3.5
Choline	0.2	0.2	0.2	0.2	0.2	0.2
Other			19.5[b]			
Caloric content (kcal/g diet)	3.86	3.71	4.61	4.61	4.61	4.61

[a] The compositions of the vitamin and mineral mixes are those recommended by the Report of the American Institute of Nutrition.[102]

[b] This 19.5% of the lipotrope-diet is composed of extracted peanut meal (12.0%), gelatin (6.0%), fibrin (1.0%), and cystine (0.5%).

Table 6
AZASERINE TREATMENT CONCURRENT WITH DIETARY MODIFICATIONS IN THE RAT

Dietary treatments	Total azaserine dose (mg/kg)	Duration of experiment (month)	Number of rats per group	Pancreatic adenomas and adenocarcinomas: Incidence (%)	Pancreatic adenomas and adenocarcinomas: Neoplasms per pancreas (mean)
AIN	0	12	16	0 (0)	0
AIN	160	12	17	12 (71)	2.4
Low fat	160	12	13	11 (85)	2.2
Saturated fat	160	12	20	15 (75)	2.4
Unsaturated fat	160	12	18	18 (100)[a]	>10

[a] Three locally invasive pancreatic adenocarcinomas.

unsaturated fat and a high level of total dietary fat. Without the minimum level of unsaturated fat, it appears that even very high levels of dietary fat will not promote breast cancer. The essential fatty acid, linoleic acid, will fulfill this requirement if fed at 3% with 17% saturated fat.[77]

Diets deficient in lipotropic factors (primarily choline and methionine) and high in fat content have been fed to rats concurrent with azaserine treatment. Shinozuka et al.[101] reported that fewer AACN were found in the pancreases of azaserine-treated rats fed a lipotrope deficient 15% fat diet. AACN were observed at 4 and 6 months. In the first 14 weeks of this study 540 mg of azaserine per kilogram were given. The latent period was too short to allow the development of cancers. We have fed a different lipotrope deficient-high fat diet to rats treated with azaserine, and observed an enhancement of pancreatic carcinogenicity.[53] This study was 12 months in duration. The reason for our divergent results is unclear.

Table 7
EFFECTS OF DIET ON INITIATION AND POSTINITIATION PHASES OF AZASERINE-INDUCED CARCINOGENESIS IN THE RAT

Initiation phase		Postinitiation phase			Pancreatic adenomas and adenocarcinomas	
Dietary treatment	Total azaserine dose (mg/kg)	Dietary treatment	Duration of experiment (month)	Number of rats per group	Incidence (%)	Neoplasma per pancreas (mean)
AIN	60	AIN	9	17	4 (24)	0.47
Saturated fat	60	AIN	9	18	2 (11)	0.11
Unsaturated fat	60	AIN	9	19	4 (21)	0.21
AIN	60	Saturated fat	9	20	3 (15)	0.20
AIN	60	Unsaturated fat	9	20	11 (55)	1.45
AIN	80	AIN	12	18	10 (56)	0.9
AIN	80	Saturated fat	12	16	11 (69)	1.3
AIN	80	Unsaturated fat	12	17	16 (94)	4.7
AIN	80	Safflower oil	12	17	16 (94)[a]	5.9

[a] Two locally invasive pancreatic adenocarcinomas.

Shinozuka et al.[101] treated with azaserine at a rate that is probably cytotoxic to the pancreatic acinar cells; whereas, we treated with a much smaller dose. Furthermore, while Shinozuka et al.[101] fed a diet of 15% fat, 10% was hydrogenated vegetable oil; whereas, our diet was 20% fat, all of which was unsaturated corn oil. As we have shown above, the unsaturated fat of the lipotrope deficient diet probably promoted the pancreatic lesions.

A preliminary report of promotion by high levels of dietary fat in the hamster/BOP model is consistent with our observations in the rat/azaserine model.[35] A doubling of the fat content in the hamster diet increased the incidence of adenocarcinomas in the female but not the male hamster. The incidence of ductular adenomas was increased in both sexes.

Raw soy bean flour is known to cause hypertrophy of the exocrine pancreas.[107,108] A heat labile protein that inhibits trypsin appears responsible for the hypertrophic effects. In the rat fed raw soy bean flour for only a few weeks, the pancreas can be two to three times as large as rats fed heat-treated soy flour. In a 2-year study of feeding raw and heat-treated soy flour to rats, McGuinness et al.[109] observed that rats fed raw soy flour developed pancreatic hypertrophy, hyperplastic nodules, and adenomatous lesions, These nodules apparently are similar to the AACN induced by azaserine.[40] Lesions first appeared at 30 weeks and by 60 weeks were seen in all rats fed raw soy flour. The first adenomas appeared at 60 weeks and by 90 weeks, 4 of 26 rats had invasive adenocarcinomas. The authors concluded that raw soy flour was a weak carcinogen or that their rats had been exposed to an unknown environmental carcinogen which the raw soy flour promoted. They regard the latter as less likely.

Enhancement of azaserine-induced pancreatic carcinogenesis has been observed in rats fed raw soy bean flour. Azaserine (5 mg/kg/week) or saline was injected for up to 24 weeks in adult rats fed raw- or heat-treated soy bean flour diets, and the number of AACN was evaluated.[110] By 19 weeks the group fed raw soy flour had significantly more AACN (>45) than in the other three groups. At 24 weeks, the number of AACN in the group fed raw soy flour was still larger (>120). The number of AACN in the azaserine-treated group fed heat-treated soy flour was three; in the saline-treated group fed raw soy flour was seven; and in the saline-treated group fed heated soy flour was zero. Similar studies by the same group have been extended up to 2 years.[109] The azaserine treatment was a once weekly i.p. injection of 5 mg/kg of body weight for life. The cumulative incidence of pancreatic adenocarcinomas in rats fed raw soy flour ranged from 14% for the saline-injected controls at 90 weeks to 65% in the azaserine-treated rats at only 75 weeks on experiment. In a similar experimental protocol, rats have been treated weekly with BHP for the first 6 months of a 16-month study.[51] Rats were fed either heated soy flour or raw soy flour diet for the entire study. Several previous experiments had already shown that BHP was not an effective pancreatic carcinogen in the rat.[41,111] In this experiment, 2 of 13 rats in the raw soy flour, BHP-treated group had pancreatic adenocarcinomas at 16 months. No adenocarcinomas were seen in the heated soy flour, BHP-treated group, or the raw soy flour saline-treated group. Furthermore, the pancreases of the raw soy flour, BHP group contained more and larger AACN than in any of the other three groups.

In the previously discussed studies, the mechanism of action of raw soy flour is not clear. Experiments have not yet been reported which indicate whether raw soy flour acts as an initiator, cocarcinogen, or a pure promoter. The question as to whether raw soy flour contains a chemical(s) which initiates pancreatic cancer, as well as leading to hyperplasia, is important but unanswered.

2. *Chemoprevention of Pancreatic Carcinogenesis*

Little work has been published concerning inhibition of pancreatic carcinogenesis either by agents acting during initiation or during postinitiation. With the availability of two well-characterized animal models previously discussed, this area should progress more rapidly.

We have published two studies concerned with chemoprevention in rats. Retinyl acetate,[25] *N*-2-hydroxyethyl retinamide, *N*-4-propionyl-oxyphenyl retinamide, and retinylidene dimedone[112] inhibited pancreatic carcinogenesis. In both studies, the rats were first initiated with multiple weekly injections of azaserine before being fed diets supplemented with retinoids. Thus, effects of the retinoids were obviously upon the postinitiation stage of carcinogenesis. This is consistent with a retardation of the progression of carcinogenesis by retinoids.[113]

We have observed that rats fed chow diets had fewer and smaller azaserine-induced pancreatic lesions compared to rats fed purified diets.[25] When compared to AIN diet, chow had no effect on the initiation of AACN by azaserine.

Subsequent experiments indicated that this was a postinitiation phenomenon. When rats were initiated over a 6-week period with multiple injections of azaserine while on AIN diet and then during the subsequent 10.5 month postinitiation phase were fed either AIN diet or chow, the incidence of adenomas and carcinomas in the chow group was significantly reduced. Both groups had AACN; however, the AACN of the chow group were approximately one quarter the size of AACN of the AIN group. The inhibitory effects of chow also have been demonstrated in the DMBA-induced breast tumor system.[114] Chow diets are chemically very complex and the mechanisms of inhibition are unknown.

III. CONCLUSIONS

Pancreatic carcinomas have been experimentally induced in four species of animals by at least 12 different chemicals. Adenocarcinomas induced in hamsters by BOP and in rats by azaserine provide the best characterized animal models for pancreatic carcinogenesis. Carcinomas appear to arise in both acinar cells and ductal cells in experimental animals, and the resulting spectrum provides a reasonable match for human tumors, although no single existing animal model adequately mimics the histologic spectrum of human pancreatic carcinoma. Organ culture of rat and human pancreas has been utilized to demonstrate in vitro transformation with induction of transplantable carcinomas. The pancreas contains inducible microsomal enzymes and can activate several carcinogens. This activity seems to be established for both acinar cells and ductal cells. The existing animal models provide opportunities for study of factors which modulate initiation and which may promote or inhibit the progression of carcinogenesis during the postinitiation phase. Dietary unsaturated fat and raw soy flour diets appear to promote pancreatic carcinogenesis while several retinoids have inhibited carcinogenesis.

ACKNOWLEDGMENTS

This research was in part supported by USPHS Fellowship F22-CA 01168 (B.D.R.), by National Cancer Institute Contract No. N01 CP 85675 (D.S.L.), and by USPHS Grants CA 20948 (J.D.Y.), CA 19410 (D.S.L.), and CA 26594 (B.D.R.). The authors wish to thank Karen Baumgartner and Linda Conrad for assistance in preparing this manuscript and Dr. J. Zurlo for her critical review.

REFERENCES

1. **MacMahon, B., Yen, S., Trichopoulos, D., Warren, K., and Nardi, G.,** Coffee and cancer of the pancreas, *N. Engl. J. Med.*, 304, 630, 1981.
2. **Lin, R. S. and Kessler, I. I.,** A multifactorial model for pancreatic cancer in man. Epidemiologic evidence, *JAMA*, 245, 147, 1981.
3. **Shedlofsky, S.,** Coffee and cancer of the pancreas (letter), *N. Engl. J. Med.*, 304, 1604, 1981.
4. **Higgins, I., Stolley, P., and Wynder, E. L.,** Coffee and cancer of the pancreas (letter), *N. Engl. J. Med.*, 304, 1605, 1981.
5. **Wynder, E. L.,** An epidemiological evaluation of the causes of cancer of the pancreas, *Cancer Res.*, 35, 2228, 1975.
6. **Blot, W. J., Fraumeni, J. F., and Stone, B. J.,** Geographic correlates of pancreas cancer in the United States, *Cancer*, 42, 373, 1978.
7. **Bell, E. T.,** Carcinoma of the pancreas. II. The relation of carcinoma of the pancreas to diabetes mellitus, *Am. J. Pathol.*, 33, 511, 1957.
8. **Maruchi, N., Brian, D., Ludwig, J., Elveback, L. R., and Kurland, L. T.,** Cancer of the pancreas in Olmsted County, Minnesota, 1935—1974, *Mayo Clin. Proc.*, 54, 245, 1979.
9. **Levin, D. L. and Connelly, R. R.,** Cancer of the pancreas. Available epidemiologic information and its implications, *Cancer*, 31, 1231, 1973.
10. **Wynder, E. L., Mabachi, K., Maruchi, N., and Fortner, J. G.,** Epidemiology of cancer of the pancreas, *J. Natl. Cancer Inst.*, 50, 645, 1973.
11. **Mack, T. M. and Paganini-Hill, A.,** Epidemiology of pancreas cancer in Los Angeles, *Cancer*, 47, 1474, 1981.
12. **Stocks, P.,** Cancer mortality in relation to national consumption of cigarettes, solid fuel, tea, and coffee, *Br. J. Cancer*, 24, 215, 1970.
13. **Mancuso, T. F. and El-Attar, A. A.,** Cohort study of workers exposed to beta-naphthylamine and benzidine, *J. Occup. Med.*, 9, 277, 1967.
14. **Paulino-Netto, A., Dreiling, D. A., and Baronofsky, I. D.,** The relationship between pancreatic calcification and cancer of the pancreas, *Ann. Surg.*, 151, 530, 1960.
15. **Burch, G. E. and Ansari, A.,** Chronic alcoholism and carcinoma of the pancreas, *Arch. Intern. Med.*, 121, 273, 1968.
16. **Berg, J. W. and Connelly, R. R.,** Updating the epidemiologic data on pancreatic cancer, *Semin. Oncol.*, 6, 275, 1979.
17. **Slye, M., Holmes, H. F., and Wells, H. G.,** The comparative pathology of carcinoma of the pancreas with report of two cases in mice, *Am. J. Cancer*, 23, 81, 1935.
18. **Rowlatt, U. F.,** Pancreatic neoplasms of rats and mice, in *Pathology of Laboratory Rats and Mice*, Cotchin, E. and Roe, F. J. C., Eds., Blackwell Scientific, Oxford, 1967, 85.
19. **Rowlatt, U. and Roe, F. J. C.,** Epithelial tumors of the rat pancreas, *J. Natl. Cancer Inst.*, 39, 18, 1967.
20. **S. Hosoda, Suzuki, H., and Suzuki, M.,** Spontaneous tumors and atypical proliferation of pancreatic acinar cells in *Mastomys (Praomys) natalensis*, *J. Natl. Cancer Inst.*, 57, 1341, 1976.
21. **Snell, K. C. and Stewart, H. L.,** Spontaneous diseases in a closed colony of *Praomys (Mastomys) natalensis*, *Bull. W. H. O.*, 52, 645, 1975.
22. **Priester, W. A.,** Data from eleven United States and Canadian colleges of veterinary medicine on pancreatic carcinoma in domestic animals, *Cancer Res.*, 34, 1372, 1974.
23. **Morris, H. P. and Eyestone, W. H.,** Tumors of the liver and urinary bladder of the dog after ingestion of 2-acetylaminofluorene, *J. Natl. Cancer Inst.*, 13, 1139, 1973.
24. **Longnecker, D. S. and Curphey, T. J.,** Adenocarcinoma of the pancreas in azaserine-treated rats, *Cancer Res.*, 35, 2249, 1975.
25. **Longnecker, D. S., Roebuck, B. D., Yager, J. D., Jr., Lilja, H. S., and Siegmund, B.,** Pancreatic carcinoma in azaserine-treated rats: induction, classification and dietary modulation of incidence, *Cancer*, 47, 1562, 1981.
26. **Dissen, J., Mills, L. R., Mainz, D. L., Black, O., Jr., and Webster, P. D., III,** Experimental induction of pancreatic adenocarcinoma in rats, *J. Natl. Cancer Inst.*, 55, 857, 1975.
27. **Bockman, D. E., Black, O., Jr., Mills, L. R., and Webster, P. D., III,** Origin of tubular complexes developing during induction of pancreatic adenocarcinoma by 7,12-dimethylbenz(a)anthracene, *Am. J. Pathol.*, 90, 645, 1978.
28. **Hayashi, Y. and Hasegawa, T.,** Experimental pancreatic tumor in rats after intravenous injection of 4-hydroxyaminoquinoline-1-oxide, *Gann*, 62, 329, 1971.
29. **Konishi, Y., Denda, A., Inui, S., Takahashi, S., and Kondo, H.,** Pancreatic carcinoma induced by 4-hydroxyaminoquinoline-1-oxide after partial pancreatectomy and splenectomy in rat, *Gann*, 67, 919, 1976.

30. **Longnecker, D. S., Curphey, T. J., Lilja, H. S., French, J. I., and Daniel, D. S.,** Carcinogenicity of a methylnitrosourea amino acid in rats, *Fed. Proc.*, 37, 231, 1978.
31. **Druckrey, H., Ivankovic, S., Bücheler, J., Preussmann, R., and Thomas, C.,** Erzeugung von Magen- und Pankreas-Krebs beim Meerschweinchen durch Methylnitroso-harnstoff und-urethan, *Z. Krebsforsch.*, 71, 167, 1968.
32. **Reddy, J. D. and Rao, M. S.,** Pancreatic adenocarcinoma in inbred guinea pigs induced by N-methyl-N-nitrosourea, *Cancer Res.*, 35, 2269, 1975.
33. **Pour, P., Salmasi, S. Z., and Runge, R. G.,** Selective induction of pancreatic ductular tumors by single doses of N-nitrosobis(2-oxopropyl)amine in Syrian golden hamsters, *Cancer Lett.*, 4, 317, 1978.
34. **Pour, P., Krüger, F. W., Althoff, J., Cardesa, A., and Mohr, U.,** Cancer of the pancreas induced in the Syrian golden hamster, *Am. J. Pathol.*, 76, 349, 1974.
35. **Pour, P. M., Runge, R. G., Birt, D., Gingell, R., Lawson, T., Nagel, D., Wallcave, L., and Salmasi, S. Z.,** Current knowledge of pancreatic carcinogenesis in the hamster and its relevance to the human disease, *Cancer*, 47, 1573, 1981.
36. **Mohr, U., Reznik, G., Emminger, E., and Lijinsky, W.,** Induction of pancreatic duct carcinomas in the Syrian hamster with 2,6-dimethyl-nitrosomorpholine, *J. Natl. Cancer Inst.*, 58, 429, 1977.
37. **Parsa, I. and Marsh, W. H.,** An *in vitro* model of pancreatic carcinoma. Morphology and *in vivo* growth, *Am. J. Pathol.*, 84, 469, 1976.
38. **Konishi, Y., Denda, A., Takahashi, S., Sunagawa, M., and Kondo, H.,** Effect of chemical carcinogens on pancreatic DNA synthesis *in vivo*, *Gann*, 67, 781, 1976.
39. **Roebuck, B. D., Lilja, H. S., Curphey, T. J., and Longnecker, D. S.,** Pathologic and biochemical effects of azaserine in inbred Wistar/Lewis rats and noninbred CD^{R}-1 mice, *J. Natl. Cancer Inst.*, 65, 383, 1980.
40. **Roebuck, B. D. and Longnecker, D. S.,** Species and rat strain variation in pancreatic nodule induction by azaserine, *J. Natl. Cancer Inst.*, 59, 1273, 1977.
41. **Longnecker, D. S. and Crawford, B. G.,** Hyperplastic nodules and adenomas of exocrine pancreas in azaserine-treated rats, *J. Natl. Cancer Inst.*, 53, 573, 1974.
42. **Yager, J. D., Jr., Roebuck, B. D., Zurlo, J., Longnecker, D. S., Weselcouch, E. O., and Wilpone, S. A.,** A single-dose protocol for azaserine initiation of pancreatic carcinogenesis in the rat, *Int. J. Cancer*, 28, 601, 1981.
43. **Pour, P., Althoff, J., Krüger, F. W., and Mohr, U.,** A potent pancreatic carcinogen in Syrian hamsters: N-nitrosobis(2-oxopropyl)amine, *J. Natl. Cancer Inst.*, 58, 1449, 1977.
44. **Pour, P., Salmasi, S., Runge, R., Gingell, R., Wallcave, L., Nagel, D., and Stepan, K.,** Carcinogenicity of N-nitrosobis(2-hydroxypropyl)amine and N-nitrosobis(2-oxopropyl)amine in MRC rats, *J. Natl. Cancer Inst.*, 63, 181, 1979.
45. **Konishi, Y., Kondo, H., Inui, S., Denda, A., Ikeda, T., and Kojima, K.,** Organotropic effect of N-bis(2-hydroxypropyl)nitrosamine: production of lung and liver tumors by its oral administration in mice, *Gann*, 69, 77, 1978.
46. **Green, U., Konishi, Y., Ketkar, M. B., and Althoff, J.,** Comparative study of the carcinogenic effect of BHP and BAP on NMRI mice, *Cancer Lett.*, 9, 257, 1980.
47. **Rao, M. S. and Pour, P.,** Development of biliary and hepatic neoplasms in guinea pigs treated with N-nitrosobis(2-oxopropyl)amine, *Cancer Lett.*, 5, 31, 1978.
48. **Rao, M. S., and Reddy, J. K.,** Carcinogenicity of 2,2′-Dihydroxy-di-*n*-propylnitrosamine in the tree shrew *(Tupaia glis)*: light and electron microscopic features of pulmonary adenomas, *J. Natl. Cancer Inst.*, 65, 835, 1980.
49. **Takahashi, M. and Pour, P.,** Spontaneous alterations in the pancreas of the aging Syrian golden hamster, *J. Natl. Cancer Inst.*, 60, 355, 1978.
50. **Gingell, R., Brunk, G., Nagel, D., and Pour, P.,** Metabolism of three radiolabeled pancreatic carcinogenic nitrosamines in hamsters and rats, *Cancer Res.*, 39, 4579, 1979.
51. **Levison, D. A., Morgan, R. G. H., Brimacombe, J. S., Hopwood, D., Coghill, G., and Wormsley, K. G.,** Carcinogenic effects of Di(2-hydroxylpropyl) nitrosamine (DHPN) in male Wistar rats: promotion of pancreatic cancer by a raw soya flour diet, *Scand. J. Gastroenterol.*, 14, 217, 1979.
52. **Cubilla, A. L. and Fitzgerald, P. J.,** Morphological patterns of primary nonendocrine human pancreas carcinoma, *Cancer Res.*, 35, 2234, 1975.
53. **Roebuck, B. D., Yager, J. D., Jr., and Longnecker, D. S.,** Dietary modulation of azaserine-induced pancreatic carcinogenesis in the rat, *Cancer Res.*, 41, 888, 1981.
54. **Longnecker, D. S., Shinozuka, H., and Dekker, A.,** Focal acinar cell dysplasia in human pancreas, *Cancer*, 45, 534, 1980.
55. **Pledger, R. A., Bates, R. R., and Saffiotti, U.,** Introduction: National Cancer Institute Pancreatic Carcinogenesis Program, *Cancer Res.*, 35, 2226, 1975.

56. **Andersson, A. and Hellerstrom, C.,** Explant culture: pancreatic islets *Methods Cell Biol.*, 21B, 135, 1980.
57. **Hay, R. J.,** The pancreatic epithelial cell *in vitro*: a possible model system for studies in carcinogenesis, *Cancer Res.*, 35, 2289, 1975.
58. **Amsterdam, A. and Jamieson, J. D.,** Studies on dispersed pancreatic exocrine cells. I. Dissociation technique and morphologic characteristics of separated cells, *J. Cell Biol.*, 63, 1037, 1974.
59. **Oliver, C.,** Isolation and maintenance of differentiated exocrine gland acinar cells *in vitro, In Vitro,* 16, 297, 1980.
60. **Zurlo, J., Longnecker, D. S., Cooney, D. A., Kuhlmann, E. T., and Curphey, T. J.,** Studies of pancreatic nodule induction and DNA damage by D-azaserine, *Cancer Lett.*, 12, 75, 1981.
61. **Zurlo, J., Yager, J. D., Jr., Longnecker, D. S., and Curphey, T. J.,** Studies on DNA damage and repair synthesis induced in rat and hamster pancreas and liver by N-nitrosobis(2-oxopropyl)amine, *Proc. Am. Assoc. Cancer Res.*, 22, 91, 1981.
62. **Zurlo, J., Curphey, T. J., Hiley, R., and Longnecker, D. S.,** Identification of 7-carboxymethylguanine in DNA from pancreatic acinar cells exposed to azaserine, *Cancer Res.*, 42, 1286, 1982.
63. **Amsterdam, A., Solomon, T. E., and Jamieson, J. D.,** Sequential dissociation of the exocrine pancreas into lobules, acini, and individual cells, in *Methods in Cell Biology*, Vol. 20, Prescott, D. M., Ed., Academic Press, New York, 1978, 361.
64. **Williams, J. A., Korc, M., and Dormer, R. L.,** Action of secretagogues on a new preparation of functionally intact, isolated pancreatic acini, *Am. J. Physiol.*, 235, E517, 1978.
65. **Stoner, G. D., Harris, C. C., Bostwick, D. G., Jones, R. T., Trump, B. F., Kingsbury, E. W., Fineman, E., and Newkirk, C.,** Isolation and characterization of epithelial cells from bovine pancreatic duct, *In Vitro,* 14, 581, 1978.
66. **Jones, R. T., Hudson, E. A., and Resaw, J. H.,** A review of *in vitro* and *in vivo* culture techniques for the study of pancreatic carcinogenesis, *Cancer,* 47, 1490, 1981.
67. **Githens, S., III, Holmquist, D. R. G., Whelan, J. F., and Ruby, J. R.,** Morphologic and biochemical characteristics of isolated and cultured pancreatic ducts, *Cancer,* 47, 1505, 1981.
68. **Parsa, I., Marsh, W. H., and Sutton, A. L.,** An *in vitro* model of human pancreas carcinogenesis: effects of nitroso compounds, *Cancer,* 47, 1543, 1981.
69. **Murrell, L. R., Germain, K. H., and Lynch, D. M.,** Survival of functional pancreatic acinar tissue in circumfusion organ culture enhanced by chemically defined medium with hydrocortisone, *Cancer Res.*, 35, 2286, 1975.
70. **Parsa, I., Marsh, W. H., and Sutton, A. L.,** An *in vitro* model of pancreas carcinogenesis: two-stage MNU-TPA effect, *Am. J. Pathol.*, 98, 649, 1980.
71. **Farber, E.,** The sequential analysis of liver cancer induction, *Biochim. Biophys. Acta,* 605, 149, 1980.
72. **Slaga, T. J., Fischer, S. M., Nelson, K., and Gleason, G. L.,** Studies on the mechanism of skin tumor promotion: evidence for several stages in promotion, *Proc. Natl. Acad. Sci. U.S.A.*, 77, 3659, 1980.
73. **Berenblum, I.,** Historical perspective, in *Carcinogenesis,* Vol. 2, Slaga, T. J., Sivak, A., and Boutwell, R. K., Eds., Raven Press, New York, 1978, 1.
74. **Peraino, C., Fry, R. J. M., and Staffeldt, E.,** Reduction and enhancement by phenobarbital of hepatocarcinogenesis induced in the rat by 2-acetyl-aminofluorene, *Cancer Res.*, 31, 1506, 1971.
75. **Pitot, H. C. and Sirica, A. E.,** The stages of initiation and promotion in hepatocarcinogenesis, *Biochim. Biophys. Acta,* 605, 191, 1980.
76. **Hopkins, G. J. and West, C. E.,** Possible roles of dietary fats in carcinogenesis, *Life Sci.*, 19, 1103, 1976.
77. **Carroll, K. K.,** Lipids and carcinogenesis, *J. Environ. Pathol. Toxicol.*, 3, 253, 1980.
78. **Reddy, B. S., Narisawa, T., Maronpot, R., Weisburger, J. H., and Wynder, E. L.,** Animal models for the study of dietary factors and cancer of the large bowel, *Cancer Res.*, 35, 3421, 1975.
79. **Bull, A. W., Soullier, B. K., Wilson, P. S., Hayden, M. T., and Nigro, N. D.,** Promotion of azoxymethanol-induced intestinal cancer by high-fat diet in rats, *Cancer Res.*, 39, 4956, 1979.
80. **Roebuck, B. D., Yager, J. D., Jr., Longnecker, D. S., and Wilpone, S. A.,** Promotion by unsaturated fat of azaserine-induced pancreatic carcinogenesis in the rat, *Cancer Res.*, 41, 3961, 1981.
81. **Adler, G., Wieger, W., and Kern, H. F.,** Amino acid transport in the rat exocrine pancreas: III. Effect of maximal and supramaximal hormonal stimulation *in vivo, Cell Tissue Res.*, 194, 447, 1978.
82. **Iwamoto, Y. and Williams, J. A.,** Inhibition of pancreatic α-aminoisobutyric acid uptake by cholecystokinin and other secretagogues, *Am. J. Physiol.*, 238, G440, 1980.
83. **Cheneval, J. P. and Johnstone, R. M.,** Changes in amino acid transport in the rat pancreas in response to fasting and feeding, *Biochim. Biophys. Acta,* 433, 630, 1976.
84. **Baril, E. F. and Potter, V. R.,** Systematic oscillation of amino acid transport in liver from rats adapted to controlled feeding schedules, *J. Nutr.*, 95, 228, 1968.

85. **Hopkins, H. A., Bonney, R. J., Walker, P. R., Yager, J. D., Jr., and Potter, V. R.,** Food and light as separate entrainment signals for rat liver enzymes, in *Advances in Enzyme Regulation,* Vol. 11, Weber, G., Ed., Pergamon Press, Oxford, 1973, 169.
86. **Perantoni, A., Berman, J. J., and Rice, J. M.,** L-azaserine toxicity in established cell lines: correlation with γ-glutamyl transpeptidase activity, *Exp. Cell Res.,* 122, 55, 1979.
87. **Harris, C. C., Autrup, H., Stoner, G., Yang, S. K., Leutz, J. C., Gelboin, H. V., Selkirk, J. K., Cannor, R. J., Barret, L. A., Jones, R. T., McDowell, E., and Trump, B. F.,** Metabolism of benzo[a]pyrene and 7,12-dimethylbenz[a]anthracene in cultured human bronchus and pancreatic duct, *Cancer Res.,* 37, 3349, 1977.
88. **Iqbal, Z. M., Varnes, M. E., Yoshida, A., and Epstein, S. S.,** Metabolism of benzo[a]pyrene by guinea pig pancreatic microsomes, *Cancer Res.,* 37, 1011, 1977.
89. **Black, O., Jr., Murrill, E., and Fanska, C.,** Metabolism of a carcinogen (7,12-dimethylbenzanthracene) in the pancreas of the Long-Evans rat, *Res. Commun. Chem. Pathol. Pharmacol.,* 33, 103, 1981.
90. **Lavigne, J.-G. and Marchand, C.,** Effects of phenobarbital pretreatment on rat pancreas, *Am. J. Physiol.,* 222, 360, 1972.
91. **Whalley, C. E., Iqbal, Z. M., and Epstein, S. S.,** In vivo and microsomal metabolism of the pancreatic carcinogen N-nitrosobis(2-oxopropyl)amine by the Syrian golden hamster, *Cancer Res.,* 41, 482, 1981.
92. **Scarpelli, D. G., Rao, M. S., Subbarao, V., Beversluis, M., Gurka, D. P., and Hollenberg, P. F.,** Activation of nitrosamines to mutagens by postmitochondrial fraction of hamster pancreas, *Cancer Res.,* 40, 67, 1980.
93. **Bolender, R. P.,** Stereological analysis of the guinea pig pancreas. I. Analytical mode and quantitative description of non-stimulated pancreatic exocrine cells, *J. Cell Biol.,* 61, 269, 1974.
94. **Nebert, D. W. and Gelboin, H. V.,** Substrate-inducible microsomal aryl hydroxylase in mammalian cell culture. I. Assay and properties of induced enzyme, *J. Biol. Chem.,* 243, 6242, 1968.
95. **Staiano, N., Everson, R. B., Cooney, D. A., Longnecker, D. S., and Thorgeirsson, S. S.,** Mutagenicity of D- and L-azaserine, 6-diazo-5-oxo-L-norleucine, and N-(N-methyl-N-nitrosocarbamoyl)-L-ornithine in the *Salmonella* test system, *Mutat. Res.,* 79, 387, 1980.
96. **Zurlo, J., Roebuck, B. D., Rutkowski, J. V., Curphey, T. J., and Longnecker, D. S.,** Effect of pyridoxal deficiency on pancreatic DNA damage and nodule induction by azaserine, *Proc. Am. Assoc. Cancer Res.,* 23, 68, 1982.
97. **Lilja, H. S., Hyde, E., Longnecker, D. S., and Yager, J. D., Jr.,** DNA damage and repair in rat tissues following administration of azaserine, *Cancer Res.,* 37, 3925, 1977.
98. **Lilja, H. S., Curphey, T. J., Yager, J. D., Jr., and Longnecker, D. S.,** Persistence of DNA damage in rat pancreas following administration of three carcinogens and/or mutagens, *Chem. Biol. Interact.,* 22, 287, 1978.
99. **Lilja, H. S., Longnecker, D. S., Curphey, T. J., Daniel, D. S., and Adams, W. E.,** Studies of DNA damage in rat pancreas and liver by 6-diazo-5-oxo-L-norleucine, ethyldiazoacetate and azaserine, *Cancer Lett.,* 12, 139, 1981.
100. **Lawson, T. A., Gingell, R., Nagel, D., Hines, L. A., and Ross, A.,** Methylation of hamster DNA by the carcinogen N-nitroso-bis(2-oxopropyl)-amine, *Cancer Lett.,* 11, 251, 1981.
101. **Shinozuka, H., Katyal, S. L., and Lombardi, B.,** Azaserine carcinogenesis: organ susceptibility change in rats fed a diet devoid of choline, *Int. J. Cancer,* 22, 36, 1978.
102. Report of the American Institute of Nutrition Ad Hoc Committee on Standards of Nutritional Studies, *J. Nutr.,* 107, 1340, 1977.
103. **Gammal, E. B., Carrol, K. K., and Plunkett, E. R.,** Effects of dietary fat on mammary carcinogenesis by 7,12-dimethylbenz(α)anthracene in rats, *Cancer Res.,* 27, 1737, 1967.
104. **Carrol, K. K. and Khor, H. T.,** Effects of level and type of dietary fat on incidence of mammary tumors induced in female Sprague-Dawley rats by 7,12-dimethylbenz(α)anthracene, *Lipids,* 6, 415, 1971.
105. **Dayton, S., Hashimoto, S., and Wollman, J.,** Effect of high-oleic and high-linoleic safflower oils on mammary tumors induced in rats by 7,12-dimethylbenz(α)anthracene, *J. Nutr.,* 107, 1353, 1977.
106. **Hopkins, G. J. and Carroll, K. K.,** Relationship between amount and type of dietary fat in promotion of mammary carcinogenesis induced by 7,12-dimethylbenz[α]anthracene, *J. Natl. Cancer Inst.,* 62, 1009, 1979.
107. **Booth, A. N., Robbins, D. J., Ribelin, W. E., and DeEds, F.,** Effect of raw soybean meal and amino acids on pancreatic hypertrophy in rats, *Proc. Soc. Exp. Biol. Med.,* 104, 681, 1960.
108. **Rackis, J. J., McGee, J. E., Gumbmann, M. R., and Booth, A. N.,** Effects of soy proteins containing trypsin inhibitors in long term feeding studies in rats, *J. Am. Oil Chem. Soc.,* 56, 162, 1979.
109. **McGuinness, E. E., Morgan, R. G. H., Levison, D. A., Hopwood, D., and Wormsley, K. G.,** Interaction of azaserine and raw soya flour on the rat pancreas, *Scand. J. Gastroenterol.,* 16, 49, 1981.
110. **Morgan, R. G. H., Levinson, D. A., Hopwood, D., Saunders, J. H. B., and Wormsley, K. G.,** Potentiation of the action of azaserine on the rat pancreas by raw soyabean flour, *Cancer Lett.,* 3, 87, 1977.

110. **Morgan, R. G. H., Levinson, D. A., Hopwood, D., Saunders, J. H. B., and Wormsley, K. G.,** Potentiation of the action of azaserine on the rat pancreas by raw soya bean flour, *Cancer Lett.*, 3, 87, 1977.
111. **Mohr, U., Reznik, G., and Pour, P.,** Carcinogenic effects of diisopropanolnitrosamine in Sprague-Dawley rats, *J. Natl. Cancer Inst.*, 58, 361, 1977.
112. **Longnecker, D. S., Curphey, T. J., Kuhlmann, E. T., and Roebuck, B. D.,** Inhibition of pancreatic carcinogenesis by retinoids in azaserine-treated rats, *Cancer Res.*, 42, 19, 1982.
113. **Sporn, M. B. and Newton, D. L.,** Chemoprevention of cancer with retinoids, *Fed. Proc.*, 38, 2528, 1979.
114. **Chan, C. P. and Dao, T. L.,** Enhancement of mammary carcinogenesis by a high-fat diet in Fischer, Long-Evans, and Sprague-Dawley rats, *Cancer Res.*, 41, 164, 1981.
115. **Roebuck, B. D.,** unpublished observations.
116. **Longnecker, D. S., Zurlo, J., Curphey, T. J., and Adams, W. E.,** Induction of pancreatic DNA damage and nodules in rats treated with N-nitrosobis(2-oxopropyl)amine and N-nitroso(2-hydroxypropyl) (2-oxopropyl)amine, *Carcinogenesis*, 3, 715, 1982.

INDEX

A

B

C

G

H

I

J

K

L

M

N

O

T

U

V

W

X